Liver Pathology: Diagnostic Challenges, Practical Considerations and Emerging Concepts

Editor

LEI ZHAO

SURGICAL PATHOLOGY CLINICS

www.surgpath.theclinics.com

Consulting Editor
JASON L. HORNICK

September 2023 • Volume 16 • Number 3

ELSEVIER

1600 John F. Kennedy Boulevard • Suite 1800 • Philadelphia, Pennsylvania, 19103-2899

http://www.theclinics.com

SURGICAL PATHOLOGY CLINICS Volume 16, Number 3
September 2023 ISSN 1875-9181, ISBN-13: 978-0-443-18218-1

Editor: Taylor Hayes
Developmental Editor: Malvika Shah

Surgical Pathology Clinics (ISSN 1875-9181) is published quarterly by Elsevier Inc., 360 Park Avenue South, New York, NY 10010. Months of issue are March, June, September, and December. Business and Editorial Office: Elsevier Inc., 1600 John F. Kennedy Blvd., Ste. 1800, Philadelphia, PA 19103-2899. Accounting and Circulation Offices: Elsevier Inc., 3251 Riverport Lane, Maryland Heights, MO 63043. Periodicals postage paid at New York, NY and at additional mailing offices. Subscription prices are $246.00 per year (US individuals), $354.00 per year (US institutions), $100.00 per year (US students/residents), $294.00 per year (Canadian individuals), $402.00 per year (Canadian Institutions), $295.00 per year (foreign individuals), $402.00 per year (foreign institutions), and $120.00 per year (international students/residents), $100.00 per year (Canadian students/residents). Foreign air speed delivery is included in all *Clinics'* subscription prices. All prices are subject to change without notice. **POSTMASTER:** Send address changes to *Surgical Pathology Clinics*, Elsevier, 3251 Riverport Lane, Maryland Heights, MO 63043. **Customer Service: 1-800-654-2452 (US). From outside the United States, call 1-314-447-8871. Fax: 1-314-447-8029. E-mail:** JournalsCustomerServiceusa@elsevier.com **(for print support)** and JournalsOnlineSupport-usa@elsevier.com **(for online support).**

Reprints. For copies of 100 or more, of articles in this publication, please contact the Commercial Reprints Department, Elsevier Inc., 360 Park Avenue South, New York, NY 10010-1710. Tel. 212-633-3874; Fax: 212-633-3820; E-mail: reprints@elsevier.com.

Surgical Pathology Clinics of North America is covered in *MEDLINE/PubMed (Index Medicus)*.

Contributors

CONSULTING EDITOR

JASON L. HORNICK, MD, PhD
Director of Surgical Pathology and
Immunohistochemistry, Brigham and Women's
Hospital, Professor of Pathology, Harvard
Medical School, Boston, Massachusetts

EDITOR

LEI ZHAO, MD, PhD
Associate Pathologist, Department of
Pathology, Brigham and Women's Hospital,
Assistant Professor, Harvard Medical School,
Boston, Massachusetts

AUTHORS

VIVEK CHARU, MD, PhD
Assistant Professor, Department of Pathology,
Stanford University School of Medicine,
Department of Medicine, Quantitative
Sciences Unit, Stanford, California

TONY EL JABBOUR, MD
Assistant Professor of Gastrointestinal and
Liver Pathology, West Virginia University,
Morgantown, West Virginia

MARIA ISABEL FIEL, MD, FAASLD
Professor, Department of Pathology, Molecular
and Cell-Based Medicine, Icahn School of
Medicine at Mount Sinai, New York,
New York

RAYMOND A. ISIDRO, MD, PhD
Assistant Attending Pathologist, Department of
Pathology, Memorial Sloan Kettering Cancer
Center, New York, New York

SANJAY KAKAR, MD
Professor, Department of Pathology, University
of California, San Francisco, San Francisco,
California

NEERAJA KAMBHAM, MD
Professor, Department of Pathology, Stanford
University School of Medicine, Stanford,
California

STEPHEN M. LAGANA, MD
Associate Professor of Pathology and Cell
Biology, NewYork-Presbyterian/Columbia
University, Irving Medical Center, New York,
New York

KATY L. LAWSON, MD
Department of Pathology and Laboratory
Medicine, David Geffen School of Medicine,
Ronald Reagan UCLA Medical Center,
University of California, Los Angeles, Los
Angeles, California

KAREN MATSUKUMA, MD, PhD
Associate Professor, Pathology and
Laboratory Medicine, University of California,
Davis, Sacramento, California

JOSEPH MISDRAJI, MD
Associate Professor, Department of
Pathology, Yale School of Medicine,
Yale New Haven Hospital, New Haven,
Connecticut

EMILIE K. MITTEN, MD
Instructor in Medicine, Harvard Medical School, Hepatologist, Brigham and Women's Hospital, Boston, Massachusetts

ATTILA MOLNAR, MD
Pathology Resident, Mount Sinai Morningside and Mount Sinai West, New York, New York

DAVID J. PAPKE JR, MD, PhD
Associate Pathologist, Department of Pathology, Brigham and Women's Hospital, Instructor in Pathology, Harvard Medical School, Boston, Massachusetts

PAIGE H. PARRACK, MD
Clinical Fellow, Harvard Medical School, Gastrointestinal Pathology Fellow, Brigham and Women's Hospital, Boston, Massachusetts

RAGINI PHANSALKAR, PhD
Department of Pathology, Stanford University School of Medicine, Stanford, California

ANNA RUTHERFORD, MD, MPH
Assistant Professor of Medicine, Harvard Medical School, Clinical Director of Hepatology, Brigham and Women's Hospital, Boston, Massachusetts

THOMAS D. SCHIANO, MD, FAASLD
Professor of Medicine, Division of Liver Diseases, Recanati-Miller Transplantation Institute, Icahn School of Medicine at Mount Sinai, New York, New York

SARAH E. UMETSU, MD, PhD
Associate Professor, Department of Pathology, University of California, San Francisco, San Francisco, California

DONGHAI WANG, MD, PhD
Clinical Assistant Professor, Department of Pathology, NYU Grossman School of Medicine, NYU Langone Health, New York, New York

HANLIN L. WANG, MD, PhD
Professor, Department of Pathology and Laboratory Medicine, David Geffen School of Medicine, Ronald Reagan UCLA Medical Center, University of California, Los Angeles, Los Angeles, California

MATTHEW M. YEH, MD, PhD
Professor, Laboratory Medicine and Pathology, University of Washington, Seattle, Washington

LEI ZHAO, MD, PhD
Associate Pathologist, Department of Pathology, Brigham and Women's Hospital, Assistant Professor, Harvard Medical School, Boston, Massachusetts

STEPHEN D. ZUCKER, MD
Associate Professor of Medicine, Harvard Medical School, Director of Hepatology, Brigham and Women's Hospital, Boston, Massachusetts

Contents

nature, however, as patients are receiving many different medications and can also have intrinsic liver disease that may be exacerbated by the systemic disorder. Some disorders have typical histologic findings that can be diagnosed on liver biopsy, whereas others will show a more nonspecific histology. Clinicians should be aware of these conditions so as to consider the performance of a liver biopsy at the most opportune time and setting to help establish the diagnosis of acute or chronic liver disease.

Oncotherapeutic agents can cause a wide range of liver injuries from elevated liver functions tests to fulminant liver failure. In this review, we emphasize newer generation of drugs including immune checkpoint inhibitors, protein kinase inhibitors, monoclonal antibodies, and hormonal therapy. A few conventional chemotherapy agents are also discussed.

Hematopoietic stem cell transplantation is used to treat a variety of hematologic malignancies and autoimmune conditions. The immunosuppressive medications as well as other therapies used both before and after transplantation leave patients susceptible to a wide spectrum of complications, including liver injury. Causes for liver damage associated with stem cell transplantation include sinusoidal obstruction syndrome, graft-versus-host disease, iron overload, and opportunistic infection. Here, the authors review the clinical and pathological findings of these etiologies of liver injury and provide a framework for diagnosis.

Pathologists face many challenges when diagnosing sclerosing biliary lesions on liver biopsy. First, histologic findings tend to be nonspecific with similar to identical features seen in numerous conditions, from benign to outright malignant. In addition, the patchy nature of many of these entities amplifies the inherent limitations of biopsy sampling. The end result often forces pathologists to issue descriptive sign outs that require careful clinical correlation; however, certain clinical, radiologic, and histologic features may be of diagnostic assistance. In this article, we review key elements of four sclerosing biliary processes whose proper identification has significant prognostic and therapeutic implications.

Although cirrhosis is one of the most common causes of portal hypertension, noncirrhotic portal hypertension can result from hemodynamic perturbations occurring in the prehepatic, intrahepatic, and posthepatic circulation. Intrahepatic portal hypertension can be further subclassified relative to the hepatic sinusoids as presinusoidal, sinusoidal, and postsinusoidal. For many of these differential diagnoses, the etiology is known but the cause of idiopathic noncirrhotic portal hypertension, recently included in porto-sinusoidal vascular disease (PSVD), remains poorly understood. Herein, we discuss the diagnostic pathological features of noncirrhotic portal hypertension, with an emphasis on PSVD.

Donghai Wang and Joseph Misdraji

Hepatic inflammatory pseudotumor (IPT) describes a mass lesion composed of fibroblasts or myofibroblasts with a dense inflammatory infiltrate comprising lymphocyte, plasma cells, and histiocytes. These lesions are presumed to be an exuberant response to an infectious organism, although in most cases the causative agent is unknown. In specific circumstances, pathologists should consider ancillary techniques to exclude specific infections, such as mycobacteria, Candida, or syphilis. IgG4-related disease may cause a plasma-cell rich IPT. Finally, true neoplasms can mimic IPTs and must be excluded with appropriate ancillary studies, including inflammatory myofibroblastic tumor, follicular dendritic cell tumor, inflammatory angiomyolipoma, Hodgkin lymphoma, and inflammatory hepatocellular carcinoma.

Sarah E. Umetsu and Sanjay Kakar

Needle core biopsies of liver lesions can be challenging, particularly in cases with limited material. The differential diagnosis for well-differentiated hepatocellular lesions includes focal nodular hyperplasia, hepatocellular adenoma, and well-differentiated hepatocellular carcinoma (HCC) in noncirrhotic liver, while dysplastic nodules and well-differentiated HCC are the primary considerations in cirrhotic liver. The first part of this review focuses on histochemical and immunohistochemical stains as well as molecular assays that are useful in the differential diagnosis. The second portion describes the features of hepatocellular adenoma subtypes and focuses on the differential diagnoses in commonly encountered clinicopathologic scenarios.

Tony El Jabbour, Attila Molnar, and Stephen M. Lagana

Intrahepatic cholangiocarcinoma is a challenge to the practicing surgical pathologist for several reasons. It is rare in many parts of the world, and thus practical exposure may be limited. Related to the fact of its rarity is the fact that more common tumors which frequently metastasize to the liver can be morphologically indistinguishable (eg, pancreatic ductal adenocarcinoma). Immunohistochemical testing is generally non-contributory in this context. Other difficulties arise from the protean morphologic manifestations of cholangiocarcinoma (ie, small duct vs. large duct) and the existence of combined cholangiocarcinoma and hepatocellular carcinoma. These, and other issues of concern to the practicing diagnostic pathologist are discussed herein.

David J. Papke Jr.

Mesenchymal neoplasms of the liver can be diagnostically challenging, particularly on core needle biopsies. Here, I discuss recent updates in neoplasms that are specific to the liver (mesenchymal hamartoma, undifferentiated embryonal sarcoma, calcifying nested stromal-epithelial tumor), vascular tumors of the liver (anastomosing hemangioma, hepatic small vessel neoplasm, epithelioid hemangioendothelioma, angiosarcoma), and other tumor types that can occur primarily in the liver (PEComa/angiomyolipoma, inflammatory pseudotumor-like follicular dendritic cell sarcoma, EBV-associated smooth muscle tumor, inflammatory myofibroblastic tumor, malignant rhabdoid tumor). Lastly, I discuss metastatic sarcomas to the liver, as well as pitfalls presented by metastatic melanoma and sarcomatoid carcinoma.

SURGICAL PATHOLOGY CLINICS

SERIES OF RELATED INTEREST

Clinics in Laboratory Medicine
http://www.labmed.theclinics.com/
Medical Clinics
https://www.medical.theclinics.com/

THE CLINICS ARE AVAILABLE ONLINE!
Access your subscription at:
www.theclinics.com

Preface

Liver Pathology: Diagnostic Challenges, Practical Considerations and Emerging Concepts

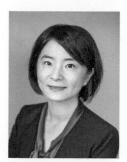

Lei Zhao, MD, PhD

Editor

With advancements in the diagnosis, surveillance, and treatment of medical liver diseases, the utility of liver biopsy has evolved significantly in recent years. In 2022, the primary purpose of tissue biopsy at the Brigham and Women's Hospital in Boston was to assess fibrosis stage (25%), autoimmune hepatitis or overlap syndrome (17.5%), fatty liver disease (14.2%), and cholestatic or hepatocellular liver injury with unknown cause (43.3%). Among the latter, many patients were suspected of having drug-/medication-induced liver injury, while some also had chronic systemic inflammatory disease. This issue of *Surgical Pathology Clinics* on Liver Pathology focuses on diagnostic criteria, differential diagnosis, practice guidelines, and challenges and pitfalls associated with these entities.

The issue begins with an update on the clinical workup and indications for medical liver diseases in contemporary practice. This update is followed by a comprehensive review of fibrosis staging systems for various chronic liver diseases. Subsequently, an extensive discussion of liver involvement in chronic systemic diseases is provided. This issue also includes a summary of SARS-CoV-2–induced liver injury. As the previous issue thoroughly covered fatty liver disease, autoimmune hepatitis, primary biliary cholangitis, and drug-induced liver injury, this issue focuses on liver complications associated with novel oncotherapeutic agents and stem cell

transplants. Selected cholangiopathies with overlapping pathologic findings and distinct clinical management are reviewed. Finally, the expanding literature and improved understanding of noncirrhotic portal hypertension and portosinusoidal vascular diseases are summarized.

Liver biopsy remains an indispensable diagnostic tool for liver masses. Here, we discuss four diagnostic challenges: well-differentiated hepatocellular tumors; adenocarcinomas; inflammatory masses; and mesenchymal tumors. Each article provides a comprehensive discussion of differential diagnosis, the utility of ancillary testing, and diagnostic challenges and pitfalls.

I am extremely grateful to all the contributors for providing a comprehensive review of their respective topics, complete with beautiful illustrations, thoughtful insights, and up-to-date concepts. I hope the readers of this issue find these references relevant, practical, and informative.

Lei Zhao, MD, PhD
Department of Pathology
Brigham and Women's Hospital
75 Francis Street
Boston, MA, 02115, USA

E-mail address:
lzhao19@bwh.harvard.edu

Surgical Pathology 16 (2023) xi
https://doi.org/10.1016/j.path.2023.04.004
1875-9181/23/© 2023 Published by Elsevier Inc.

How Hepatologists Use Liver Biopsy in the Evaluation of Liver Disease?

Emilie K. Mitten, MD, Anna Rutherford, MD, MPH*

KEYWORDS

- Abnormal liver tests • Liver biopsy • Hepatic steatosis • Hepatic fibrosis • Liver fibrosis

Key points

- Liver biopsy is an integral part of the evaluation of abnormal liver tests and underlying liver disease.
- The utility of liver biopsy in diagnosis and management varies among etiologies of liver disease.
- Liver biopsy is particularly useful when multiple diagnoses with differing management strategies are being considered and when results from noninvasive fibrosis assessments are conflicting.

ABSTRACT

This article focuses on how hepatologists view the role of liver biopsy in diagnosis, assessment, and management of chronic and acute liver disease, and its variable use among different etiologies of liver disease and in the evaluation of liver fibrosis.

THE ROLE OF LIVER BIOPSY IN CLINICAL PRACTICE

Hepatologists consider liver biopsy to be an integral part of the evaluation of abnormal liver tests or underlying liver disease, the evaluation of abnormal liver imaging, the assessment of hepatic fibrosis, and occasionally, the evaluation of acute hepatitis, acute liver injury, or acute liver failure.

Alanine aminotransferase (ALT), aspartate aminotransferase (AST), alkaline phosphatase (ALP), and bilirubin are markers of liver injury and should be referred to as liver tests or chemistries. The two best markers of liver function are albumin and prothrombin time (PT), the latter of which is often reported as the international normalized ratio (INR).[1] Hepatocellular liver injury is defined as a pronounced elevation of AST and ALT levels as compared to ALP, whereas cholestatic liver injury is defined as a pronounced elevation in ALP as compared to AST and ALT. Mixed liver injury refers to the elevation of AST, ALT, and ALP. The R ratio (**Box 1**),[1] which is calculated by dividing the proportion of ALT elevation by the proportion of ALP elevation, can help distinguish between hepatocellular, cholestatic, or mixed liver injury.[1,2]

When evaluating abnormal liver tests or suspected underlying liver disease, a hepatologist will start with a careful liver-focused history, including medications, supplements, recent antibiotics or new medications in the last 6 months, alcohol intake, metabolic risk factors, risk factors for viral hepatitis, and personal and family history of liver disease and autoimmune disease. They will perform a targeted physical exam, including the percussion and palpation of the liver and spleen; inspection of the skin for jaundice, spider angiomata, and palmar erythema; and inspection of the chest and abdominal wall for gynecomastia, caput medusae, and a fluid wave. While considering the pattern of liver

Drs E.K. Mitten and A. Rutherford do not have any commercial or financial conflicts of interest related to this article.

Harvard Medical School and Division of Gastroenterology, Hepatology & Endoscopy at Brigham & Women's Hospital, 75 Francis Street, Boston, MA 02115, USA

* Corresponding author. Division of Gastroenterology, Hepatology & Endoscopy, Brigham & Women's Hospital, 75 Francis Street, ASB II, Boston, MA 02115.

E-mail address: arutherford@bwh.harvard.edu

Box 1
The R ratio[1] helps to differentiate between hepatocellular and cholestatic liver injury

$$R \text{ ratio} = \frac{(\text{patient's ALT/upper limit of normal of ALT})}{(\text{patient's ALP/upper limit of normal of ALP})}$$

An R ratio of >5 indicates hepatocellular injury
An R ratio of <2 indicates cholestatic injury
An R ratio of 2–5 indicates a mixed pattern of injury

injury (hepatocellular, cholestatic, or mixed), as well as the history and physical exam, the hepatologist will perform serologic evaluation, including viral hepatitis studies, autoimmune studies, and screening tests for metabolic liver disease (iron studies, alpha-1 antitrypsin level, ceruloplasmin), as well as imaging of the liver (Fig. 1).

If there is no clear etiology or cause of abnormal liver tests or underlying liver disease, or if there are several possible diagnoses being considered, the hepatologist will discuss a liver biopsy with the patient. In one study, liver biopsy for the evaluation of unexplained liver test abnormalities identified a cause in 84% of patients, yielded normal liver tissue in 13%, and was nondiagnostic in 3%.[3] Liver biopsies can be performed percutaneously, via a transjugular approach, via an endoscopic approach, and intra-operatively. A percutaneous biopsy, usually done with guidance by computed tomography (CT) or ultrasound (US), is the most common type of liver biopsy performed. If a patient has significant thrombocytopenia, coagulopathy, or ascites, which might increase the risk of bleeding or infection with percutaneous biopsy, or if additional information such as hepatic venous pressure gradient (HVPG) or hepatic venography is

warranted, the transjugular approach is preferred. Liver biopsy via endoscopic ultrasound (EUS) may be done in combination with other endoscopic tests, including elastography, direct portal vein pressure measurements, assessment of the biliary tree, and management of varices.[4]

Another indication for a liver biopsy is to further evaluate abnormal findings on liver imaging, such as coarse hepatic echotexture on US or nodular liver contour on any type of abdominal imaging, including US, CT, and magnetic resonance imaging (MRI). Coarse hepatic echotexture most often reflects hepatic steatosis, hepatic fibrosis, or both, and distinctions between these can be clinically relevant.[5] Nodular liver contour commonly indicates underlying cirrhosis; however, there are several alternate diagnoses, such as nodular regenerative hyperplasia, congestive hepatopathy, chronic Budd Chiari syndrome, hepatic metastasis, and pseudocirrhosis, all of which have very different clinical implications and may only be distinguished by liver biopsy.

If the etiology of elevated liver tests or underlying liver disease is clear with the above evaluation and does not require a liver biopsy, a hepatologist will perform an assessment of liver fibrosis. The degree of liver fibrosis predicts the risk of future hepatic

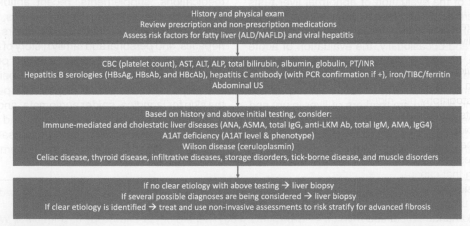

Fig. 1. Evaluation of elevated liver tests or underlying liver disease. A1AT, alpha-1 antitrypsin; ALD, alcohol-associated liver disease; ALP, alkaline phosphatase; ALT, alanine aminotransferase; AMA, antimitochondrial antibody; ANA, antinuclear antibody; anti-LKM, anti-liver kidney microsome type 1 antibody; ASMA, anti-smooth muscle antibody; AST, aspartate aminotransferase; CBC, complete blood count; HBcAb, hepatitis C core antibody; HBsAb, hepatitis B surface antibody; HBsAg, hepatitis B surface antigen; IgG, immunoglobulin G; IgG4, IgG subclass 4; IgM, immunoglobulin M; NAFLD, nonalcoholic liver disease; PT/INR, prothrombin time/international normalized ratio; TIBC, total iron binding capacity; US, ultrasound.

complications and guides management, including identifying those with advanced fibrosis who will need hepatocellular carcinoma screening and variceal screening. While liver biopsy is still regarded as the gold standard for fibrosis staging, noninvasive assessment of fibrosis (using serum tests and/or imaging modalities) is widely used in clinical practice now[6] and recommended for fibrosis risk stratification in the setting of chronic liver diseases.[7]

Hepatologists often use a combination of serologic testing and elastography, when available, to noninvasively assess liver fibrosis. Serologic markers of fibrosis can be direct or indirect. Direct markers of fibrosis reflect extracellular matrix turnover (eg, hyaluronic acid, procollagen types I and III), whereas indirect markers reflect hepatic function (eg, platelet count, coagulation studies, and hepatic aminotransferases). Commonly used, nonpatented, low-cost serum biomarker tests (which utilize markers of hepatic function) include the fibrosis-4 (FIB-4) index and the AST to platelet ratio index (APRI). Commonly used, commercially available serum biomarker tests that incorporate markers of matrix turnover include FibroTest/FibroSURE, Hepascore, and FIBROSpect. These tests are good at distinguishing between minimal liver fibrosis and advanced fibrosis, but those with indeterminate results require further testing; in addition, these panels contain components that are not liver-specific, and that can be affected by systemic inflammation. Cross-sectional imaging can demonstrate anatomic features of advanced liver disease, such as hepatic nodularity, caudate lobe hypertrophy, or signs of portal hypertension, but they are not sufficient to detect earlier stages of liver fibrosis. Transient elastography (by US or MRI) estimates liver stiffness by sending mechanical waves through hepatic tissue and measuring propagation speed. The degree of liver stiffness correlates with the degree of liver fibrosis for different etiologies of liver disease. US elastography is most commonly used, as it is widely available, quick, and portable, and it has been validated in large populations.[8] However, MRI elastography has higher accuracy, especially in patients with obesity and/or ascites.[9]

Liver biopsy is used to stage liver fibrosis if noninvasive means of assessing liver fibrosis yield conflicting results, or if the patient has an underlying condition that cannot be adequately assessed with noninvasive tests. For example, transient elastography is unable to distinguish between hepatic congestion and liver fibrosis, therefore congestive hepatopathy results in very elevated liver stiffness measurements, even in the absence of underlying fibrosis.

How often a liver biopsy is required or used in the diagnosis, assessment, or management of a chronic liver disease varies with each etiology of liver disease. Autoimmune hepatitis (AIH) requires a liver biopsy for diagnosis. Primary biliary cholangitis (PBC), sclerosing cholangitis, and noncirrhotic portal hypertension usually require a liver biopsy, whereas alcohol-associated liver disease (ALD), nonalcoholic fatty liver disease (NAFLD), hereditary hemochromatosis (HH), Wilson disease, and alpha-1 antitrypsin (A1AT) deficiency liver disease less commonly require liver biopsy. Diagnosis of chronic viral hepatitis, including hepatitis B (HBV), hepatitis C (HCV), and hepatitis D (HDV) rarely requires a liver biopsy. The evaluation of acute hepatitis, acute liver injury (ALI), or acute liver failure (ALF) is usually based on history and exam as well as serologic testing and imaging. However, a liver biopsy may be obtained in the setting of ALI/ALF if the etiology remains unclear, if the suspected etiology is a liver disease that relies on biopsy for diagnosis (such as autoimmune hepatitis), or if liver biopsy and diagnosis might alter management (such as prompting liver transplant evaluation in acute liver failure from Wilson disease).

AUTOIMMUNE HEPATITIS

AIH is an immune-mediated liver disease in which loss of self-tolerance to hepatic autoantigens leads to hepatic inflammation, necrosis, and fibrosis. It occurs in adults and children, predominately female, of all ages, races, and ethnicities. The most common symptoms of AIH are fatigue, myalgias, and arthralgias. Around 25% to 35% of patients with AIH are asymptomatic, in which case, workup occurs after the incidental detection of abnormal liver tests. Patients with AIH may present with chronic hepatitis, cirrhosis (present in up to one-third of patients at the time of diagnosis), acute hepatitis, or acute liver failure. Associated extrahepatic autoimmune diseases (autoimmune thyroiditis, rheumatoid arthritis, systemic lupus erythematosus, celiac disease, inflammatory bowel disease, vitiligo, and type 1 diabetes mellitus) may also be present.[1,10]

According to the American Association for the Study of Liver Diseases (AASLD) 2019 guidelines and the European Association for the Study of the Liver (EASL) 2015 guidelines, the diagnosis of AIH requires a liver biopsy.[10,11] The diagnosis requires compatible histologic findings (eg, interface hepatitis, plasma cell infiltration, lobular hepatitis, and centrilobular necrosis) in addition to elevated serum aminotransferase levels, elevated serum immunoglobulin G (IgG) level and/or positive circulating autoantibodies, and exclusion of diseases that may resemble AIH (such as viral hepatitis). The most common antibodies in AIH are antinuclear antibody (ANA) and anti-smooth muscle antibody (ASMA) in type 1 autoimmune hepatitis (seen in adults and children), and anti-liver kidney microsome type 1 antibody (anti-LKM) in type 2 autoimmune hepatitis (seen mainly in children). Up to 20% of patients have seronegative AIH; liver biopsy is especially important in these patients. The International Autoimmune Hepatitis Group (IAIHG) published a scoring system for the diagnosis of AIH in 1993 (and a simplified version in 2008, used more in research than clinical practice), that requires liver biopsy for diagnosis.[10]

In addition to evaluating for typical histologic features of AIH, grading necro-inflammatory activity, and staging fibrosis, a liver biopsy can also help to identify overlapping or concurrent liver diseases, such as primary biliary cholangitis (PBC), primary sclerosing cholangitis (PSC), and nonalcoholic fatty liver disease (NAFLD).[10] Diagnosis of overlapping liver disease is important, as it can affect overall management strategy and prognosis.

Histologic findings and autoantibodies are similar in AIH and drug-induced AIH-like injury; therefore, clinical history is most helpful when drug-induced AIH-like injury is suspected. Most importantly, there should be an association between drug exposure and onset of liver injury. However, the latency interval is variable; onset of drug-induced AIH-like injury may occur in 1 week to 12 months after drug exposure. Many medications have been associated with drug-induced AIH-like injury, including minocycline, nitrofurantoin, infliximab, and adalimumab. While less than 20% of cases of AIH are acute in onset, greater than 60% of cases of drug-induced AIH-like injury are acute in presentation. Hypersensitivity reactions (such as fever, rash, and eosinophilia) are unusual in AIH but seen in up to 30% of patients with drug-induced AIH-like injury. HLA DRB1*03:01 or DRB1*04:01 haplotypes are common in AIH whereas there are no HLA haplotypes associated with drug-induced AIH-like injury. Concurrent autoimmune diseases and cirrhosis at the time of presentation are seen in a significant percentage of those with AIH (15%–45% and 30%, respectively), but both are rare in those with drug-induced AIH-like injury. Differentiating the two disease processes is important, as the treatment and prognosis are different. Initial treatment for AIH consists of immunosuppression with a glucocorticoid and an antimetabolite. Initial treatment for drug-induced AIH-like injury consists of withdrawal of culprit medication followed by close monitoring to ensure the normalization of liver biochemistries; if the laboratory tests do not improve, or if the laboratory abnormalities are significant (serum aminotransferase levels >3-fold ULN or total bilirubin >2-fold ULN), glucocorticoid therapy can be considered. Up to 60% to 85% of patients with AIH relapse after withdrawal of immunosuppression; in contrast, relapse after withdrawal of immunosuppression in drug-induced AIH is rare.[10,12]

Once the diagnosis of AIH is established, liver biopsy can also play a role in assessing response to therapy and risk of relapse. Initial histologic assessment at the time of diagnosis plays a role in determining the most appropriate glucocorticoid therapy; budesonide is often preferred over prednisone (or prednisolone), but should be avoided in cirrhosis and acute severe AIH. Once biochemical remission (defined by the normalization of AST, ALT, and IgG) is achieved, glucocorticoid therapy is slowly tapered and a steroid-sparing agent such as azathioprine, mycophenolate or tacrolimus is initiated for maintenance. If unable to achieve biochemical remission or taper glucocorticoids, a repeat liver biopsy may be needed to re-confirm the diagnosis and exclude new etiologies of liver injury. In patients who have been in biochemical remission for at least 2 years, withdrawal of immunosuppression can be considered. A repeat liver biopsy to assess for histologic remission is always recommended in children and often recommended in adults prior to the withdrawal of immunosuppression; those who are not in histologic remission are more likely to relapse off immunosuppression. Once immunosuppression is withdrawn, liver biochemistries are monitored to assess for relapse. Relapse may or may not require repeat liver biopsy, depending on the clinical confidence in the diagnosis of relapse and the likelihood of a new type of liver injury.[10]

Because a patient with AIH may need to undergo numerous liver biopsies to assist with the optimization of immunosuppression and to assess for the risk of relapse prior to the withdrawal of immunosuppression, there are ongoing efforts to develop noninvasive biomarkers that predict risk of relapse and/or serve as early markers for relapse. For example, serum adenosine deaminase (ADA) levels appear to correlate with histologic disease severity at presentation, while serum TGF- ß1 levels appear to correlate with active histologic disease, even in the setting of biochemical remission.[13] However, such markers have not yet been validated for clinical practice.

PRIMARY BILIARY CHOLANGITIS

PBC is a chronic cholestatic liver disease that arises in the setting of immune-mediated injury to (and destruction of) the small intralobular bile ducts. PBC occurs almost exclusively (>90%) in females, who are most often in middle age (age 30–60) at the time of diagnosis. Patients may be symptomatic or asymptomatic at the time of diagnosis; however, among those without symptoms, 35% to 90% will become symptomatic over a median of 2 to 4 years from diagnosis. The most common symptoms are fatigue and pruritis.[1,14] Hepatomegaly and xanthomas may be detected on exam. Symptoms of associated extrahepatic autoimmune diseases, such as Sjogren's syndrome and scleroderma, may also be present. Natural history studies done prior to the introduction of ursodeoxycholic acid (UDCA) demonstrate that most patients with PBC experience progressive fibrosis; in this setting, the median time from diagnosis to the development of advanced fibrosis (>/ = F3) was 2 years. However, since the introduction of UDCA, the rate of progression to cirrhosis has significantly decreased.[14]

The workup of cholestatic liver disease begins with imaging to exclude bile duct stenosis or obstruction, including large duct sclerosing cholangitis. As described in the AASLD 2019 guidelines, the diagnosis of PBC is based on the presence of at least two of three criteria, which include: (1) biochemical evidence of cholestasis with elevated ALP activity; (2) presence of antimitochondrial antibody (AMA); and (3) histopathologic evidence of nonsuppurative cholangitis and destruction of small or medium-sized bile ducts on liver biopsy. Of note, circulating AMA is detected in greater than 95% of patients with PBC and is thought to play a role in disease pathogenesis. An elevated immunoglobulin M (IgM), while not part of the diagnostic criteria, may support the diagnosis of PBC. Those with AMA-negative PBC require liver biopsy to make the diagnosis, although some argue that the diagnosis can still be made without histology if other highly specific antibodies (such as antibodies to sp100, gp210, anti-kelch-like 12, and anti-hexokinase 1) are present.[14] Liver biopsy should also be considered in atypical patients (eg, a young male) and those with a history of inflammatory bowel disease (IBD) to improve diagnostic certainty.

While mild aminotransferase elevations are common in PBC, liver biopsy is recommended in patients with ALT > 5-fold ULN, as this may indicate concomitant AIH or other liver diseases. Scoring systems have been developed for the diagnosis of AIH-PBC overlap, the most common of which is the Paris Criteria. If liver histology is consistent with both PBC and AIH, treatment may include both UDCA and immunosuppression. In general, liver histology takes priority over the presence of disease-specific autoantibodies; for example, a patient with a positive AMA without histologic evidence of PBC should be treated like AIH.[14]

Weight-based UDCA is first-line therapy for PBC. Treatment response is assessed through liver biochemistries. Biochemical response to UDCA should be determined at 12 months after the initiation of therapy. Liver biopsy is not necessary prior to the initiation of second-line therapy, but may be considered if the initial diagnosis is in question. Initial response to UDCA followed by subsequent worsening of liver biochemistries should prompt the consideration of AIH or other liver disease.[14]

Noninvasive tests, such as elastography, have largely replaced liver biopsy to monitor for the progression of fibrosis or the development of portal hypertension. Elastography has been used to risk stratify patients with PBC; higher stiffness is associated with higher risk of decompensation, death, and LT.[14]

SCLEROSING CHOLANGITIS

Sclerosing cholangitis refers to the inflammation and scarring of the bile ducts. It may occur in the setting of a primary progressive fibroinflammatory disease of the bile ducts, termed primary sclerosing cholangitis (PSC), or it may occur secondary to another disease process, referred to as secondary sclerosing cholangitis. A diagnosis of PSC requires the exclusion of secondary sclerosing cholangitis. Etiologies of secondary sclerosing cholangitis include chronic bacterial cholangitis, recurrent pyogenic cholangitis (hepatolithiasis), ischemic cholangiopathy, recurrent pancreatitis, surgical biliary trauma, cholangiocarcinoma, diffuse hepatic metastases, mast cell cholangiopathy, eosinophilic cholangitis, HIV/AIDS-associated cholangiopathy, and IgG4 disease. Many of these etiologies can be ruled out by clinical history, cross-sectional imaging, and cholangiography. MRCP has become the preferred method of cholangiography in suspected PSC without a dominant stricture. However, ERCP remains an important diagnostic modality, especially when bile duct brushings or biopsy are needed to diagnose cholangiocarcinoma or IgG4-associated sclerosing cholangitis.[15] It should be noted that IgG4-associated sclerosing cholangitis is likely a separate entity, rather than a subtype of PSC. A history of autoimmune pancreatitis should raise clinical suspicion for IgG4-sclerosing cholangitis. All patients with newly diagnosed sclerosing cholangitis should have serum IgG4 level checked at the time of presentation to exclude IgG4 disease, which is managed differently than PSC.[16]

The pathogenesis of PSC is not fully understood, but it is likely immune mediated. It is estimated that up to two-thirds of patients with PSC have IBD, usually ulcerative colitis (UC)[15]; among PSC patients with UC, there is a male predominance, whereas PSC patients without UC, there is a slight female predominance. The clinical course is highly variable. PSC may be aysymptomatic, but most common symptoms are fatigue and pruritis. PSC can result in complications including bile duct obstruction, cholangitis, cholangiocarcinoma, and decompensated cirrhosis. Large duct PSC usually involves both the intrahepatic and extrahepatic ducts, although a subset of patients (<25%) may have only intrahepatic involvement. Large duct PSC does not require liver biopsy for diagnosis; once other causes of sclerosing cholangitis are excluded, cholestatic liver biochemistries and characteristic multifocal strictures and segmental dilations on cholangiogram are sufficient. The multifocal strictures in PSC are classically short and alternate with normal or slightly dilated segments, producing a "beaded" pattern on cholangiogram. It has been demonstrated that 60% of patients with PSC have an elevated IgG and up to 50% of patients with PSC have circulating autoantibodies, which are most commonly atypical proteinase-3 antineutrophil cytoplasmic antibodies (p-ANCA) but also ANA and ASMA. However, the presence or absence of these serologic findings is not part of the diagnostic criteria for PSC.[16]

While large duct PSC generally does not require a liver biopsy for diagnosis, there are some exceptions. First, a liver biopsy is indicated if there is clinical suspicion of IgG4-related disease or if serum IgG4 levels are elevated. Histopathology in IgG4-related disease demonstrates a dense lymphoplasmacytic infiltrate rich in IgG4 + plasma cells.[17] As mentioned above, the diagnosis of IgG4-related disease is important, as this condition is best treated with immunosuppression (whereas PSC does not respond to immunosuppression). Second, a liver biopsy is indicated in the setting of disproportionate aminotransferase elevations, as this raises suspicion for AIH-PSC overlap. Criteria for the diagnosis of AIH-PSC overlap syndrome include the presence of typical features of AIH, the absence of AMA, and evidence of large-duct PSC by endoscopic or magnetic resonance cholangiography or evidence of small-duct PSC based on "onion skinning" periductal fibrosis on histology.[10]

In contrast to large duct PSC, a diagnosis of small duct PSC requires a liver biopsy. Small duct PSC represents only about 5% of all cases of PSC. This variant presents with cholestatic liver biochemistries and normal appearance of the bile ducts on cholangiogram.[16]

There is no established therapy for PSC. UDCA is associated with biochemical improvement, but not definitively associated with clinical improvement. Case series suggest that oral vancomycin may improve biochemistries and symptoms.

Glucocorticoids, antimetabolites, and calcineurin inhibitors have not been shown to be beneficial.[16] Patients with large duct PSC require frequent screening for colon cancer and cholangiocarcinoma.

NONCIRRHOTIC PORTAL HYPERTENSION OF UNCLEAR ETIOLOGY

NCPH is defined as elevated portal pressure, meaning a hepatic-venous or porta-caval pressure gradient exceeding 5 mm Hg, in the absence of cirrhosis.[18] NCPH is associated with a number of different, often extra-hepatic or systemic, diseases. Traditionally, NCPH is classified by the site of vascular resistance: pre-hepatic, hepatic (pre-sinusoidal, sinusoidal, or post-sinusoidal), or post-hepatic (**Fig. 2**).[18–22]

Liver biopsy is indicated in all cases of suspected NCPH to exclude cirrhosis and to evaluate for specific etiologies of NCPH. Liver biopsy can reveal specific patterns of injury, including pre-sinusoidal, sinusoidal, and post-sinusoidal injury. Transjugular liver biopsy with hemodynamic measurements is also helpful in characterizing the type of NCPH.[18–22]

The management of NCPH mainly consists of optimizing therapy for the underlying disease and managing complications of portal hypertension.[18–22]

ALCOHOL-ASSOCIATED LIVER DISEASE

Alcohol-associated liver disease (ALD) includes a spectrum of clinical presentations (including asymptomatic liver test elevations, mild or severe alcoholic hepatitis, and compensated or decompensated cirrhosis) and histologic findings (**Fig. 3**).[9,23–25] ALD is associated with alcohol use disorder (AUD), defined as drinking behavior that results in negative consequences and symptoms. The incidence of AUD and ALD is increasing in the US. While only 10% to 20% of patients with ALD will develop cirrhosis,[9,25] ALD is now the most common indication for liver transplant and etiology of liver-related death in the US. Furthermore, the burden of ALD is likely underestimated, as ALD may contribute to accelerated liver injury in other chronic liver diseases (including chronic viral hepatitis, NAFLD, and hemochromatosis).[23,26,27]

ALD is frequently diagnosed by abnormal liver tests or abnormal liver imaging (fatty- or cirrhotic-appearing liver), as greater than 90% of patients with ALD are asymptomatic or have nonspecific symptoms such as fatigue.[9] Proposed criteria for the diagnosis of ALD include harmful alcohol use (>2 drinks/d in females and >3 drinks/d in men) during the past 12 months or longer; liver disease

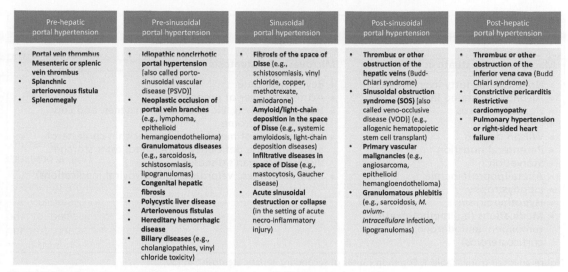

Fig. 2. Etiologies of noncirrhotic portal hypertension.[18–22] (Figure adapted from "Table 1: Causes of non-cirrhotic portal hypertension" in [18].)

manifested by abnormal liver biochemistries, imaging showing steatosis or cirrhosis, and/or clinical signs of cirrhosis; elevated AST and ALT (usually <400 IU/L with AST/ALT ratio >1); and exclusion of other causes of liver disease.[9] Of note, positive autoantibodies (such as ANA and ASMA) and hypergammaglobulinemia (particularly elevated IgA) are common in ALD, especially in the setting of advanced liver disease.[28,29] ANA and ASMA antibody titers in ALD are typically much lower than those seen in AIH.[29]

Liver biopsy is not routinely used for the diagnosis of ALD.[23,27] However, exceptions arise in the setting of alcoholic hepatitis (AH), and in the setting of positive (especially high-titer) autoantibodies. Alcohol

use can be assessed through clinical history. In addition, alcohol biomarkers, such as urine ethyl glucuronide (ETG), urine ethyl sulfate (ETS), and serum phosphatidylethanol (PEth), can detect moderate to significant alcohol use (over the past 24–72 hours with ETG and ETS and up to 14–28 days with PEth).[23] Alternative etiologies for steatosis (**Table 1**)[30] and cirrhosis can be ruled out by clinical history and laboratory tests. Hepatic fat can be assessed and/or quantified by noninvasive means (such as the controlled attenuation parameter on US elastography, or more accurately, the proton density fat fraction on MRI). Similarly, hepatic fibrosis can be assessed by noninvasive means, including US or MRI elastography as well as serum

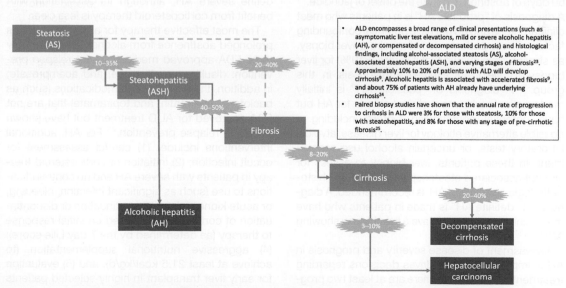

Fig. 3. The natural history of alcohol-associated liver disease (ALD).[9,23–25] (Figure adapted from "Figure 1: Natural history of alcohol-associated liver disease" in [23].)

Table 1
Etiologies of hepatic steatosis[30]

Macrovesicular steatosis	Microvesicular steatosis
• Nonalcoholic fatty liver disease • Alcohol-associated liver disease • Hepatitis C virus • Celiac disease • Wilson disease • Parenteral nutrition • Starvation • Abetalipoproteinemia • Lipodystrophy • Hypothyroidism • Medications (eg, methotrexate, tamoxifen, amiodarone, corticosteroids)	• Reye's syndrome • Acute fatty liver of pregnancy • HELLP (Hemolysis, Elevated Liver enzymes, and Low Platelets) syndrome • Inborn errors of metabolism (eg, lecithin-cholesterol acyltransferase deficiency, cholesterol ester storage disease, Wolman's disease) • Medications (eg, valproate, antiretroviral medications)

Figure adapted from "Table 1. Common causes of secondary hepatic steatosis" in [30].

fibrosis markers, such as the FibroTest/FibroSURE.[9,23] Steatohepatitis, which is associated with increased risk of cirrhosis as compared to simple steatosis, is a histologic finding that can only be diagnosed with liver biopsy.[27]

Alcoholic hepatitis (AH) is a clinical syndrome characterized by rapid onset of jaundice and liver-related complications. Most patients with AH have underlying cirrhosis (75%); therefore, in its severe form, AH is best described as an acute-on-chronic liver failure (ACLF).[24] The National Institute on Alcohol Abuse and Alcoholism (NIAAA) consensus definition for clinical diagnosis of AH is: serum total bilirubin greater than 3.0 mg/dL; AST greater than 50 IU/L, AST and ALT less than 400 IU/L, and AST/ALT greater than 1.5; onset of jaundice within the past 8 weeks; heavy consumption of alcohol (>40 g/d in females or >60 g/d in males) for at least 6 months; and less than 60 days of abstinence before the onset of jaundice.[31] A diagnosis of "probable AH" is in patients who meet clinical criteria and do not have potential confounding factors. These patients do not require a liver biopsy, as studies have shown that it is rare (<10%) for liver biopsy to yield an alternative diagnosis in this group.[31] A diagnosis of "possible AH" is initially made patients who meet clinical criteria for AH but have potential confounding factors including a possible alternative etiology for liver disease, atypical laboratory tests, or uncertain alcohol use assessment. In these patients, liver biopsy to assess for alcohol-associated steatohepatitis (ASH), the histopathologic correlate of AH, is recommended. A diagnosis of "definite AH" is made in patients who have meet clinical criteria and have a liver biopsy showing ASH.[23,24,26,31]

Assessment of disease severity and prognosis in AH is important, as this drives decisions regarding treatment options. While there are at least two prognostic scores that incorporate histologic findings, namely the Alcoholic Hepatitis Histologic Score (AHHS) and the gene-signature plus MELD (gs-MELD) scoring system, the 2019 AASLD guidelines recommend using lab-based prognostic scores to determine prognosis in AH.[23] The Maddrey discriminant function (MDF), derived from a clinical trial comparing corticosteroids to placebo for the treatment of AH and later modified to predict short-term mortality in AH, is commonly used to assess for disease severity and associated prognosis. An MDF of at least 32 defines severe AH (which is associated with 30%–50% mortality at 28 days), while an MDF of less than 32 identifies those with mild/moderate AH. Those with an MDF score of at least 32 may benefit from corticosteroid therapy; in contrast, the risks of corticosteroid therapy are felt to outweigh the benefits in those with MDF less than 32. A MELD score greater than 20 has also been used to define severe AH, although its association with benefit from corticosteroid therapy is less clear.[9,23]

The most effective therapy for all forms of ALD is prolonged abstinence from alcohol. There are now three FDA-approved medications for relapse prevention: disulfiram, naltrexone, and acamprosate; in addition, there are several medications (such as baclofen, gabapentin, and topiramate) that are not FDA approved for AUD treatment but have shown benefit in relapse prevention.[23] For AH, additional interventions include: (1) careful assessment for occult infection; (2) initiation of corticosteroid therapy in patients with severe AH and no contraindications to use (such as significant infection, bleeding, or acute kidney injury) (3) continuation or discontinuation of corticosteroids based on initial response to therapy (as determined by the 7 day Lille score); (4) aggressive nutritional supplementation (to achieve at least 21.5 kcal/kg/d); and (5) evaluation for early liver transplant in highly selected patients with severe AH.[23]

NONALCOHOLIC FATTY LIVER DISEASE

Nonalcoholic fatty liver disease (NAFLD) is defined by the presence of steatosis (on imaging or in more than 5% of hepatocytes on biopsy) in association with metabolic risk factors and in the absence of excessive alcohol consumption or other chronic liver diseases.[30,32] Obesity, type II diabetes mellitus (T2DM), and dyslipidemia are highly prevalent in those with NAFLD, and these conditions increase the risk of developing NAFLD.[30] Like ALD, NAFLD encompasses a broad spectrum of histologic findings, including steatosis or nonalcoholic fatty liver (NAFL), nonalcoholic steatohepatitis (NASH), varying stages of fibrosis, and is associated with heterogenous disease progression and clinical outcomes.[30,32]

The prevalence of NAFLD in the general population, estimated through noninvasive means, is about 25% globally and 35% in the US.[33,34] It has been estimated that 90% of those undergoing bariatric surgery, 80% of those with obesity, 45% to 65% of those with T2DM, and 50% of those with dyslipidemia have NAFLD.[33,35] The prevalence of NAFLD is also higher in older adults, men more than women and in the Hispanic population as compared to non-Hispanic white population in the US.[30] Fibrosis progresses at a faster rate in NASH as compared to NAFL.[36] The prevalence of NASH is more difficult to assess, as this is a histologic finding, and therefore, can only be diagnosed by liver biopsy. Prior estimates suggested that the prevalence of NASH was about 1% to 7% globally and 3% to 5% in the US.[33,35] However, a large prospective cohort study of asymptomatic middle-aged adults in the US, the prevalence of NASH was 14% in the general population and 48% in those with biopsy-confirmed NAFLD.[34] Similarly, the prevalence of fibrosis in NAFLD appears to be higher than previously estimated. In the same study, clinically significant fibrosis (>F2) was seen in 20% of those with biopsy-confirmed NAFLD (NAFL + NASH) and 35% of those with biopsy-confirmed NASH; F3 fibrosis was found in 6% and 10%, respectively.[34]

Less than 10% of patients with NAFLD develop complications of cirrhosis or HCC during the 10 to 20 years after diagnosis (Fig. 4),[32,36–38] and the leading causes of death in NAFLD are cardiovascular disease followed by extrahepatic malignancy.[30] However, given the high prevalence of NAFLD, decompensated NAFLD cirrhosis is now the second leading indication (first among women) for liver transplant in US adults.[39,40] NAFLD is now the third most common cause of HCC in the US, and NAFLD-associated HCC tends to have worse outcomes than HCC related to other liver diseases.[30] Fibrosis is the most important prognostic marker for liver-related outcomes and mortality in NAFLD, and poor outcomes increase incrementally with fibrosis stage.[32,41]

There are no specific recommendations from the U.S. Preventive Services Task Force (USPSTF) or AASLD to screen for NAFLD in the general population or even in at-risk populations. In contrast, the EASL recommends noninvasive screening for NAFLD in patients with metabolic risk factors.[42,43] The 2018 AASLD practice guidance does recommend maintaining a high index of suspicion for NAFLD in patients with T2DM and assessing the likelihood of advanced fibrosis in these patients with noninvasive risk-stratification tools, such as the FIB-4 index, the NAFLD fibrosis score (NFS), or elastography.[30] In addition, AASLD recommends further workup for any incidental finding of steatosis on imaging[30]; as it has been estimated (using FIB-4 and NFS) that 10% to 15% of these patients may already have advanced fibrosis.[5,44] Similarly, patients with abnormal liver chemistries and metabolic risk factors should be evaluated for NAFLD.[30] In 2021, the American Gastroenterological Association (AGA) published a "Clinical Care Pathway" for the risk stratification of patients with NAFLD. In this algorithm, it is recommended that clinicians screen for NAFLD (using history, laboratory tests, and noninvasive fibrosis assessment via FIB-4) in those at high risk, including those with T2DM, those with two or more metabolic risk factors, and those with incidental finding of steatosis or abnormal liver biochemistries.[7]

Like ALD, most cases of NAFLD do not require liver biopsy for diagnosis, as steatosis can be assessed through noninvasive testing (as described later in discussion) and other liver diseases can be excluded through history and serologic testing. However, serologic testing to exclude other causes of liver disease can be challenging in NAFLD, as abnormal tests may occur even when NAFLD is the only underlying liver disease. A mild elevation in ferritin is common in NAFLD and does not necessarily reflect hepatic iron deposition. HFE testing and MRI quantification of iron may aid in assessing the likelihood of hemochromatosis, but in the setting of very elevated ferritin and transferrin saturation (or presence of the C282Y HFE mutation), a liver biopsy may be considered to evaluate for the presence and extent of iron overload.[30,45] Similarly, autoantibodies, especially ANA and ASMA, may be present in NAFLD. Titers are commonly low level, although one study found that ANA greater than 1:160 and ASMA greater than 1:40 were present in 21% of 864 subjects with NAFLD in the NASH clinical research registry; furthermore, NAFLD subjects with these high titers did not have any atypical

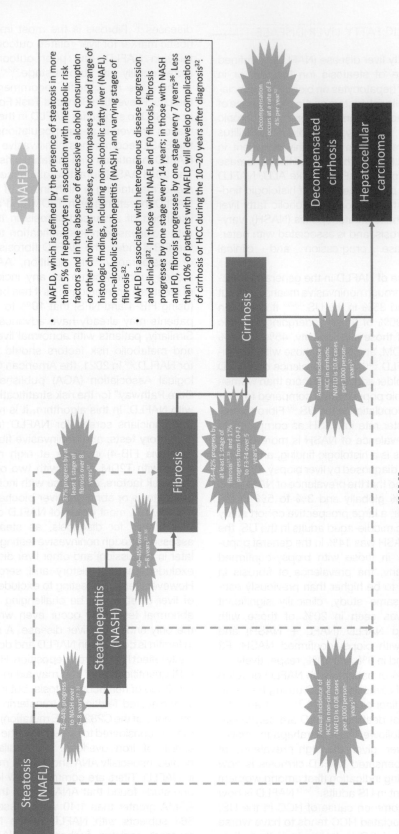

NAFLD

NAFLD, which is defined by the presence of steatosis in more than 5% of hepatocytes in association with metabolic risk factors and in the absence of excessive alcohol consumption or other chronic liver diseases, encompasses a broad range of histologic findings, including non-alcoholic fatty liver (NAFL), non-alcoholic steatohepatitis (NASH), and varying stages of fibrosis[32].

- NAFLD is associated with heterogenous disease progression and clinical[32]. In those with NAFL and F0 fibrosis, fibrosis progresses by one stage every 14 years; in those with NASH and F0, fibrosis progresses by one stage every 7 years[36]. Less than 10% of patients with NAFLD will develop complications of cirrhosis or HCC during the 10–20 years after diagnosis[32].

Steatosis (NAFL)

42–44% progress to NASH over 6–8 years[37,38]

Steatohepatitis (NASH)

40–45% over 5–8 years[37,38]

37% progress by at least 1 stage of fibrosis over 8 years[37]

Fibrosis

34–42% progress by at least 1 stage of fibrosis[7,38] and 17% progress from F0-F2 to F3-F4 over 5 years[38]

Cirrhosis

Annual incidence of HCC in non-cirrhotic NAFLD is 0.08% cases per 1000 person-years[3]

Annual incidence of HCC in cirrhotic NAFLD is 10.6 cases per 1000 person-years[3]

Decompensation occurs at a rate of 3-4% per year[3]

Decompensated cirrhosis

Hepatocellular carcinoma

Fig. 4. The natural history of nonalcoholic fatty liver disease (NAFLD). [32,36-38]

histologic features or advanced disease.[46] Liver biopsy may be considered in patients with positive autoantibodies or other features concerning for AIH (such as aminotransferases >5x ULN, high globulins, or a high total protein to albumin ratio).[30]

Given the high prevalence of NAFLD, the increased risk of disease progression in the setting of NASH (as opposed to NAFL), and the increased risk of liver-related mortality and HCC in the setting of advanced fibrosis, there have been efforts to noninvasively assess the degree of steatosis, the presence of NASH, and the extent of fibrosis. Steatosis can be accurately quantified through MRI (either spectroscopy or proton density fat fraction) or by the continuous attenuation parameter (CAP) obtained during transient elastography. In contrast to steatosis, the ability to predict NASH through noninvasive measures is limited. Elevated liver enzymes, which can be a marker of liver injury, are insensitive for the diagnosis of NASH; in one study, 38% of those with normal ALT had biopsy-proven NASH or advanced fibrosis, and 53% of those with elevated ALT had no NASH or advanced fibrosis.[47] There is active investigation into circulating biomarkers (such as cleaved cytokeratin-18 fragment) that be associated with NASH, but none are used in clinical practice at this time.[30] Thus, liver biopsy remains the only way to accurately identify NASH. Noninvasive assessment of fibrosis, which is the most important prognostic marker in NAFLD, is very well validated in NAFLD. The most common tools include clinical scoring systems (such as FIB-4 index and NFS), proprietary serum biomarkers (such as the Enhanced Liver Fibrosis panel and FibroTest/FibroSURE), and elastography (by US or MRI).[30,45,48,49]

In summary, liver biopsy is not usually necessary to evaluate for steatosis or fibrosis in NAFLD, but it is important in ruling out alternative etiologies of liver disease, assessing for fibrosis in those with indeterminate, disparate, or unexpected results on noninvasive testing, and assessing for steatohepatitis in those who would most benefit from this diagnostic and prognostic information.[30,45] Currently, therapeutics for NAFLD are limited. Weight loss remains the mainstay of therapy (body weight loss of 3%–5% to improve steatosis and 7%–10% to improve NASH and fibrosis), as well as aggressive control of risk factors associated with cardiovascular disease. However, additional therapeutics do not currently exist for simple steatosis. For patients with biopsy-proven NASH, vitamin E therapy (in nondiabetics without cirrhosis), pioglitazone (in nondiabetics and diabetics without decompensated cirrhosis), and semaglutide (in nondiabetics and diabetics) can be considered.[30,45]

HEREDITARY HEMOCHROMATOSIS

HH is a genetic disorder that leads to excessive iron deposition in tissues (including liver, pancreas, heart, joints, skin) and subsequent dysfunction (such as cirrhosis, diabetes, congestive heart failure, arthralgias, skin hyper-pigmentation, and/or porphyria cutanea tarda). HH is distinguished from secondary causes of iron overload by genetic testing and clinical history, and is most prevalent in those of northern European ancestry.[50] Mutations in the HFE gene, which influences hepcidin expression, account for greater than 90% of all cases of HH. The most common mutations in the HFE gene include C282Y, H63D, and S65C. About 80% to 85% of patients with HH are C282Y homozygotes. The prevalence of C282Y homozygosity is 1 in 250 in white populations. Interestingly, the C282Y HFE mutation has highly variable penetrance (only 70% of C282Y homozygotes develop iron overload, eg. elevated ferritin) and expressivity (only 10% of C282Y homozygotes develop organ damage due to iron overload). Compound heterozygotes (C282Y/H63D or C282Y/S65C) may also develop iron overload in tissues. The C282Y/wild-type genotype is very common (prevalence of 1 in 10 in white populations); it may result in elevated serum iron markers, but it is not associated with iron overload in tissues. There are also non-HFE forms of HH caused by mutations in genes that encode other regulatory components of iron homeostasis, such as transferrin receptor 2 (TfR2), ferroportin (SLC40A1), hepcidin (HAMP), and hemojuvelin (HJV); these non-HFE mutations account for less than 5% of all cases of HH.[50]

If genetic testing reveals the C282Y homozygosity or compound heterozygosity, the diagnosis of HH is established (although concurrent liver disease must still be excluded). C282Y homozygotes and compound heterozygotes with both normal liver enzymes and ferritin less than 1000 ug/L are unlikely to have cirrhosis and can be treated with therapeutic phlebotomy to reduce iron stores (and ultimately prevent end-organ damage). C282Y homozygotes and compound heterozygotes with abnormal liver enzymes or ferritin greater than 1000 ug/L may have more advanced liver disease. Serum ferritin appears to be the most significant predictor of advanced fibrosis in C282Y homozygotes, yet its specificity is limited (Bacon and colleagues, 2011). In the setting of abnormal liver enzymes or ferritin greater than 1000 ug/L, 2011 AASLD guidelines and 2017 American College of Gastroenterology (ACG) guidelines recommend liver biopsy to quantify hepatic iron overload and stage fibrosis.[1,50] However, recent studies have shown good correlation between hepatic iron content on liver biopsy and hepatic iron content estimated by MRI techniques (proton transverse relaxation time)[50]; thus, while liver biopsy remains the gold standard to quantify iron overload and assess fibrosis, MRI has gained clinical acceptance as a noninvasive and reliable alternative.[51] Furthermore, MRI can be used to monitor response to therapy, assess for concurrent steatosis, and screen for HCC in those with fibrosis.[51]

WILSON DISEASE

Wilson disease is a rare autosomal recessive disorder, caused by a defective ATP7B copper transporter protein, that results in excess hepatic and systemic copper deposition. The prevalence is 30 per 1 million worldwide.[1,52,53]

Wilson disease is highly variable in presentation, and most commonly presents between ages 5 and 40 as liver disease and/or neuropsychiatric disease. Liver disease from Wilson may be detected during workup for persistently elevated AST and ALT, hepatomegaly, or fatty liver on imaging. It may present as cirrhosis (with or without portal hypertension and decompensation), acute hepatitis, or acute liver failure.[52,53]

Wilson disease can often be diagnosed through clinical assessment and noninvasive tests, but a liver biopsy may be needed if the clinical signs and noninvasive tests are indeterminate or if there is suspicion for alternative or additional liver diseases.[53] The Working Party at the 8th International Meeting on Wilson disease in Leipzig 2001 proposed a diagnostic score that incorporates multiple indicators, including the presence of Kayser-Fleischer rings, the presence of neurologic symptoms, the presence of Coombs-negative hemolytic anemia, low serum ceruloplasmin, elevated urinary copper, elevated hepatic copper assessment, and positive *ATP7B* mutation analysis. A score of at least 4 establishes the diagnosis, a score of 3 indicates that the diagnosis is possible (and more tests should be performed), while a score of 2 or less makes the diagnosis unlikely.[53]

While there are no pathognomonic histologic findings for Wilson disease, careful clinicopathologic correlation may facilitate early diagnosis of Wilson disease when clinical symptoms are not well developed. Depending on the clinical situation, liver biopsy to assess the stage of fibrosis and to measure hepatic copper concentration remains important.[53] In contrast to hemochromatosis, genetic testing remains expensive and less accessible.[53]

ALPHA-1 ANTITRYPSIN DEFICIENCY

A1ATD is the most common genetic cause of liver disease in children, but a rare cause of liver disease in adults. The gene encoding A1AT is SERPINA1; it has autosomal codominant expression.[54] A1AT, which is synthesized in and secreted by the liver, is a serine protease inhibitor (Pi) that protects elastin in lung tissue from excessive destruction by neutrophil elastase.[54] Different mutations in SERPINA1 result in the accumulation of misfolded A1AT protein in hepatocytes (which may lead to chronic liver disease) and/or reduced systemic circulation of A1AT (which may lead to emphysema). The most common pathologic mutations associated with A1ATD liver disease are the Z and S alleles; the M allele is the wild-type allele.[1,54]

The PiZZ phenotype and the less common compound heterozygote PiSZ phenotype result in severe A1AT deficiency (serum A1AT levels are usually <15% in ZZ and 35% in SZ of levels seen in MM). However, clinical presentation associated with PiZZ phenotype is highly variable. It may present in childhood as acute cholestatic liver disease or fulminant hepatitis and progress to end-stage liver disease. It may also present in adulthood with a more indolent course; liver enzymes are often only minimally elevated and progressive liver disease is often not recognized until complications from portal hypertension or cirrhosis (including HCC) arise. Risk factors for the progression of A1ATD liver disease include male sex, older age (>50 years), viral hepatitis, diabetes, and chronic alcohol use.[54]

As recommended in the 2020 AASLD update, screening for A1ATD is recommended in all patients with unexplained liver enzyme elevations as well as those with cryptogenic cirrhosis or HCC. Screening is also recommended in those with a family history of A1AT mutations or rare manifestations of A1ATD (such as necrotizing panniculitis). Screening for A1ATD is also part of the workup for neonatal cholestasis and hepatitis. Screening includes both serum A1AT level (nephelometry) and A1AT phenotypic testing (isoelectric focusing for M, Z, and S alleles). For the PiSZ and PiMZ phenotypes, liver biopsy is helpful in determining whether mutant A1AT protein is contributing to liver disease (eg, detection of the pathognomic PAS-positive, diastase-resistant inclusions in hepatocytes) and whether concurrent liver disease is present.[54,55]

In contrast to lung disease associated with A1ATD (which can be treated with IV enzyme replacement therapy), there is currently no approved therapy to prevent or treat liver disease associated with A1ATD, aside from LT (which effectively restores normal A1AT levels). Management of concurrent liver disease (such as viral hepatitis, NAFLD, ALD) that may accelerate disease progression is recommended.[55] Once diagnosed, yearly elastography to monitor for advanced fibrosis/cirrhosis is recommended in the 2020 AASLD guidelines. Therapies under investigation for A1ATD liver disease aim to enhance the protective mechanisms (for detecting and destroying misfolded proteins in the ER of hepatocytes) and reduce the production of mutant A1AT. Clinical trial data for fazirsiran, an RNA interference therapy designed to reduce the synthesis of the mutant Z-AAT protein, appear promising.[56]

SUMMARY

Hepatologists consider liver biopsy to be an integral part of the evaluation of abnormal liver tests or underlying liver disease. The necessity of liver biopsy in diagnosis and management varies among etiologies of liver disease. Liver biopsy is particularly useful when multiple diagnoses with different management strategies are being considered and when results from noninvasive fibrosis assessments are conflicting.

REFERENCES

1. Kwo PY, Cohen SM, Lim JK. ACG Clinical Guideline: Evaluation of Abnormal Liver Chemistries. Am J Gastroenterol 2017;112(1):18–35.
2. Kalas MA, Chavez L, Leon M, et al. Abnormal liver enzymes: A review for clinicians. World J Hepatol 2021;13(11):1688–98.
3. Khalifa A, Rockey DC. The utility of liver biopsy in 2020. Curr Opin Gastroenterol 2020;36(3):184–91.
4. Obaitan I, Saxena R, Al-Haddad MA. EUS Guided Liver Biopsy. Techniques and Innovations in Gastrointestinal Endoscopy 2022;24(1):66–75.
5. Wright AP, Desai AP, Bajpai S, et al. Gaps in recognition and evaluation of incidentally identified hepatic steatosis. Dig Dis Sci 2015;60(2):333–8.
6. Tana MM, Muir AJ. Diagnosing Liver Fibrosis and Cirrhosis: Serum, Imaging, or Tissue? Clin Gastroenterol Hepatol 2018;16(1):16–8.
7. Kanwal F, Shubrook JH, Adams LA, et al. Clinical Care Pathway for the Risk Stratification and Management of Patients With Nonalcoholic Fatty Liver Disease. Gastroenterology 2021;161(5):1657–69.
8. Lim JK, Flamm SL, Singh S, et al. American Gastroenterological Association Institute Guideline on the Role of Elastography in the Evaluation of Liver Fibrosis. Gastroenterology 2017;152(6):1536–43.
9. Singal AK, Mathurin P. Diagnosis and Treatment of Alcohol-Associated Liver Disease: A Review. JAMA 2021;326(2):165–76.
10. Mack CL, Adams D, Assis DN, et al. Diagnosis and Management of Autoimmune Hepatitis in Adults and Children: 2019 Practice Guidance and Guidelines From the American Association for the Study of Liver Diseases. Hepatology 2020;72(2):671–722.
11. EASL Clinical Practice Guidelines: Autoimmune hepatitis. J Hepatol 2015;63(4):971–1004.
12. Bjornsson E, Talwalkar J, Treeprasertsuk S, et al. Drug-induced autoimmune hepatitis: clinical characteristics and prognosis. Hepatology 2010;51(6):2040–8.
13. Harrington C, Krishnan S, Mack CL, et al. Noninvasive biomarkers for the diagnosis and management of autoimmune hepatitis. Hepatology 2022. https://doi.org/10.1002/hep.32591.
14. Lindor KD, Bowlus CL, Boyer J, et al. Primary Biliary Cholangitis: 2018 Practice Guidance from the American Association for the Study of Liver Diseases. Hepatology 2019;69(1):394–419.
15. Lindor KD, Kowdley KV, Harrison ME, et al. ACG Clinical Guideline: Primary Sclerosing Cholangitis. Am J Gastroenterol 2015;110(5):646–59, [quiz: 660].
16. Chapman R, Fevery J, Kalloo A, et al. Diagnosis and management of primary sclerosing cholangitis. Hepatology 2010;51(2):660–78.
17. Miyabe K, Zen Y, Cornell LD, et al. Gastrointestinal and Extra-Intestinal Manifestations of IgG4-Related Disease. Gastroenterology 2018;155(4):990–1003 e1.
18. Semela D. Systemic disease associated with noncirrhotic portal hypertension. Clin Liver Dis 2015;6(4): 103–6.
19. Schouten JN, Garcia-Pagan JC, Valla DC, et al. Idiopathic noncirrhotic portal hypertension. Hepatology 2011;54(3):1071–81.
20. Etzion O, Koh C, Heller T. Noncirrhotic portal hypertension: An overview. Clin Liver Dis 2015;6(3):72–4.
21. Vuppalanchi R, Mathur K, Pyko M, et al. Liver Stiffness Measurements in Patients with Noncirrhotic Portal Hypertension-The Devil Is in the Details. Hepatology 2018;68(6):2438–40.
22. Sarin SK, Khanna R. Non-cirrhotic portal hypertension. Clin Liver Dis 2014;18(2):451–76.
23. Crabb DW, Im GY, Szabo G, et al. Diagnosis and Treatment of Alcohol-Associated Liver Diseases: 2019 Practice Guidance From the American Association for the Study of Liver Diseases. Hepatology 2020;71(1): 306–33.
24. Gougol A, Clemente-Sanchez A, Argemi J, et al. Alcoholic Hepatitis. Clin Liver Dis 2021;18(2): 90–5.
25. Parker R, Aithal GP, Becker U, et al. Natural history of histologically proven alcohol-related liver disease: A systematic review. J Hepatol 2019;71(3):586–93.
26. Bertha M, Choi G, Mellinger J. Diagnosis and Treatment of Alcohol-Associated Liver Disease: A Patient-Friendly Summary of the 2019 AASLD Guidelines. Clin Liver Dis 2021;17(6):418–23.
27. Singal AK, Bataller R, Ahn J, et al. ACG Clinical Guideline: Alcoholic Liver Disease. Am J Gastroenterol 2018;113(2):175–94.
28. Lian M, Hua J, Sheng L, et al. Prevalence and significance of autoantibodies in patients with alcoholic liver disease. J Dig Dis 2013;14(7):396–401.
29. McFarlane IG. Autoantibodies in alcoholic liver disease. Addict Biol 2000;5(2):141–51.

30. Chalasani N, Younossi Z, Lavine JE, et al. The diagnosis and management of nonalcoholic fatty liver disease: Practice guidance from the American Association for the Study of Liver Diseases. Hepatology 2018;67(1): 328–57.

31. Crabb DW, Bataller R, Chalasani NP, et al. Standard Definitions and Common Data Elements for Clinical Trials in Patients With Alcoholic Hepatitis: Recommendation From the NIAAA Alcoholic Hepatitis Consortia. Gastroenterology 2016;150(4):785–90.

32. Powell EE, Wong VW-S, Rinella M. Non-alcoholic fatty liver disease. Lancet 2021;397(10290):2212–24.

33. Younossi ZM, Koenig AB, Abdelatif D, et al. Global epidemiology of nonalcoholic fatty liver disease-Meta-analytic assessment of prevalence, incidence, and outcomes. Hepatology 2016;64(1):73–84.

34. Harrison SA, Gawrieh S, Roberts K, et al. Prospective evaluation of the prevalence of non-alcoholic fatty liver disease and steatohepatitis in a large middle-aged US cohort. J Hepatol 2021;75(2):284–91.

35. Younossi ZM, Golabi P, de Avila L, et al. The global epidemiology of NAFLD and NASH in patients with type 2 diabetes: A systematic review and meta-analysis. J Hepatol 2019;71(4):793–801.

36. Singh S, Allen AM, Wang Z, et al. Fibrosis progression in nonalcoholic fatty liver vs nonalcoholic steatohepatitis: a systematic review and meta-analysis of paired-biopsy studies. Clin Gastroenterol Hepatol 2015;13(4):643–54.e1-9, [quiz: e39-40].

37. McPherson S, Hardy T, Henderson E, et al. Evidence of NAFLD progression from steatosis to fibrosing-steatohepatitis using paired biopsies: implications for prognosis and clinical management. J Hepatol 2015;62(5):1148–55.

38. Kleiner DE, Brunt EM, Wilson LA, et al. Association of Histologic Disease Activity With Progression of Nonalcoholic Fatty Liver Disease. JAMA Netw Open 2019;2(10):e1912565.

39. Wong RJ, Aguilar M, Cheung R, et al. Nonalcoholic steatohepatitis is the second leading etiology of liver disease among adults awaiting liver transplantation in the United States. Gastroenterology 2015;148(3):547–55.

40. Noureddin M, Vipani A, Bresee C, et al. NASH Leading Cause of Liver Transplant in Women: Updated Analysis of Indications For Liver Transplant and Ethnic and Gender Variances. Am J Gastroenterol 2018;113(11):1649–59.

41. Taylor RS, Taylor RJ, Bayliss S, et al. Association Between Fibrosis Stage and Outcomes of Patients With Nonalcoholic Fatty Liver Disease: A Systematic Review and Meta-Analysis. Gastroenterology 2020; 158(6):1611–25.e12.

42. Pandyarajan V, Gish RG, Alkhouri N, et al. Screening for Nonalcoholic Fatty Liver Disease in the Primary Care Clinic. Gastroenterol Hepatol 2019;15(7):357–65.

43. European Association for the Study of the L, European Association for the Study of D, European Association for the Study of O. EASL-EASD-EASO Clinical Practice Guidelines for the management of non-alcoholic fatty liver disease. J Hepatol 2016; 64(6):1388–402.

44. Kontrick AV, VanWagner LB, Yeh C, et al. Hepatic Steatosis: An Incidental Finding That Deserves Attention. Acad Emerg Med 2021;28(5):578–81.

45. Younossi ZM, Noureddin M, Bernstein D, et al. Role of Noninvasive Tests in Clinical Gastroenterology Practices to Identify Patients With Nonalcoholic Steatohepatitis at High Risk of Adverse Outcomes: Expert Panel Recommendations. Am J Gastroenterol 2021;116(2): 254–62.

46. Vuppalanchi R, Gould RJ, Wilson LA, et al. Clinical significance of serum autoantibodies in patients with NAFLD: results from the nonalcoholic steatohepatitis clinical research network. Hepatol Int 2012;6(1): 379–85.

47. Verma S, Jensen D, Hart J, et al. Predictive value of ALT levels for non-alcoholic steatohepatitis (NASH) and advanced fibrosis in non-alcoholic fatty liver disease (NAFLD). Liver Int 2013;33(9):1398–405.

48. Imajo K, Kessoku T, Honda Y, et al. Magnetic Resonance Imaging More Accurately Classifies Steatosis and Fibrosis in Patients With Nonalcoholic Fatty Liver Disease Than Transient Elastography. Gastroenterology 2016;150(3):626–37.e7.

49. Castellana M, Donghia R, Guerra V, et al. Fibrosis-4 Index vs Nonalcoholic Fatty Liver Disease Fibrosis Score in Identifying Advanced Fibrosis in Subjects With Nonalcoholic Fatty Liver Disease: A Meta-Analysis. Am J Gastroenterol 2021;116(9):1833–41.

50. Bacon BR, Adams PC, Kowdley KV, et al. American Association for the Study of Liver D. Diagnosis and management of hemochromatosis: 2011 practice guideline by the American Association for the Study of Liver Diseases. Hepatology 2011;54(1):328–43.

51. Golfeyz S, Lewis S, Weisberg IS. Hemochromatosis: pathophysiology, evaluation, and management of hepatic iron overload with a focus on MRI. Expert Rev Gastroenterol Hepatol 2018;12(8):767–78.

52. Roberts EA, Schilsky ML. Diagnosis and treatment of Wilson disease: An update. Hepatology 2008; 47(6):2089–111. https://doi.org/10.1002/hep.22261.

53. European Association for Study of L. EASL Clinical Practice Guidelines: Wilson's disease. J Hepatol 2012;56(3):671–85.

54. Narayanan P, Mistry PK. Update on Alpha-1 Antitrypsin Deficiency in Liver Disease. Clin Liver Dis 2020;15(6):228–35.

55. Strnad P, Buch S, Hamesch K, et al. Heterozygous carriage of the alpha1-antitrypsin Pi*Z variant increases the risk to develop liver cirrhosis. Gut 2019;68(6):1099–107.

56. Strnad P, Mandorfer M, Choudhury G, et al. Fazirsiran for Liver Disease Associated with Alpha1-Antitrypsin Deficiency. N Engl J Med 2022;387(6):514–24.

Practical Guide, Challenges, and Pitfalls in Liver Fibrosis Staging

Karen Matsukuma, MD, PhD[a],*, Matthew M. Yeh, MD, PhD[b]

KEYWORDS

- Liver • Liver biopsy • Cirrhosis • Liver fibrosis • Staging system • Fibrosis regression
- Hepatic repair complex

Key Points

- Choosing the most appropriate staging system depends on the pattern of liver injury and local practices. When in doubt, choosing a simple, well-recognized system and providing a microscopic description of the fibrosis pattern is best. Including the staging system in the diagnostic line is imperative.

- Fibrosis regression occurs in most liver diseases. As the number of effective pharmacologic therapies for liver diseases increases, recognition of fibrosis regression will become essential in the clinical setting.

- The Beijing system is a simple system that classifies advanced liver fibrosis into progressive, regressive, or indeterminate for regression/progression. It focuses on the quality of fibrous septa as an indicator of the directionality of injury/tissue remodeling and has been shown to correlate with fibrosis regression in hepatitis B.

- Markers of chronic cholestasis (eg, orcein stain, cytokeratin 7 stain) improve prognostication when included in staging systems for primary biliary disease.

- Glutamine synthetase staining can be helpful for identifying the central zone in cases in which presence of aberrant arterioles and ductules is suspected.

ABSTRACT

Liver fibrosis staging has many challenges, including the large number of proposed staging systems, the heterogeneity of the histopathologic changes of many primary liver diseases, and the potential for slight differences in histologic interpretation to significantly affect clinical management. This review focuses first on fibrosis regression. Following this, each of the major categories of liver disease is discussed in regard to (1) appropriate fibrosis staging systems, (2) emerging concepts, (3) current clinical indications for liver biopsy, (4) clinical decisions determined by fibrosis stage, and (5) histologic challenges and pitfalls related to staging.

OVERVIEW

One of the pivotal aspects in biopsy assessment of liver fibrosis is knowing which staging system to apply. It is important to recognize that each major category of liver disease (eg, viral hepatitis, fatty liver disease, primary biliary disease, congestive hepatopathy) develops fibrosis in a specific sequence albeit with diverse patterns. As such, application of earlier proposed staging systems (Ishak,[1] Batts-Ludwig,[2] METAVIR[3]), which are based on features of chronic viral hepatitis, does not provide the most clinically useful information in every situation. Another key component of liver fibrosis assessment is understanding the clinical stakes of the fibrosis stage in the context of the

[a] University of California Davis, Pathology and Laboratory Medicine, 4400 V Street, Sacramento, CA 95817, USA; [b] University of Washington Medical Center - Montlake, Box 356100, 1959 NE Pacific Street, Seattle, WA 98195, USA
* Corresponding author. University of California Davis, Pathology and Laboratory Medicine, 4400 V Street, Sacramento, CA 95817.
E-mail address: kmatsukuma@ucdavis.edu

Surgical Pathology 16 (2023) 457–472
https://doi.org/10.1016/j.path.2023.04.002

Box 1
Hepatic repair complex

Scar/fibrosis	Delicate perforated septa
	Isolated thick collagen fibers (eg, undigested remnants of septa)
	Periportal fibrous spikes
Vascular remodeling	Portal tract remnants (eg, portal tracts with minimal collagen, attenuated or absent portal venules)
	Hepatic vein remnants containing prolapsed hepatocytes
	Aberrant hepatic veins (eg, hepatic veins in close proximity to portal tracts)
Parenchymal regeneration	Hepatocyte clusters within portal tracts or splitting septa
	Minute regenerative nodules (or hepatocyte "buds")

underlying disease process. For example, a diagnosis of advanced fibrosis (eg, bridging) in a patient with congestive hepatopathy may preclude cardiac transplant. Although histologic criteria must be consistently applied, pathologists frequently encounter liver biopsies with fibrosis patterns that straddle 2 stages or show features that would seem pertinent but are not accounted for in the relevant staging system. In these situations, understanding the clinical consequences of the fibrosis stage aids in the development of a pathology interpretation that is clinically meaningful.

This review first focuses on fibrosis regression, a key concept relevant to all major liver diseases, particularly as the list of effective therapies grows. Following this, each of the major categories of liver disease is discussed in regard to (1) appropriate fibrosis staging systems, (2) emerging concepts, (3) current clinical indications for liver biopsy, (4) clinical decisions determined by fibrosis stage, and (5) histologic challenges and pitfalls related to staging.

FIBROSIS REGRESSION

One of the major phenomena now recognized to affect essentially all major categories of liver disease is the concept of fibrosis regression. Controversial at the time of its initial histologic description more than 2 decades ago, the concept of fibrosis regression has slowly gained widespread acceptance. Even still, it is infrequently documented in pathology reports, possibly due to pathologists'

lack of familiarity with its numerous and relatively subtle histologic features.

In their seminal article, Wanless and colleagues[4] documented the dramatic and near complete regression of cirrhosis in a patient treated with lamivudine for hepatitis B. The investigators additionally defined the specific histologic features that they attributed to fibrosis regression, a constellation of findings they termed the "hepatic repair complex" and demonstrated that these features could be found in explants of end-stage liver disease due to alcohol, hepatitis B, hepatitis C, and primary biliary cholangitis. The "hepatic repair complex" refers to the following 8 histologic findings: (1) delicate perforated septa, (2) isolated thick collagen fibers, (3) periportal fibrous spikes, (4) portal tract remnants (eg, portal tracts with minimal collagen and attenuated or absent portal venules), (5) hepatic vein remnants containing prolapsed hepatocytes, (6) aberrant hepatic veins (eg, hepatic veins in close proximity to portal tracts), (7) hepatocyte clusters within portal tracts or splitting septa, and (8) minute regenerative nodules (or hepatocyte "buds") (Box 1, Fig. 1). These parameters can be conceptually organized into 3 categories of tissue injury or repair: scar/fibrosis, vascular remodeling, and parenchymal regeneration.[5]

Since then, numerous studies have provided evidence supporting the existence of fibrosis regression.[6-11] In clinical practice, the concept of fibrosis regression was significantly bolstered in 2017 by Sun and colleagues[12] who proposed a novel fibrosis classification system, the Beijing classification, based on the proportion of liver demonstrating features of regression. This system is applicable to specimens with at least bridging fibrosis and focuses on the quality of fibrous septa as in indicator of the directionality of the injury/tissue remodeling process. Liver specimens are classified into 3 fibrosis categories: predominantly progressive, predominantly regressive, and indeterminate (Table 1, Fig. 2). Predominantly progressive fibrosis is defined as having greater than 50% of the fibrous septa showing wide, loosely arranged collagen fibers that demonstrate a mixture of pale and dense blue fibers on trichrome stain and at least moderately prominent inflammatory cells, macrophages, and ductular reaction. Predominantly regressive fibrosis is defined as having greater than 50% of fibrous septa composed of thin, compact stroma (similar to the delicate perforated septa of the hepatic repair complex) with intense trichrome staining and minimal inflammatory infiltrates or ductular reaction. Indeterminate (for fibrosis progression or regression) is defined as showing a mixture of progressive and regressive features, for which no pattern predominates.

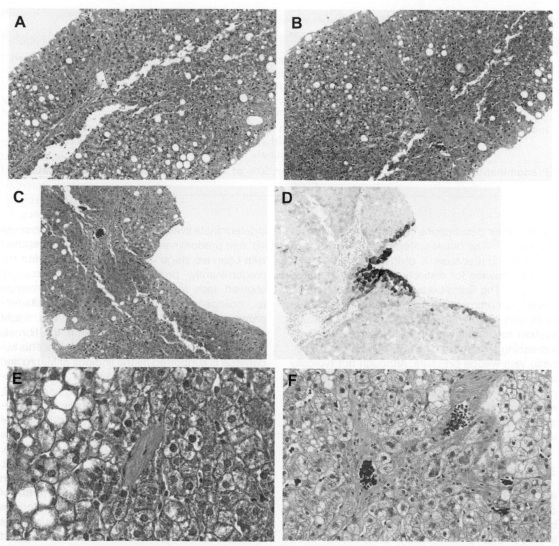

Fig. 1. The hepatic repair complex. (*A, B*) Delicate septa; with perforation (panel *A*). (*C, D*) Aberrant hepatic vein. Portal fibrosis with bridging and adjacent hepatic/central vein (panel *C*). Glutamine synthetase stain highlights hepatic/central vein (panel *D*). (*E*) Isolated thick collagen fiber. (*F*) Hepatocytes within portal tracts, a feature of parenchymal regeneration. Trichrome stain, except as noted. All images digitally scanned at 40X.

Applying this classification system to 71 paired hepatitis B liver biopsies before and after antiviral therapy, the investigators demonstrated that 53% of posttreatment predominantly regressive specimens were associated with a downstage in at least one Ishak stage. In addition, of the remaining posttreatment predominantly regressive specimens, all but 1 (2%) showed a downstage in cirrhosis substage by Laennec classification (discussed further later), despite remaining at the same Ishak stage. These findings strongly support the concept of fibrosis regression, demonstrate regression in the setting of cirrhosis, and perhaps most importantly provide a simple tool for its recognition.

CHRONIC HEPATITIS

STAGING SYSTEMS

Chronic hepatitis (eg, hepatitis C, hepatitis B, autoimmune hepatitis) is the prototypic liver condition for which most well-known staging systems were designed, including Knodell,[13] Scheuer,[14] META-VIR, Ishak,[1] Batts-Ludwig,[2] and Laennec.[15] The METAVIR system was developed for hepatitis C research, and although infrequently used in diagnostic pathology, the American Association for the Study of Liver Diseases (AASLD) practice guidance statements on hepatitis B and hepatitis C have adopted METAVIR terminology (eg, A0-3,

Table 1
Beijing classification system of advanced fibrosis

Predominantly progressive	More than 50% of septa showing broad, loosely aggregated collagen fibers Mix of light and dark staining fibers on trichrome stain Moderate to marked cellularity (inflammatory cells, macrophages, ductular reactions)
Indeterminate	Uncertain mix of progressive and regressive scarring When neither progression nor regression seems to predominate
Predominantly regressive	More than 50% of septa showing thin, compact acellular fibers

F0-4) in their descriptions of hepatitis activity and fibrosis.[16,17] The Ishak system is frequently used for research because it divides fibrosis into 6 stages, allowing for distinction of subtle changes (Table 2). The Batts-Ludwig system, which has 4 stages, is commonly used in clinical practice due to its simplicity. The Laennec system is a 3-stage system for stratifying cirrhosis (stages 4A–C, in increasing severity) and notably correlates with hepatic vein wedge pressure. Although not typically used in the clinical setting, the Laennec system is particularly useful to assess for late-stage fibrosis regression in research.[12,17] Another classification system for late-stage fibrosis is the Beijing system (discussed later).

EMERGING CONCEPTS

In their 2021 study of hepatitis C explants, Fiel and colleagues[18] characterized cirrhotic livers using both the Beijing and Laennec systems and showed that predominantly progressive livers correlated perfectly with Laennec stage 4C;

indeterminate livers correlated with Laennec stage 4B; and predominantly regressive livers correlated with Laennec stage 4A. They also noted that the predominantly progressive/Laennec 4C livers showed less interpatient variation with regard to collagen:parenchyma ratio (ie, collagen-proportionate area) and suggested this might indicate an upper physiologic limit for fibrosis accumulation and potential for regression. This hypothesis is supported by the findings of Mauro and colleagues[19] who found that none of 27 posttransplant cirrhotic patients with recurrent hepatitis C, sustained viral response after therapy, and Laennec 4C fibrosis showed histologic evidence of regression (defined as a decrease of at least one METAVIR stage) on posttreatment biopsy, whereas 69% of Laennec 4B and 78% of Laennec 4A patients did. Furthermore, histologic regression inversely correlated with clinical features of advanced liver disease (increased hepatic vein wedge pressure, pretherapy liver-related adverse events). Taken together, these studies suggest that Laennec substage may be a clinically relevant

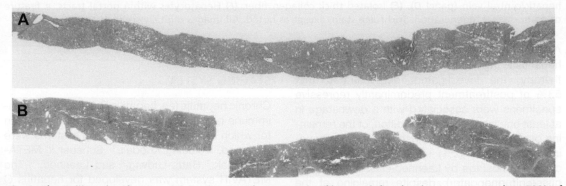

Fig. 2. The Beijing classification. (A) Predominantly progressive fibrosis, defined as having greater than 50% of the fibrous septa showing wide collagen bands that demonstrate a mixture of pale and dense blue fibers on trichrome stain and moderately prominent inflammatory cells, macrophages, and ductular reaction. (B) Predominantly regressive fibrosis, defined as having greater than 50% of delicate fibrous septa, with intense trichrome staining and minimal inflammatory infiltrates or ductular reaction. Trichrome stain. All images digitally scanned at 40X.

Table 2
Well-known fibrosis staging systems

Ishak	0	No fibrosis
	1	Fibrous expansion of some portal areas, with or without short fibrous septa
	2	Fibrous expansion of most portal areas, with or without short fibrous septa
	3	Fibrous expansion of some portal areas, with occasional portal to portal bridging
	4	Fibrous expansion of portal areas, with marked bridging, portal to portal and portal to central
	5	Marked bridging with occasional nodules (incomplete cirrhosis)
	6	Cirrhosis, probable, or definite
Batts-Ludwig	0	No fibrosis; normal connective tissue
	1	Portal fibrosis; fibrous portal expansion
	2	Periportal fibrosis; periportal or rare portal-portal septa
	3	Septal fibrosis; fibrous septa with architectural distortion, no obvious cirrhosis
	4	Cirrhosis
Laennec	4A	Nodules enclosed by thin fibrous septa
	4B	Nodules enclosed by broad fibrous septa
	4C	Very broad fibrous septa with more than half of the biopsy composed of micronodules
METAVIR	F0	No fibrosis
	F1	Portal fibrosis without septa (stellate enlargement of portal tracts without septa)
	F2	Portal fibrosis with few septa (enlargement of portal tracts with rare septa)
	F3	Portal fibrosis with numerous septa without cirrhosis
	F4	Cirrhosis

histologic endpoint that may warrant inclusion in the pathology report. Indeed, as asserted by Fiel's group, given the likely lower potential for regression of Laennec 4C cirrhosis, such patients may be at greater risk of hepatic decompensation and thus require closer follow-up.[18]

CLINICAL INDICATIONS FOR BIOPSY

Given the effectiveness of direct-acting antivirals for the treatment of hepatitis C, most of the patients with confirmed hepatitis C infection are eligible for treatment. The current AASLD practice guidance statement for hepatitis C indicates that liver biopsy is not required to initiate treatment of hepatitis C, as pretreatment assessment for cirrhosis can be performed via noninvasive tests (eg, elastography, serologic tests).[17] As such, biopsies for hepatitis C are no longer as common as they once were.

For hepatitis B, treatment decisions are more complex and based on whether there is evidence of at least portal fibrosis with rare septa on biopsy (METAVIR F2), severe inflammation (METAVIR A3), elevated alanine transferase level, and/or detectable hepatitis B virus DNA. The current AASLD practice guidance statement for hepatitis B recommends liver biopsy to evaluate histologic disease severity in select circumstances, such as in patients older than 40 years with a long duration of infection and evidence of low-level viral replication—for consideration of therapy.[16] Biopsy is particularly valuable in this setting because studies have found that liver stiffness measurements in patients with hepatitis B reflect a combination of necroinflammatory activity and fibrosis and thus can misrepresent extent of fibrosis.[20,21]

CRITICAL CLINICAL DECISIONS DETERMINED BY FIBROSIS STAGE

As mentioned earlier, for hepatitis B, evidence of at least portal fibrosis with few septa (METAVIR F2) is an indication for antiviral therapy. Screening for hepatocellular carcinoma by ultrasound every 6 months is indicated for adults with cirrhosis who have hepatitis C or are hepatitis B surface antigen (HBsAg)-positive and for children who are HBsAg-positive and have at least bridging fibrosis.[16,17]

HISTOLOGIC CHALLENGES AND PITFALLS

Fibrosis staging systems for viral hepatitis and other forms of chronic hepatitis such as autoimmune hepatitis are generally easy to apply once a staging system is selected. One major pitfall is overinterpretation of the trichrome stain in portal tracts that contain significant inflammation (Fig. 3). Pale blue staining in portal and periportal areas that contain dense inflammatory infiltrates does not reflect pathologic fibrosis. Comparison of the tinctorial quality of the trichrome stain in those areas with that in uninflamed portal tracts

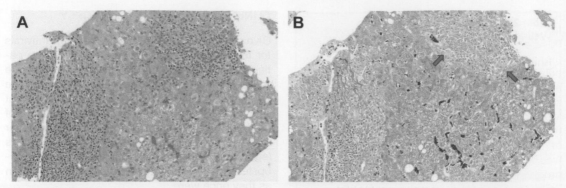

Fig. 3. Portal tract inflammation can cause overestimation of portal fibrosis. (*A*) Moderate portal inflammation with interface activity; hematoxylin and eosin stain. (*B*) True portal fibrosis stains intense blue on trichrome stain (*yellow arrows*). In contrast, stromal expansion induced by inflammation of the portal tract is pale blue (*blue arrows*). All images digitally scanned at 40X.

or the hepatic capsule, which should be intensely blue (ie, mature collagen), can be helpful.

NONALCOHOLIC STEATOHEPATITIS

STAGING SYSTEMS

It is well established that nonalcoholic steatohepatitis (NASH) is a risk factor for the development of cirrhosis.[22] In NASH, lipid droplets and ballooned hepatocytes classically accumulate in the centrilobular area where oxygen tension is lower. Because both steatosis and hepatocyte ballooning result in expansion of the hepatocyte cytoplasm, these changes lead to compression of the sinusoids and space of Disse. The ensuing hypoxia activates the local hepatic stellate cells and ultimately results in centrizonal fibrosis.[23] In NASH, fibrosis may also develop within portal tracts and eventually bridge portal and central zones. Because of this unique pattern of progression, a novel fatty liver-specific staging system was first proposed by Brunt and colleagues.[24] This system and 2 other systems subsequently derived from it (Kleiner and colleagues,[25] Bedossa and colleagues[26]) have been the most widely used systems for staging NASH both in research and clinical practice (**Table 3**).

EMERGING CONCEPTS

In the last few years, 2 large clinical trials have been conducted to evaluate drugs targeting NASH-related cirrhosis.[27,28] Although both studies showed no effect of the interventions, 16% of these cirrhotic patients showed a spontaneous decrease in fibrosis by modified Ishak criteria.[29] Importantly, this group also demonstrated a significantly lower frequency of adverse liver-related events, underscoring the clinical significance of

this histologic change. A concurrent observational study by the Nonalcoholic Steatohepatitis Clinical Research Network found that 34% of patients with NASH at all stages of fibrosis showed a spontaneous decrease in fibrosis stage and that 33% of patients with baseline cirrhosis showed spontaneous fibrosis regression to bridging fibrosis.[30] Although these observations do not shed light on the underlying causes of the fibrosis regression, they do strongly support the existence of fibrosis regression in the setting of NASH.

Another important emerging concept in the histologic characterization of NASH is the significance of perivenular ductular reaction. Ductular reaction, a proliferation of ductules in response to biliary or severe hepatocellular injury, has long been appreciated in the periportal zone in NASH and other chronic liver diseases. However, more recently ductular reaction has been documented in the centrilobular zone in association with NASH.[31,32] In addition, in a subset of central zones, arterioles and abnormal sinusoidal vascularization are also found. In their study, Zhao and colleagues used a combination of CK7 and glutamine synthetase stains to highlight the ductules

Table 3 Brunt staging system	
0	No fibrosis
1	Zone 3 perisinusoidal fibrosis, focal or extensive
2	Zone 3 perisinusoidal fibrosis with focal or extensive periportal fibrosis
3	Zone 3 perisinusoidal fibrosis and portal fibrosis with focal or extensive bridging fibrosis
4	Cirrhosis

and central zones, respectively, and documented the presence of perivenular ductular reaction in 90% of (pre-cirrhotic) NASH liver biopsies. They also showed that the overall frequency of perivenular ductular reaction in a given liver biopsy (as a proportion of the total number of centrilobular zones) correlated strongly with fibrosis stage. More importantly, in the longitudinal portion of their study, they demonstrated that the frequency of perivenular ductular reaction in the initial biopsy was the only histologic feature that correlated with progression of fibrosis on subsequent biopsy. Thus, perivenular ductular reaction may be an important prognostic marker of progression.

CLINICAL INDICATIONS FOR BIOPSY

Although nonalcoholic fatty liver disease (NAFLD) (encompassing simple steatosis and NASH) can result in hepatomegaly, in most cases it does not result in clinical symptoms, and it may only come to clinical attention during routine screening of liver function tests or as an incidental finding on imaging workup for other conditions. Imaging results showing hepatic steatosis are an indication for biopsy (to evaluate for advanced fibrosis) in those patients with high-risk factors (eg, significant alcohol use, diabetes mellitus, elevated body mass index, older age) or elevated liver function tests.[33] In addition, biopsy is considered in patients undergoing bariatric surgery to evaluate for the presence and severity of NASH[34] and in patients with suspected NAFLD in whom alternative causes or other (superimposed) chronic liver disease is a possibility.[33]

CRITICAL CLINICAL DECISIONS DETERMINED BY FIBROSIS STAGE

Patients with NAFLD are typically encouraged to adopt lifestyle modifications (eg, weight loss, exercise, alcohol abstinence), regardless of presence or absence of fibrosis. Patients with biopsy-proven NASH with fibrosis may be offered pharmacologic therapy (eg, pioglitazone, vitamin E). Those with evidence of cirrhosis require screening for esophageal varices and for hepatocellular carcinoma.[33]

HISTOLOGIC CHALLENGES AND PITFALLS

Overstaining of the trichrome stain can contribute to accentuation of the sinusoids in the central zone, a pitfall that can mimic pericellular fibrosis (Fig. 4A). True sinusoidal fibrosis should be intense blue on trichrome stain and has the same staining intensity as the collagen surrounding large native bile ducts. Evidence of concomitant hepatocyte

injury and/or distortion of the hepatic plate architecture will also typically be present. In addition, reactive fibrous tissue surrounding lobular lipogranulomas containing lymphocytes and Kupffer cells can mimic centrilobular sinusoidal fibrosis, particularly at low magnification (Fig. 4B, C).[35] On higher magnification, the presence of a lipid droplet and Kupffer cells is usually readily apparent. The staining intensity of the fibrous tissue within the lipogranuloma will also be less intense than that of mature collagen.

One caveat for the use of glutamine synthetase for identification of central zones (discussed earlier) is that areas of fibrosis can show loss of metabolic zonation (eg, loss or reversal of the normal glutamine synthetase expression pattern).[36,37] Attention to the degree of local fibrosis as well as to the background liver pattern (eg, alternating portal tracts and central venules) can aid in identification of these aberrations.

PRIMARY BILIARY CHOLANGITIS

STAGING SYSTEMS

Because primary biliary cholangitis (PBC) is a duct-centered autoimmune process, fibrosis begins in the portal tract. With progression, inflammation and hepatic injury extend from the portal tracts and lead to parenchymal collapse, replacement by fibrous septa, and ultimately development of cirrhosis. Early PBC-specific staging systems developed by Scheuer[38] in 1967 and by Ludwig and colleagues[39] in 1978 incorporated features of both inflammation and fibrosis. These publications were extremely valuable for characterizing the histologic features of the disease. However, the staging systems were not validated clinically at their inception. In 2006, a unique staging system that included fibrosis along with bile duct loss and use of orcein stain to identify chronic cholestasis was proposed by Nakanuma and colleagues[40] (Table 4). These 3 features (fibrosis, bile duct loss, orcein-positive granules) strongly correlated with one another when analyzed against biochemical markers of PBC. Because PBC is notoriously heterogeneous, the investigators intentionally chose to include these covariable features in the stage calculation in an additive fashion as a means to abrogate the effect of biopsy heterogeneity. Importantly, this system was clinically validated, and its performance was shown to exceed that of the other systems.[41] In addition, this staging system could predict cirrhosis-related complications (eg, esophageal varices, ascites, hepatic encephalopathy), even in the absence of histologic cirrhosis. It is worth noting that several studies

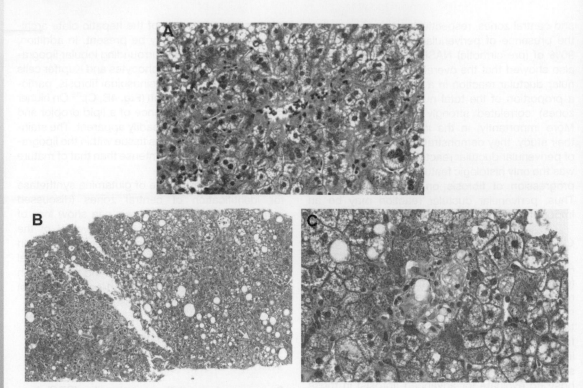

Fig. 4. Pitfalls of staging of nonalcoholic fatty liver disease. (*A*) Overstained trichrome can accentuate the sinusoids around the central vein. Note the trichrome staining around the sinusoids is more pale than that around the central vein. (*B, C*) Lipogranulomas can mimic zone 3 fibrosis. The lipogranuloma (*orange arrow*) stains less intensely than true pericellular fibrosis (*yellow arrow*) (panel *B*). On higher power magnification, the lipid droplet, macrophages, and inflammation are apparent (panel *C*). Trichrome stain. All images digitally scanned at 40X.

support the superiority of orcein stain over fibrosis assessment for prognostication of PBC and primary sclerosing cholangitis (PSC).[43–45] However, the requirement for orcein staining (which is not universally available) and poor interobserver agreement[42] have been obstacles to widespread adoption of the Nakanuma system. A simplified version that removes the requirement for orcein staining was published in 2013.[46] Although easier to use, it retains components that represent conceptual deviations from other well-recognized staging systems, specifically the following: (1) no stage 0 exists, such that even in the absence of any of the defined stage-specific lesions, a liver biopsy is scored as stage 1, and (2) it incorporates features other than fibrosis (eg, bile duct loss) in the determination of stage.

Because the relative rarity of biopsies for PBC makes adoption of a complex staging system more prone to confusion and poor reproducibility, in the clinical setting it may be more advantageous to use the Batts-Ludwig or other commonly recognized portal-based staging system. Of note, however, both the Scheuer and Ludwig systems are still used clinically. The more complex Nakanuma system is frequently used in clinical trials and retrospective studies in which validating histologic endpoints is one of the goals of the study. Regardless of staging system used, specifying the staging system in the diagnosis line is imperative.

EMERGING CONCEPTS

In 2020 Bowlus and colleagues[47] published results of a substudy of a large clinical trial on the use of obeticholic acid for patients with PBC (who did not respond or could not tolerate first-line therapy with ursodeoxycholic acid). Of 17 patients with paired biopsies before and 3 years after obeticholic acid treatment, greater than 70% showed stable or decreased fibrosis, bile duct loss, and ductular proliferation. Furthermore, morphometric analysis of collagen character and quantity as single features and aggregately showed a statistically significant improvement (p < 0.002, for combined score) after treatment. This study supports the use of obeticholic acid therapy and suggests that an even

Table 4 Nakanuma staging system for primary biliary cholangitis	
Fibrosis	
0	Absent or limited to portal tracts
1	Periportal fibrosis (incomplete septa)
2	Bridging fibrosis (complete septa) with lobular distortion
3	Cirrhosis (extensive fibrosis and regenerative nodules)
Bile duct loss	
0	Absent
1	<1/3 of portal tracts
2	<2/3 of portal tracts
3	>2/3 of portal tracts
Chronic cholestasis (based on presence of orcein-positive granules)	
0	Absent
1	<1/3 of periportal areas
2	<2/3 of periportal areas
3	>2/3 of periportal areas
Stage[a]	Sum of fibrosis, bile duct loss, and chronic cholestasis scores
1	0
2	1–3
3	4–6
4	7–9

[a] Revised stage classification from Nakanuma et al., 2010.

greater subset of patients with PBC can be effectively treated by pharmacotherapy.

CLINICAL INDICATIONS FOR BIOPSY

Because serologic evidence of antimitochondrial antibody and a compatible biochemical profile (eg, alkaline phosphatase at least 1.5 times normal, aminotransferases less than 5 times normal) is sufficient to make the diagnosis of PBC,[48] the biopsy rate for suspected PBC is low. Clinical concern for antimitochondrial antibody (AMA)-negative PBC, comprising approximately 10% of all PBC cases, has traditionally been an indication for biopsy; however, discovery of other PBC-specific autoantibodies (eg, sp100, gp210, anti-Kelch-like 12, anti-hexokinase 1) has now made diagnosis of a subset of AMA-negative PBC cases possible without liver biopsy.[48] As such, liver biopsies for diagnosis of PBC are infrequent.

CRITICAL CLINICAL DECISIONS DETERMINED BY FIBROSIS STAGE

At present, clinical decisions in regard to PBC do not rely on histologic evaluation of fibrosis stage. Although not all patients respond to first-line therapy with ursodeoxycholic acid, liver biopsy is not indicated for monitoring therapy, and instead, transient elastography has been advocated as a means to risk stratify patients.[48] Although risk of hepatocellular carcinoma is less than that associated with viral hepatitis, it has been noted that men with PBC have an increased risk. As such, a diagnosis of cirrhosis or any man with a diagnosis of PBC (regardless of fibrosis stage) is an indication for cross-sectional imaging every 6 months.[48]

HISTOLOGIC CHALLENGES AND PITFALLS

The main challenge for staging PBC is to choose a fibrosis staging system that can be applied consistently within one's practice and that is readily understood by the hepatologists who will be receiving the report. As described earlier, a well-recognized portal-based staging system may be preferable for ease of use and to decrease the possibility of misinterpretation of the pathology report. One caveat for the use of the Scheuer and Ludwig systems is that Scheuer also published a staging system for chronic hepatitis,[14] and Ludwig also published a staging system for PSC[49,50] (discussed later), making it necessary to specify which Scheuer or Ludwig staging system is being referenced.

PRIMARY SCLEROSING CHOLANGITIS

STAGING SYSTEMS

The first staging system specifically designed for PSC was published by Ludwig, initially in 1981[49] and in further detail in 1984.[50] This staging system, known as the Ludwig staging system for PSC, included histologic features of duct obstruction and fibrosis. Although not validated at the time of its inception, more recently it has been shown to correlate with relevant clinical endpoints.[45] Because of the common biliary obstructive nature of primary sclerosing cholangitis and PBC, the Nakanuma staging system, originally developed for PBC, has also been applied to PSC. Importantly, the Nakanuma system has been shown to correlate better with occurrence of transplant and liver-related events in PSC compared with other systems, such as the Ludwig system for PSC and the Ishak system.[44,45] Of note, unlike other chronic liver diseases, indications for transplant in PSC include not only decompensated

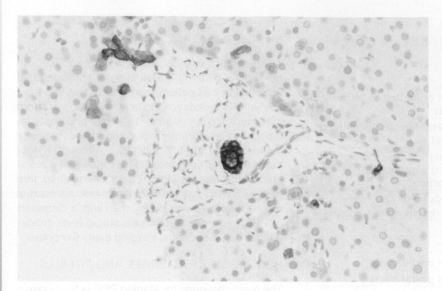

Fig. 5. Cytokeratin 7 stain can highlight chronic cholestasis. Expression of cytokeratin 7 in periportal hepatocytes is a marker of chronic cholestasis. Image digitally scanned at 40X.

cirrhosis but also biliary conditions including cholangitis, pruritis, and cholangiocarcinoma. This distinction is one of the rationales for inclusion of additional clinical endpoints (eg, time to transplant, transplant-free survival) beyond liver-related complications (eg, ascites, esophageal varices) in studies that assess the value of histologic staging systems for the prognostication of PSC.

Because biopsies for PSC are relatively uncommon in most clinical practices, use of a well-recognized system (eg, Batts-Ludwig) may be the best approach. However, as noted earlier, the PSC-specific system developed by Ludwig and the Nakanuma system for PBC are clinically validated for PSC and are also in clinical use.

EMERGING CONCEPTS

In 2022 Sjoblom and colleagues[51] proposed a novel PSC-specific scoring system, the PSC histoscore, which consists of 8 semiquantitative features classified as either grade (hepatitis, cholangitis, portal inflammation, periportal edema) or stage (fibrosis, bile duct loss, chronic cholestasis assessed on cytokeratin 7 stain, ductular reaction). They used this system to evaluate a series of 300 PSC liver biopsies and correlated findings with a compound endpoint that included occurrence of transplant, cholangiocarcinoma, or death. They found that both the grade and stage of the PSC histoscore and the total PSC histoscore (grade plus stage) had a higher predictive value for the compound clinical endpoint compared with a modified version of the Nakanuma system that used CK7 stain in lieu of orcein stain as a measure of chronic cholestasis. Unfortunately, a true

head-to-head comparison of the Nakanuma system and the PSC histoscore was not performed, limiting the strength of this conclusion. However, the PSC histoscore is more user friendly because it relies on the more widely available cytokeratin 7 stain rather than orcein stain for assessment of chronic cholestasis (**Fig. 5**).

CLINICAL INDICATIONS FOR BIOPSY

PSC is typically diagnosed by the presence of biochemical evidence of persistent or fluctuating cholestasis and characteristic imaging findings on MRI and/or molecular resonance cholangio-pancreatography (MRCP); this is because noninvasive imaging is adequately specific,[52] and histologic findings particularly in the early stages can be patchy and nonspecific due to heterogeneity of the disease. Liver biopsy is indicated, however, for suspicion of small duct disease (which lacks significant imaging findings) or to evaluate for suspected PSC-autoimmune hepatitis overlap.

Because no effective therapy for PSC currently exists, the AASLD recommends that all PSC patients be considered for participation in clinical trials.[52] In this setting, liver biopsies may be required for confirmation of the diagnosis or evaluation of histologic endpoints. For scientific consistency, central review by a study pathologist will typically be performed after the local interpretation has been completed.

CRITICAL CLINICAL DECISIONS DETERMINED BY FIBROSIS STAGE

Although histologic fibrosis stage is prognostic in PSC,[44,45,51] the AASLD does not recommend liver biopsy for the purpose of staging. Instead, liver stiffness measurements by transient or magnetic resonance elastography have been clinically validated and are recommended surrogates for fibrosis assessment. In addition, risk stratification models (eg, UK-PSC, Amsterdam-Oxford, SCOPE 2020) based on age, laboratory data, clinical history, and/or imaging are used to assist with determining appropriate follow-up and management.[52]

As with other liver diseases, surveillance for hepatocellular carcinoma is initiated when there is histologic (or other) evidence of cirrhosis. Patients with PSC also have increased risk of cholangiocarcinoma and gallbladder carcinoma, a risk that is independent of extent of fibrosis. Therefore, annual screening by MRI or MRCP is recommended for all patients with PSC, except those with small-duct PSC or who are younger than 18 years.[52]

HISTOLOGIC CHALLENGES AND PITFALLS

PSC is an extremely heterogeneous disease,[53] in which high-grade strictures can lead to uneven distribution of fibrosis in the liver. Even in the same location within the liver, biopsies may show a difference of 1 or even 2 fibrosis stages.[54] Although sampling variability is beyond the control of the pathologist, any observed intrabiopsy heterogeneity can be included as additional descriptive information in the pathology report, as has been advocated for congestive hepatopathy[55] (discussed later). Regarding histologic pitfalls, periductal collagen in larger portal tracts that normally have a thicker collar of collagen can be mistaken for periductal/concentric fibrosis (Fig. 6 A, B). Evidence of cholangiocyte injury within the duct and irregular layering of thin bands of collagen around the bile duct support true periductal fibrosis and should be included as portal fibrosis (Fig. 6C, D).

CONGESTIVE HEPATOPATHY

STAGING SYSTEMS

Congestive hepatopathy is the result of right heart failure, including valvular defects, congenital heart disease, and constrictive pericarditis. The classic pattern of injury is sinusoidal dilatation with centrilobular fibrosis; this can progress to portal and bridging fibrosis and less commonly cirrhosis. Portal fibrosis can be particularly evident in Fontan patients.[56,57]

Although different scoring systems have been developed to describe fibrosis due to congestive hepatopathy,[58–61] the congestive hepatic fibrosis score proposed by Dai and colleagues[59] in 2014 and subsequently validated by Bosch and colleagues[37] is currently the most widely applied (Table 5).[55,60–63] Importantly, this scoring system has been demonstrated to correlate with clinical indicators of chronic volume and pressure overload (eg, right atrial pressure, right atrial dilatation, and left atrial dilatation).[37,59]

EMERGING CONCEPTS

Fibrosis in congestive hepatopathy is frequently heterogeneous. Underscoring this, a recent study by Dhall and colleagues[55] demonstrated that 26% of liver biopsies from patients with congestive hepatopathy showed a 2-stage discrepancy in fibrosis in different parts of the same core biopsy. In addition, nodular regenerative hyperplasia, a potential mimic of cirrhotic nodules, was frequently observed (20%) and was not associated with significant fibrosis. These findings highlight the complexity of fibrosis scoring in congestive hepatopathy. To account for this, the study's investigators recommend reporting both the predominant fibrosis stage and the secondary pattern (along with its relative abundance) if geographic heterogeneity of 2 stages or more is present in a biopsy.

In 2019, Silva-Sepulveda and colleagues proposed a revised fibrosis staging system for patients with Fontan anatomy.[61] Their system, termed the modified Ishak congestive hepatic fibrosis score, incorporates the centrilobular-focused pattern of the congestive hepatic fibrosis score with the more discrete definitions of evolving septal fibrosis and early cirrhosis of the Ishak system. In this study, the Ishak, congestive hepatic fibrosis, and modified Ishak congestive hepatic fibrosis scores performed equivalently in regard to clinical measures of hepatic congestion. Although the modified system provides more granular detail regarding the extent of advanced fibrosis and may better account for the progression of fibrosis in patients with Fontan anatomy, it awaits validation of its superiority for clinical decision-making.

CLINICAL INDICATIONS FOR BIOPSY

Although a combination of clinical and imaging findings may be sufficient to diagnose chronic venous outflow obstruction (including congestive hepatopathy), biopsy may be performed for confirmation of the diagnosis and/or to exclude other causes, particularly as these patients can present with a cholestatic chemistry profile.[64]

For assessment of fibrosis, biopsy remains the gold standard because in the setting of passive congestion, imaging may indicate a nodular liver even in the absence of cirrhosis. In addition, liver

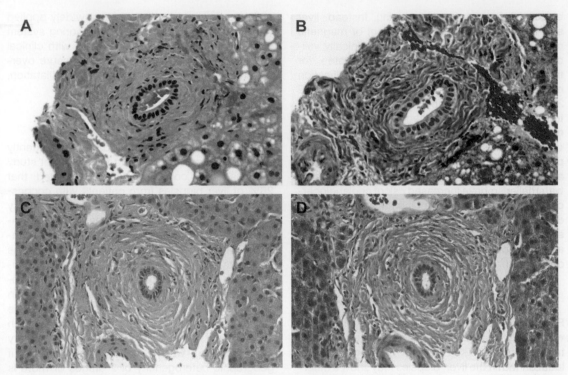

Fig. 6. Large bile tracts have thicker collagen collars that can mimic periductal fibrosis. (*A, B*) Normal portal tract. (*C, D*) Periductal fibrosis in a patient with primary sclerosing cholangitis. Hematoxylin and eosin (*A, C*). Trichrome (*B, D*).

stiffness measurements can reflect both congestion and fibrosis, and biochemical surrogates do not correlate with fibrosis stage.[65]

In patients with Fontan anatomy, transjugular liver biopsy may be performed as part of a surveillance protocol[63] or selectively performed when clinical signs of cirrhosis are present and/or the magnetic resonance elastography score is greater than 5 kPa (which correlates with significant bridging).[61] In addition, in both Fontan and non-Fontan congestive hepatopathy, liver biopsy may

Table 5	
Congestive hepatic fibrosis score	
0	No fibrosis
1	Central zone fibrosis
2A	Central zone fibrosis and mild portal fibrosis, with accentuation at central zone
2B	At least moderate portal fibrosis and central zone fibrosis, with accentuation at portal zone
3	Bridging fibrosis
4	Cirrhosis

be performed to assess severity of liver fibrosis as a part of the evaluation for heart or combined heart-liver transplant.[66,67]

CRITICAL CLINICAL DECISIONS DETERMINED BY FIBROSIS STAGE

For cardiac transplant evaluation, advanced fibrosis (eg, bridging) and cirrhosis can affect a patient's chances of transplant.[66] Indeed, in regard to liver biopsy for cardiac transplant evaluation, some investigators have concluded that due to the known heterogeneity of the disease and the potential consequences for the patient, caution should be taken when considering a histologic diagnosis of cirrhosis.[58]

HISTOLOGIC CHALLENGES AND PITFALLS

Similar to NASH, aberrant arterioles and ductules near central zones have been described in the setting of chronic venous outflow obstruction due to a variety of causes, including congestive hepatopathy.[36] These aberrant arterioles and ductules are common (ie, present in >70% of cases), and their frequency increases with stage of fibrosis. Because these findings can lead to misinterpretation of central zones as portal tracts, errors in fibrosis staging can result. These aberrant arterioles and ductules can be challenging to distinguish from true portal tracts on hematoxylin and eosin–stained sections, and use of glutamine synthetase stain to highlight central zones can be extremely helpful.

An additional challenge related to fibrosis staging in congestive hepatopathy is the disproportionate number of transjugular liver biopsies that can be received, particularly in patient care settings where Fontan surveillance by cardiac catheterization includes liver biopsy. These biopsies can be smaller, more fragmented, and contain fewer portal tracts than percutaneous biopsies.[68] Reviewing additional serial sections of the biopsy and utilization of glutamine synthetase stain for identification of central zones can be helpful in this regard.

SUMMARY

Staging fibrosis in liver biopsies is challenging for many reasons, including the large number of staging systems that have been proposed, the well-established heterogeneity of most primary liver diseases, and the potential clinical significance of slight differences in interpretation (eg, stage discrepancies). In current clinical practice, however, familiarity with only a few staging systems is generally necessary: (1) a portal-based staging system for chronic hepatitis (eg, Batts-Ludwig), (2) the Brunt classification for NAFLD, and (3) the congestive hepatic fibrosis score. Although disease heterogeneity is a somewhat intractable problem from a liver biopsy standpoint, identification of intrabiopsy heterogeneity can be communicated in the pathology report. Should there be a discrepancy between clinical, imaging, and histologic impressions of disease severity, a descriptive comment on the heterogeneity of the specimen can highlight the possibility of sampling error. Knowledge of the clinical consequences of fibrosis stage in the context of the disease process can help the pathologist focus on answering the specific question the biopsy is meant to address rather than on assignment to a numerical category that is minimally defined (although still an essential element of the pathology report). In this regard, direct communication with the hepatologist can also be extremely valuable.

In the last few years, the number and efficacy of therapeutic options for primary liver disease have increased significantly. Although this increase will undoubtedly diminish the need for liver biopsies, those that are received will be more apt to show features of regression. Thus, recognition of the histologic features of regression is likely to become essential in the clinical setting. Also looking forward, recent developments in digital pathology and artificial intelligence have demonstrated the power of computational tools to reliably and perhaps more accurately discriminate different stages in chronic liver disease using morphologic features not captured in current staging systems[69–71]; this in turn has provided new insights into the evolution of fibrosis progression and treatment-induced fibrosis regression in NASH.[70,71] Such tools may assist pathologists staging liver fibrosis in the future, although further studies are certainly warranted.

COMMERCIAL OR FINANCIAL CONFLICTS OF INTEREST AND FUNDING SOURCES

The authors have nothing to disclose.

REFERENCES

1. Ishak K, Baptista A, Bianchi L, et al. Histological grading and staging of chronic hepatitis. J Hepatol 1995;22(6):696–9.
2. Batts KP, Ludwig J. Chronic hepatitis. An update on terminology and reporting. Am J Surg Pathol 1995; 19(12):1409–17.
3. Intraobserver and interobserver variations in liver biopsy interpretation in patients with chronic hepatitis C. The French METAVIR Cooperative Study Group. Hepatology 1994;20(1):15–20.
4. Wanless IR, Nakashima E, Sherman M. Regression of human cirrhosis. Morphologic features and the genesis of incomplete septal cirrhosis. Arch Pathol Lab Med 2000;124(11):1599–607.
5. Theise ND, Jia J, Sun Y, et al. Progression and regression of fibrosis in viral hepatitis in the treatment era: the Beijing classification. Mod Pathol 2018;31(8):1191–200.
6. Poynard T, McHutchison J, Manns M, et al. Impact of pegylated interferon alfa-2b and ribavirin on liver fibrosis in patients with chronic hepatitis C. Gastroenterology 2002;122(5):1303–13.
7. Czaja AJ, Carpenter HA. Decreased fibrosis during corticosteroid therapy of autoimmune hepatitis. J Hepatol 2004;40(4):646–52.
8. Falize L, Guillygomarc'h A, Perrin M, et al. Reversibility of hepatic fibrosis in treated genetic hemochromatosis: a study of 36 cases. Hepatology 2006;44(2):472–7.
9. Chang TT, Liaw YF, Wu SS, et al. Long-term entecavir therapy results in the reversal of fibrosis/cirrhosis and continued histological improvement in patients with chronic hepatitis B. Hepatology 2010;52(3): 886–93.
10. D'Ambrosio R, Aghemo A, Rumi MG, et al. A morphometric and immunohistochemical study

to assess the benefit of a sustained virological response in hepatitis C virus patients with cirrhosis. Hepatology 2012;56(2):532–43.

11. Marcellin P, Gane E, Buti M, et al. Regression of cirrhosis during treatment with tenofovir disoproxil fumarate for chronic hepatitis B: a 5-year open-label follow-up study. Lancet 2013;381(9865): 468–75.

12. Sun Y, Zhou J, Wang L, et al. New classification of liver biopsy assessment for fibrosis in chronic hepatitis B patients before and after treatment. Hepatology 2017;65(5):1438–50.

13. Knodell RG, Ishak KG, Black WC, et al. Formulation and application of a numerical scoring system for assessing histological activity in asymptomatic chronic active hepatitis. Hepatology 1981;1(5):431–5.

14. Scheuer PJ. Classification of chronic viral hepatitis: a need for reassessment. J Hepatol 1991;13(3): 372–4.

15. Kutami R., Girgrah N., Wanless I.R., et al., The Laennec grading system for assessment of hepatic fibrosis: validation by correlation with wedged hepatic vein pressure and clinical features (Abstract 992), Hepatology, 32(4) pt 2 of 2, 2000, 407A.

16. Terrault NA, Lok ASF, McMahon BJ, et al. Update on prevention, diagnosis, and treatment of chronic hepatitis B: AASLD 2018 hepatitis B guidance. Hepatology 2018;67(4):1560–99.

17. Ghany MG, Morgan TR, Panel A-IHCG. Hepatitis C Guidance 2019 update: American Association for the study of liver diseases-infectious diseases society of america recommendations for testing, managing, and treating hepatitis C virus infection. Hepatology 2020;71(2):686–721.

18. Zhang X, Schiano TD, Doyle E, et al. A comparative study of cirrhosis sub-staging using the Laennec system, Beijing classification, and morphometry. Mod Pathol 2021;34(12):2175–82.

19. Mauro E, Crespo G, Montironi C, et al. Portal pressure and liver stiffness measurements in the prediction of fibrosis regression after sustained virological response in recurrent hepatitis C. Hepatology 2018;67(5):1683–94.

20. Ji D, Chen Y, Shang Q, et al. unreliable estimation of fibrosis regression during treatment by liver stiffness measurement in patients with chronic hepatitis B. Am J Gastroenterol 2021;116(8):1676–85.

21. Jia J, Hou J, Ding H, et al. Transient elastography compared to serum markers to predict liver fibrosis in a cohort of Chinese patients with chronic hepatitis B. J Gastroenterol Hepatol 2015;30(4):756–62.

22. Caldwell S, Argo C. The natural history of nonalcoholic fatty liver disease. Dig Dis 2010;28(1): 162–8.

23. Scorletti E, Carr RM. A new perspective on NAFLD: Focusing on lipid droplets. J Hepatol 2022;76(4): 934–45.

24. Brunt EM, Janney CG, Di Bisceglie AM, et al. Nonalcoholic steatohepatitis: a proposal for grading and staging the histological lesions. Am J Gastroenterol 1999;94(9):2467–74.

25. Kleiner DE, Brunt EM, Van Natta M, et al. Design and validation of a histological scoring system for nonalcoholic fatty liver disease. Hepatology 2005;41(6): 1313–21.

26. Bedossa P, Poitou C, Veyrie N, et al. Histopathological algorithm and scoring system for evaluation of liver lesions in morbidly obese patients. Hepatology 2012;56(5):1751–9.

27. Harrison SA, Abdelmalek MF, Caldwell S, et al. Simtuzumab is ineffective for patients with bridging fibrosis or compensated cirrhosis caused by nonalcoholic steatohepatitis. Gastroenterology 2018; 155(4):1140–53.

28. Harrison SA, Wong VW, Okanoue T, et al. Selonsertib for patients with bridging fibrosis or compensated cirrhosis due to NASH: results from randomized phase III STELLAR trials. J Hepatol 2020;73(1):26–39.

29. Sanyal AJ, Anstee QM, Trauner M, et al. Cirrhosis regression is associated with improved clinical outcomes in patients with nonalcoholic steatohepatitis. Hepatology 2022;75(5):1235–46.

30. Kleiner DE, Brunt EM, Wilson LA, et al. Association of histologic disease activity with progression of nonalcoholic fatty liver disease. JAMA Netw Open 2019;2(10):e1912565.

31. Gill RM, Belt P, Wilson L, et al. Centrizonal arteries and microvessels in nonalcoholic steatohepatitis. Am J Surg Pathol 2011;35(9):1400–4.

32. Zhao L, Westerhoff M, Pai RK, et al. Centrilobular ductular reaction correlates with fibrosis stage and fibrosis progression in non-alcoholic steatohepatitis. Mod Pathol 2018;31(1):150–9.

33. Chalasani N, Younossi Z, Lavine JE, et al. The diagnosis and management of nonalcoholic fatty liver disease: practice guidance from the American association for the study of liver diseases. Hepatology 2018;67(1):328–57.

34. Cusi K, Isaacs S, Barb D, et al. American association of clinical endocrinology clinical practice guideline for the diagnosis and management of nonalcoholic fatty liver disease in primary care and endocrinology clinical settings: co-sponsored by the american association for the study of liver diseases (AASLD). Endocr Pract 2022;28(5):528–62.

35. Brunt EM. Alcoholic and nonalcoholic steatohepatitis. Clin Liver Dis 2002;6(2):399–420, vii.

36. Krings G, Can B, Ferrell L. Aberrant centrizonal features in chronic hepatic venous outflow obstruction: centrilobular mimicry of portal-based disease. Am J Surg Pathol 2014;38(2):205–14.

37. Bosch DE, Koro K, Richards E, et al. Validation of a congestive hepatic fibrosis scoring system. Am J Surg Pathol 2019;43(6):766–72.

38. Scheuer P. Primary biliary cirrhosis. Proc R Soc Med 1967;60(12):1257–60.

39. Ludwig J, Dickson ER, McDonald GS. Staging of chronic nonsuppurative destructive cholangitis (syndrome of primary biliary cirrhosis). Virchows Arch A Pathol Anat Histol 1978;379(2):103–12.

40. Hiramatsu K, Aoyama H, Zen Y, et al. Proposal of a new staging and grading system of the liver for primary biliary cirrhosis. Histopathology 2006;49(5): 466–78.

41. Kakuda Y, Harada K, Sawada-Kitamura S, et al. Evaluation of a new histologic staging and grading system for primary biliary cirrhosis in comparison with classical systems. Hum Pathol 2013;44(6): 1107–17.

42. Nakanuma Y, Zen Y, Harada K, et al. Application of a new histological staging and grading system for primary biliary cirrhosis to liver biopsy specimens: Interobserver agreement. Pathol Int 2010;60(3): 167–74.

43. Chan AW, Chan RC, Wong GL, et al. Evaluation of histological staging systems for primary biliary cirrhosis: correlation with clinical and biochemical factors and significance of pathological parameters in prognostication. Histopathology 2014;65(2): 174–86.

44. de Vries EM, Verheij J, Hubscher SG, et al. Applicability and prognostic value of histologic scoring systems in primary sclerosing cholangitis. J Hepatol 2015;63(5):1212–9.

45. de Vries EM, de Krijger M, Farkkila M, et al. Validation of the prognostic value of histologic scoring systems in primary sclerosing cholangitis: An international cohort study. Hepatology 2017;65(3):907–19.

46. Harada K, Hsu M, Ikeda H, et al. Application and validation of a new histologic staging and grading system for primary biliary cirrhosis. J Clin Gastroenterol 2013;47(2):174–81.

47. Bowlus CL, Pockros PJ, Kremer AE, et al. Long-term obeticholic acid therapy improves histological endpoints in patients with primary biliary cholangitis. Clin Gastroenterol Hepatol 2020;18(5):1170–1178 e6.

48. Lindor KD, Bowlus CL, Boyer J, et al. Primary biliary cholangitis: 2018 practice guidance from the American association for the study of liver diseases. Hepatology 2019;69(1):394–419.

49. Ludwig J, Barham SS, LaRusso NF, et al. Morphologic features of chronic hepatitis associated with primary sclerosing cholangitis and chronic ulcerative colitis. Hepatology 1981;1(6):632–40.

50. LaRusso NF, Wiesner RH, Ludwig J, et al. Current concepts. Primary sclerosing cholangitis. N Engl J Med 1984;310(14):899–903.

51. Sjoblom N, Boyd S, Kautiainen H, et al. Novel histological scoring for predicting disease outcome in primary sclerosing cholangitis. Histopathology 2022;81(2):192–204.

52. Bowlus CL, Arrive L, Bergquist A, et al. AASLD practice guidance on primary sclerosing cholangitis and cholangiocarcinoma. Hepatology 2022. https://doi.org/10.1002/hep.32771.

53. Portmann B, Zen Y. Inflammatory disease of the bile ducts-cholangiopathies: liver biopsy challenge and clinicopathological correlation. Histopathology 2012;60(2):236–48.

54. Olsson R, Hagerstrand I, Broome U, et al. Sampling variability of percutaneous liver biopsy in primary sclerosing cholangitis. J Clin Pathol 1995;48(10): 933–5.

55. Dhall D, Kim SA, Mc Phaul C, et al. Heterogeneity of fibrosis in liver biopsies of patients with heart failure undergoing heart transplant evaluation. Am J Surg Pathol 2018;42(12):1617–24.

56. Schwartz MC, Sullivan L, Cohen MS, et al. Hepatic pathology may develop before the Fontan operation in children with functional single ventricle: an autopsy study. J Thorac Cardiovasc Surg 2012; 143(4):904–9.

57. Johnson JA, Cetta F, Graham RP, et al. Identifying predictors of hepatic disease in patients after the Fontan operation: a postmortem analysis. J Thorac Cardiovasc Surg 2013;146(1):140–5.

58. Louie CY, Pham MX, Daugherty TJ, et al. The liver in heart failure: a biopsy and explant series of the histopathologic and laboratory findings with a particular focus on pre-cardiac transplant evaluation. Mod Pathol 2015;28(7):932–43.

59. Dai DF, Swanson PE, Krieger EV, et al. Congestive hepatic fibrosis score: a novel histologic assessment of clinical severity. Mod Pathol 2014;27(12): 1552–8.

60. Surrey LF, Russo P, Rychik J, et al. Prevalence and characterization of fibrosis in surveillance liver biopsies of patients with Fontan circulation. Hum Pathol 2016;57:106–15.

61. Silva-Sepulveda JA, Fonseca Y, Vodkin I, et al. Evaluation of fontan liver disease: correlation of transjugular liver biopsy with magnetic resonance and hemodynamics. Congenit Heart Dis 2019;14(4): 600–8.

62. Horvath B, Zhu L, Allende D, et al. Histology and glutamine synthetase immunoreactivity in liver biopsies from patients with congestive heart failure. Gastroenterology Res 2017;10(3):182–9.

63. Patel ND, Sullivan PM, Sabati A, et al. Routine surveillance catheterization is useful in guiding management of stable fontan patients. Pediatr Cardiol 2020;41(3):624–31.

64. Pai RK, Hart JA. Aberrant expression of cytokeratin 7 in perivenular hepatocytes correlates with a cholestatic chemistry profile in patients with heart failure. Mod Pathol 2010;23(12):1650–6.

65. Goldberg DJ, Surrey LF, Glatz AC, et al. Hepatic fibrosis is universal following fontan operation, and

severity is associated with time from surgery: a liver biopsy and hemodynamic study. J Am Heart Assoc 2017;6(5). https://doi.org/10.1161/JAHA.116.004809.

66. Mehra MR, Canter CE, Hannan MM, et al. The 2016 International society for heart lung transplantation listing criteria for heart transplantation: a 10-year update. J Heart Lung Transplant 2016;35(1):1–23.

67. Reardon LC, DePasquale EC, Tarabay J, et al. Heart and heart-liver transplantation in adults with failing Fontan physiology. Clin Transplant 2018;32(8): e13329.

68. Cholongitas E, Quaglia A, Samonakis D, et al. Transjugular liver biopsy: how good is it for accurate histological interpretation? Gut 2006;55(12):1789–94.

69. Xu S, Wang Y, Tai DCS, et al. qFibrosis: a fully-quantitative innovative method incorporating histological features to facilitate accurate fibrosis scoring in animal model and chronic hepatitis B patients. J Hepatol 2014;61(2):260–9.

70. Heinemann F, Gross P, Zeveleva S, et al. Deep learning-based quantification of NAFLD/NASH progression in human liver biopsies. Sci Rep 2022; 12(1):19236.

71. Naoumov NV, Brees D, Loeffler J, et al. Digital pathology with artificial intelligence analyses provides greater insights into treatment-induced fibrosis regression in NASH. J Hepatol 2022; 77(5):1399–409.

Systemic Disease and the Liver-Part 1
Systemic Lupus Erythematosus, Celiac Disease, Rheumatoid Arthritis, and COVID-19

Maria Isabel Fiel, MD[a], Thomas D. Schiano, MD[b],*

KEYWORDS

- Liver biopsy • Rheumatoid arthritis • COVID 19 • SARS-CoV-2 infection • Celiac disease
- Fatty liver • Nodular regenerative hyperplasia • Systemic lupus erythematosus

Key points

- Patients with systemic diseases often have abnormal linver chemistry tests with a broad-based differential diagnosis, which may include drug-induced liver injury, infection, liver hypo-perfusion, and worsening of an underlying chronic liver disease.
- Liver chemistry tests can sometimes rise and fall in parallel with the activity of an underlying collagen vascular disease.
- A liver biopsy may at times show nonspecific findings and not yield a definitive diagnosis, so the clinician should be aware of the clinical settings in which a liver biopsy may be helpful.
- Nodular regenerative hyperplasia is a common cause of non-cirrhotic portal hypertension and is most often idiopathic, but is a histologic feature found in many collagen vascular and systemic diseases.
- There is a large armamentarium of medications that patients use in the setting of systemic diseases that themselves can lead to liver injury and then abnormal liver chemistry tests.

ABSTRACT

The development of liver dysfunction in patients having various systemic diseases is common and has a broad differential diagnosis, at times being the initial manifestation of the disorder. Liver injury associated with systemic lupus erythematosus is heterogeneous and may present with nonspecific histology. Differentiating autoimmune hepatitis from lupus hepatitis is challenging on histologic grounds alone. Other systemic diseases that may present mostly with nonspecific findings are rheumatoid arthritis and celiac disease. More recently COVID-19 cholangiopathy and secondary sclerosing cholangitis have become increasingly recognized as distinct liver conditions. Many patients may also have intrinsic liver disease or may develop drug-induced liver injury from the treatment of the systemic disease. Timely identification of the cause of the liver dysfunction is essential and liver biopsy may help the clinician in diagnosis and management.

OVERVIEW

The development of abnormal liver chemistry tests is a frequent sequela of many systemic diseases and infections. For instance, common infections such as influenza and COVID-19 may be

[a] Department of Pathology, Molecular and Cell-Based Medicine, Icahn School of Medicine at Mount Sinai, One Gustave Levy Place, New York, NY 10029, USA; [b] Division of Liver Diseases, Recanati-Miller Transplantation Institute, Icahn School of Medicine at Mount Sinai, One Gustave Levy Place-Box 1104, New York, NY 10029, USA
* Corresponding author.
E-mail address: thomas.schiano@mountsinai.org

Surgical Pathology 16 (2023) 473–484
https://doi.org/10.1016/j.path.2023.04.003

associated with a nonspecific elevation of amino-transferases, while infectious mononucleosis can cause a cholestatic pattern. Patients undergoing general surgical procedures may develop abnormal liver biochemistries related to anesthesia and the surgical procedure itself. In collagen vascular diseases, liver biochemistries may rise and fall in parallel with the activity of the underlying rheumatological disorder. Liver biopsies in these settings may show nonspecific hepatitis.

Elucidation of the etiology of abnormal liver tests in patients having systemic diseases can be difficult because of the many different insults that impact the liver. Patients may often have intrinsic liver disease, such as nonalcoholic fatty liver disease (NAFLD) and chronic viral hepatitis that is contributing to their medical co-morbidities. Some liver diseases such as primary biliary cholangitis are associated with other diseases, for instance celiac disease, that it causes liver disease. Drug-induced liver injury (DILI) is another confounder in these patients as often the medications they are receiving to treat the extrahepatic disease may be hepatotoxic. Patients may also be using complimentary alternative medications (CAM) which can lead to liver dysfunction. Liver biopsies thus are sometimes necessary to help guide medical management.

Many conditions are associated with nonspecific liver histologic findings while others will have more typical histology, and thus aid the clinician in their decision-making process. The following article describes some of these disorders and suggests when a liver biopsy may be helpful. This is not meant to be an exhaustive review of these entities but rather it is meant to highlight the importance of liver histology with clinical correlation in patients having some systemic diseases that can affect the liver.

SYSTEMIC LUPUS ERYTHEMATOSUS

Systemic lupus erythematosus (SLE) affects many organs, including the liver. Although liver injury is acknowledged as part of SLE, it is not part of the diagnostic criteria for SLE.[1,2] Liver injury in SLE is common and heterogeneous with a wide spectrum of findings, ranging from nonspecific liver biochemistry abnormalities mostly in the form of aminotransferase elevation to rare cases of fulminant hepatic failure.[3–9] Although liver injury has several different types of patterns, the majority of liver biopsies show no histologic findings or only a mild nonspecific histology and the precise pathology may be obscure.[3,6,10,11] Rarely, advanced liver disease and cirrhosis may be the initial presentation.[12] Up to half of patients with SLE are reported to develop liver disease at some point during the disease course. Some patients may present with liver injury preceding the diagnosis of SLE while others may manifest with liver involvement at an average of 5 years after initial diagnosis.[10] Most liver injury that occurs is seen in patients already having coexisting liver disease such as viral hepatitis, fatty liver, and DILI.[2,6] Medications to treat SLE can cause DILI. Numerous studies have shown that steatosis is the most common histologic presentation and has been reported to be present in up to 73% of patients with SLE.[13] The mainstay of therapy is steroids, which can cause nonalcoholic fatty liver disease (NAFLD) while non-steroidal anti-inflammatory drugs (NSAIDS), azathioprine and methotrexate can cause nonspecific hepatitis and chronic liver disease (CLD).[2,4,14] It is estimated that DILI has an incidence of 30% in patients with SLE.[15] Most of the hepatic injuries occurring in SLE are secondary causes which can lead to CLD and cirrhosis, with lupus hepatitis (LH) considered to be the only primary SLE-related disease involving the liver.[2,6,16,17] Overlaps between SLE and autoimmune hepatitis (AIH) or SLE and primary biliary cholangitis (PBC) can occur.[18] AIH in SLE has an estimated incidence between 5% and 10% while the incidence of PBC in SLE is between 2.5% and 5%.[11,19] Of note, the diagnosis of SLE-AIH overlap should fulfill both American College of Rheumatology and International autoimmune hepatitis Group Criteria.[11]

LUPUS HEPATITIS

SLE-related hepatitis (lupus hepatitis) affects 3% to 8% of patients with SLE.[20] In some cases, LH may not be clinically apparent. In a large study conducted in China, a prevalence of 9.3% was found with a significantly greater prevalence in those patients having active disease versus those without (11.8% vs 3.2%).[21] Histologically, LH may be nonspecific and can show mild hepatitis involving both lobular and portal zones. The inflammation is typically mild consisting predominantly of an infiltrate of lymphocytes (Fig. 1). The underlying etiology of LH is complement activation and vasculitis.[13,15,22] The main differential diagnosis is autoimmune hepatitis (AIH) because both entities have elevated IgG and positive ANA.[16,23,24] Liver biopsy will help distinguish LH from AIH because the latter will show a prominent population of plasma cells and a greater degree of interface activity.[24,25] The presence of hepatocyte rosettes and significant fibrosis may also support the diagnosis of AIH over that of LH.[24] Serum anti-ribosomal P autoantibody titer has a higher

Fig. 1. Lupus hepatitis. The portal tract shows a mild mononuclear infiltrate consisting predominantly of lymphocytes. Mild interface hepatitis is noted. H&E, original magnification x20.

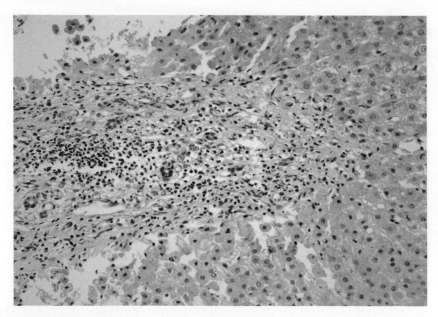

positive rate in LH compared to other SLE -elated liver disorders including AIH, and thus may be a useful marker for LH.[5,11,26] Immunohistochemical staining demonstrates positive deposition of auto-antibodies. C1q particularly has been shown to be positive in treatment-naïve patients with SLE as compared to those who have undergone treatment for SLE and as in those with other liver diseases.[21] This therefore may assist in establishing the diagnosis of SLE versus other secondary disorders.[21] Response to the treatment of LH with corticosteroids is typically rapid, as also occurs with most cases of AIH.[15]

VASCULAR DISORDERS

Patients with SLE have increased susceptibility to pro-thrombotic disorders.[27,28] Intrahepatic vessels may have immune complex deposition leading to inflammation and the initiated coagulation cascade results in thrombosis.[3] The presence of anti-cardiolipin antibodies places patients at risk for thrombosis, including of the hepatic vessels. The obliteration of blood vessels, particularly the portal veins, can result in obliterative portal venopathy (OPV) with secondary changes of nodular regenerative hyperplasia (NRH).[29] NRH is also found in patients having other collagen vascular diseases and patients may present with noncirrhotic portal hypertension.[3,6] Imaging studies may show a nodular liver, which can mistakenly lead to a clinical diagnosis of cirrhosis.[30,31] Biopsy will show diffuse nodular transformation with nodules comprised of thickened hepatocyte plates with the portal tract in the center of the nodule, and in the periphery of the nodule there are atrophic hepatocytes.[31,32] **(Fig. 2)** Changes of NRH may be subtle and the diagnosis may be easily missed.[3,32]

Liver Biopsy Recommended in Systemic Lupus Erythematosus

In order to ascertain the specific cause of abnormal liver tests in SLE, a liver biopsy may be necessary. The most common finding is steatosis, mainly as a result of steroid therapy.[6] Liver biopsy may be very helpful in distinguishing LH from AIH. Clinical and laboratory presentations are similar but the histology in LH is mild, nonspecific, and the inflammatory infiltrate is mainly lymphocytic, as compared to AIH in which plasma cells are the predominant infiltrate, with accompanying features of greater interface activity and the presence of hepatocyte rosettes. When patients with SLE present with low platelets, splenomegaly, and variceal bleeding, strong consideration of NRH should be entertained and liver biopsy will aid in establishing the diagnosis. Because patients with SLE are receiving multiple medications, including those that are known to cause DILI with some leading to CLD, progression to significant fibrosis and even cirrhosis, liver biopsy may helpful in identifying these patients in a timely fashion.

CELIAC DISEASE

Celiac disease is a systemic disorder that can affect other organs other than the small intestine and may affect the colon, thyroid, skin, pancreas, and liver.[33,34] In the liver, the common manifestation is isolated aminotransferase elevation.[34]

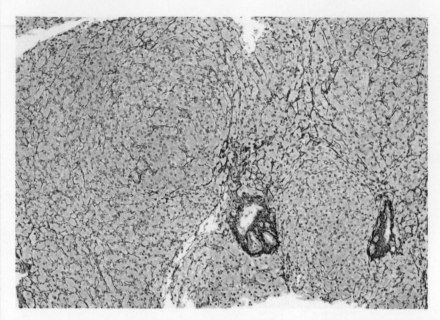

Fig. 2. Nodular regenerative hyperplasia. Diffuse nodular transformation may be seen with nodules composed of two-cell thick plates and are bordered by atrophic hepatocyte plates. These changes are better highlighted on a reticulin stain. Original magnification x10.

Abnormal aminotransferases in untreated celiac disease may rise and fall with dietary discretion. It can cause direct liver damage or may be associated with other autoimmune conditions such as AIH and PBC, which have their own intrinsic histologic features that confound liver biopsy interpretation[35–37] The prevalence of celiac disease in patients with autoimmune hepatitis is estimated to be 3.5%, which is much higher than the 0.5% to 1% prevalence seen in the general population.[35,38] Overall solid organ cancer risk is also higher in patients with celiac disease with a hazard ratio of 6.89; (95% CI 2.18 to 21.75) while the risk

of small intestinal cancer development is also higher (HR 6.89; 95% CI, 2.18–21.75; $P = .001$).[39] Liver injury attributed to celiac disease is loosely termed "cryptogenic liver disease."[40] While celiac disease commonly affects the liver, liver biopsy is not necessary to establish the diagnosis of celiac hepatitis or liver disease.

Liver disease in celiac disease can range from mild to severe hepatitis and is termed celiac hepatitis.[41] Celiac hepatitis is characterized by portal and periportal inflammation and lobular inflammation.[42] (Fig. 3) The inflammatory infiltrates are typically mononuclear and consist of mature lymphocytes

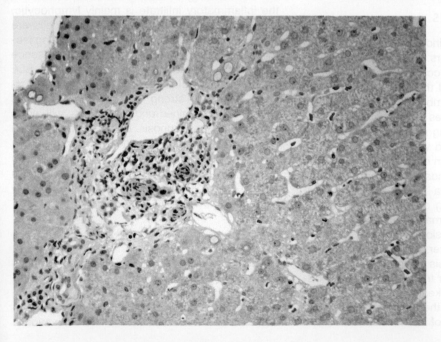

Fig. 3. Celiac hepatitis. A portal tract shown has a mild mononuclear infiltrate consisting mostly of mature lymphocytes. No interface activity is noted. There is no fibrosis and the architecture is preserved. H&E, original magnification x20.

with the architecture remaining preserved. These histologic features are, however, nonspecific. Other liver biopsy findings include steatosis, Kupffer cell hyperplasia and fibrosis and, rarely, cirrhosis.[43] Some reports indicate that intraepithelial lymphocytes in interlobular bile ducts (similar to those seen in the small intestine) may be present. Reversibility of the histologic changes of "celiac hepatitis" can occur with strict dietary compliance.[44] Celiac disease is in the differential diagnosis of NAFLD.[45] It should be clinically suspected in a patient having a liver biopsy for abnormal liver chemistries that shows portal inflammation or hepatic fibrosis of unknown etiology, or in patients having "lean" NAFLD.[45]

RHEUMATOID ARTHRITIS

Rheumatoid arthritis (RA) is an autoimmune disease that primarily affects the joints and causes damage to cartilage and bone. RA has variable clinical expression with approximately 70% of patients being women.[46] The prevalence of RA is estimated to be 0.5% to 1% in the general population.[47] Genetic factors play a role in disease susceptibility with the most commonly associated gene being HLA-DRB1. Genetic factors also play an important role in the treatment of RA because certain enzyme activity related to drug metabolism is pertinent with the use of methotrexate and azathioprine.[46] RA is characterized by the presence of autoantibodies such as rheumatoid factor (RF) and anti-cyclic citrullinated peptide (CCP). Extra-articular involvement is not common, but up to 50% of patients with RA have abnormal liver biochemistry tests. In a large population study in Denmark, liver disease was estimated to occur in 1.39 per 1000 person-years with an estimated 0.22 per 1000 person-years occurrence of cirrhosis.[48] As with many collagen vascular diseases, liver tests (typically aminotransferases) may rise and fall in parallel with activity of the underlying disease. A liver biopsy performed at this time might show very nonspecific findings and not be conclusive which the clinician must be aware of. Abnormal liver enzymes are often attributed to hepatotoxicity from the therapies for RA, especially methotrexate, which is the first line of therapy.[49] In previous studies, the existence or development of any liver fibrosis was of particular concern because of the potential development of cirrhosis.[48–50] However, in a cross-sectional study using transient elastography in 319 patients with RA treated with methotrexate, the prevalence of fibrosis was low.[51] Another non-invasive imaging study (ARFI) showed no increased risk of liver fibrosis in patients with RA treated with methotrexate.[47]

DILI from other medications used to treat RA is common. These medications include TNF inhibitors, rituximab, and tocilizumab.[52] Concomitant autoimmune diseases can also occur. In 2% to 4% of patients with autoimmune disease, RA can also be found.[53,54] Overall, RA can be found in 5% of patients having any type of autoimmune disease such as AIH, PBC, and PSC.[53]

Felty syndrome is a rare complication of RA presenting with the triad of arthritis, splenomegaly, and neutropenia.[54] Liver abnormalities are common with 2/3 of patients suffering from Felty syndrome having hepatomegaly and more than half having at least one abnormal liver biochemistry test.[54]

Histology

Hepatotoxicity is a well-recognized complication in patients receiving methotrexate therapy.[48] The most common histologic findings in RA are mild portal chronic inflammation, scattered hepatocyte necrosis, and fatty liver.[55–57] (Fig. 4) Nuclear variability (pleomorphism) is also associated with methotrexate therapy.[56,57] NASH was reported in a group of patients with psoriasis treated with methotrexate who underwent liver biopsy.[58] In patients with RA, fibrosis is rare and routine liver biopsy prior to starting methotrexate therapy is not necessary; progression to cirrhosis has not been reported. In a large Japanese study with well-characterized patients with RA, fibrosis was found in 24/846 (2.8%) with a mean cumulative methotrexate dose of 2.48 g.[59] There were 32 patients who underwent liver biopsy with 22/32 demonstrating non-alcoholic steatohepatitis (NASH)-like histology with 13 of the 22 (59%) having advanced fibrosis.[59] Although cases of "≥stage 3" fibrosis cases of cirrhosis were not identified, a NASH-like histology was noted in this group of patients with RA with persistently elevated aminotransferases. Seven of the 32 biopsies showed nonalcoholic fatty liver and three showed interface hepatitis.[59]

Liver dysfunction is common in patients with RA who develop Felty syndrome. In a large autopsy study, Wanless reported 35% of patients with Felty syndrome having abnormal liver tests were found to have nodular regenerative hyperplasia (NRH).[60] NRH has also been reported in patients with RA without Felty syndrome.[61] Sinusoidal lymphocyte infiltration may also be found.[62] Overall, the histologic findings in RA are heterogeneous and include fatty liver with a NASH-like histology, fibrosis occurring in different liver compartments, and mild portal or lobular inflammation. Concomitant DILI, particularly from methotrexate, which may also show similar histologic changes, should be considered when evaluating liver biopsies from patients with RA. NASH-like histology in patients on methotrexate is considered to be the

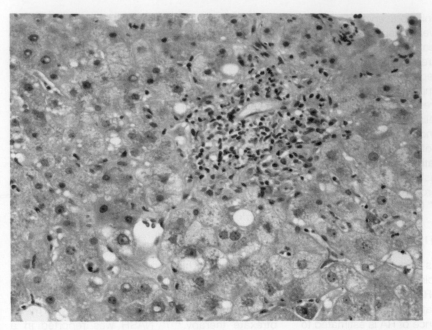

Fig. 4. Nonspecific liver injury in rheumatoid arthritis. As shown in this photomicrograph, mild portal chronic inflammation, scattered hepatocyte necrosis and apoptosis, and mild steatosis may be seen in patients with rheumatoid arthritis. In addition, nuclear variability (pleomorphism) as shown in this photo is also associated with methotrexate therapy. H&E, Original magnification, x20.

basis for the development of fibrosis in RA.[63] Liver biopsy may be necessary in some cases to demonstrate the liver damage caused by methotrexate.[59,63]

COVID-19

While the respiratory tract remains the primary target of SARS-CoV-2 infection, other organs may be affected, including the hepatobiliary system.[64–66] The mechanisms related to injury are unknown but it is believed they are due to direct and indirect pathogenic injury from SARS-CoV-2, the induction of a cytokine storm during COVID-19 infection, increased inflammatory mediators, endothelial dysfunction, and coagulation abnormalities.[66–69] Increased infiltrates of inflammatory cells in multiple organs are noted.[66,70,71] Although the angiotensin-converting enzyme 2 receptors for SARS-CoV-2 are highly expressed in cholangiocytes, studies have shown that SARS-CoV-2 is capable of directly infecting hepatocytes.[72] Various hepatic manifestations and complications are associated with COVID-19 and may range from mild liver dysfunction to hepatic failure and many investigators believe that severe liver injury is a reflection of severe SARS-CoV-2 infection.[73,74]

COVID-19 Liver Injury and Hepatitis

In addition to the hypoxic damage to the liver resulting from respiratory compromise, direct liver injury from SARS-CoV-2 may occur and hepatocytes may undergo necrosis and apoptosis.[67,74] (Fig. 5) A systematic review of 603 severe/fatal COVID-19 cases that included 75 studies showed

that the incidence of hepatitis was 21%.[71] In a postmortem study of patients with COVID-19 from China, liver histology showed ballooning and necrosis of hepatocytes, steatosis, as well as portal and lobular inflammation.[74] Severe liver injury as shown on liver biopsy from two patients demonstrated prominent apoptotic hepatocytes throughout the lobule, severe bile duct damage, endotheliitis, and mixed portal and lobular inflammation (Fig. 6); using in-situ hybridization SARS-CoV-2 viral particles were identified.[67] Rare cases of acute liver failure caused by SARS-CoV-2 have also been reported.[75] In addition, endothelial cells may become infected leading to sinusoidal endothelial cell dysfunction that contributes to liver injury.[76] This may be the underlying mechanism predisposing the liver to developing thromboses in portal veins and terminal hepatic venules.[70] Additional findings may include steatosis and sinusoidal dilatation.[70,74] Confounding conditions leading to liver injury include DILI (remdesivir is one such medication), underlying chronic liver disease (CLD), and hemodynamic changes including congestive hepatopathy as well as hypo-perfusion.[77,78] Patients with CLD may experience acute-on-chronic liver failure (ACLF) and have a relatively higher mortality rate as compared to those without CLD.[68]

POST-COVID-19 CHOLANGIOPATHY

SARS-CoV-2-associated cholangiopathy is increasingly being recognized.[79] The first series of three patients with COVID-19 recovering from

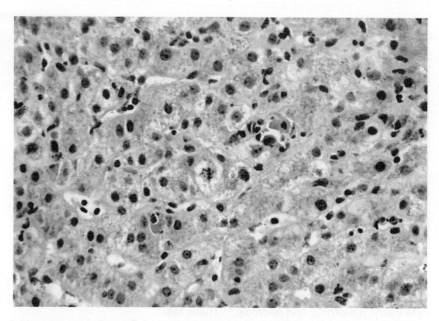

Fig. 5. COVID liver injury. Photomicrograph showing scattered apoptotic bodies, which may be the only manifestation of liver injury in patients with COVID-19. H&E, original magnification x40.

severe infection and developing cholangiopathy confirmed by histology was first reported in New York.[80] Another series described 12 patients presenting with clinical signs of cholestasis, four of whom had liver biopsies.[81] Both series showed histology similar to acute and/or chronic large duct obstruction, with no definitive bile duct lesions demonstrated on imaging.[80,81] The cholangiopathy occurred on average approximately 118 days after the onset of COVID-19.[81] While some patients who develop post-COVID-19 cholangiopathy may improve, others may progress and lead to liver failure and the need for transplantation.[82] With prolonged cholangiopathy, progressive cholestasis and bile duct loss with biliary fibrosis develop.[80,83] Cholestatic liver disease therefore is considered to be a long-term sequela of COVID-19.[83,84]

Liver histology shows changes typical of biliary injury and large duct obstruction, such as portal edema, ductular reaction, portal inflammation, and cholestasis.[80,82,83,85] (Fig. 7) Both

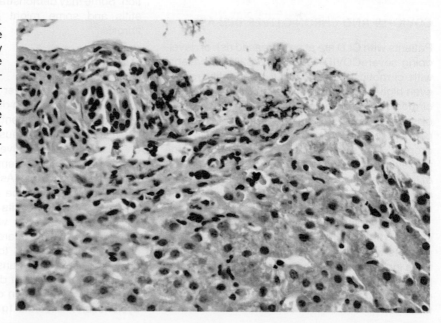

Fig. 6. COVID liver injury. Severe bile duct damage and microvascular injury may be seen. Note the cholangiocytes are hyperchromatic and have irregular shapes while the endothelial lining of the adjacent portal vein is starting to slough off. H&E, original magnification x40.

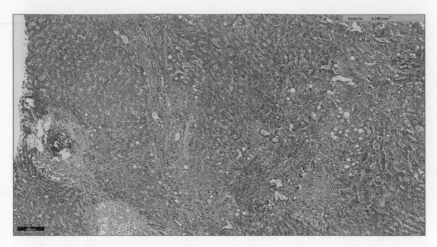

Fig. 7. COVID cholangiopathy. Portal tracts are expanded by fibrosis with fibrous septa. Bile ducts are damaged and frequently show periductal fibrosis. The lumina of the ductules are dilated. In periportal zones, occasional bile infarcts may be present. H&E, original magnification x10.

canalicular and ductular cholestasis are seen. Interlobular bile ducts show extensive cholangiocyte injury, apoptosis, and necrosis.[82] These features show some resemblance to the histology seen in secondary sclerosing cholangitis in critically-ill patients (SSC-CIP).[86] However, features that are unique in COVID-19 cholangiopathy as described by Roth and colleagues include microangiopathy, which is characterized by endothelial swelling with luminal narrowing of hepatic arteries and portal vein endophlebitis, and cholangiocytes showing prominent cytoplasmic vacuolization.[80] Other histologic features that may be seen are lymphocytic infiltrates, hepatocyte dropout, acidophilic bodies, lytic necrosis, bile infarcts, feathery degeneration and cholate stasis.[82]

COVID-19 AND CHRONIC LIVER DISEASE

Patients with CLD are at an increased risk of developing severeCOVID-19.[87] Up to 32% of patients with cirrhotic may die and the mortality rate is even higher at 51% in those with decompensated cirrhosis.[77,78,88] Studies have shown that the risk of severe COVID-19 increases with NAFLD independent of the presence of the metabolic syndrome.[89] A study showed that although the presence of NAFLD was shown to be a predictor of liver injury, it was not found to negatively impact morbidity and mortality in patients with severe COVID-19.[90]

It may be difficult to distinguish the histology of COVID-19 injury from the intrinsic liver disease in patients with CLD. Additional confounding conditions include DILI, ischemic injury, and congestive hepatopathy since COVID-19 liver injury as described in the previous section may have similar features.[77,91]

COVID-19 AND VACCINATION-INDUCED AUTOIMMUNE HEPATITIS

Several case reports have documented an increase in liver enzymes after vaccination to SARS-CoV-2.[92,93] These cases document an acute hepatitis along with positive autoimmune serology following SARS-CoV-2 vaccination.[93–95] The underlying mechanism is unclear and is believed to be molecular mimicry and bystander activation in predisposed individuals.[95] The infiltrate is composed mainly of activated cytotoxic CD8 T cells with SARS-CoV-2 specificity.[94] Along with the enriched CD8 T cells, CD4 T cells, B cells, plasma cells, and myeloid cells are also present.[94] Liver histology shows a pan-lobular distribution of the immune cells with relatively uniform distribution. Some may demonstrate severe interface hepatitis and some might even show significant fibrosis.[93]

SUMMARY

The development of liver dysfunction in patients having various systemic diseases has a broad differential diagnosis. Patients may have intrinsic liver disease as a primary cause of abnormal liver biochemistries. Or the native liver condition may be exacerbated by the systemic illness or the medications used to treat it. Associated liver diseases may develop or can be a consequence of the systemic disorder or its therapies. This is an ever-changing process with the advent of new therapies and newly-characterized diseases such as complications due to COVID-19. The liver dysfunction may be transient or be more longstanding with the risk of development of liver failure. Timely identification of the cause of the liver dysfunction is essential to help prevent worsening liver disease, and to guide the clinician in making the appropriate management decisions. Liver biopsy and the close collaboration of the pathologist and clinician is critical in helping guide this process.

REFERENCES

1. Aringer M, Costenbader K, Daikh D, et al. 2019 European League Against Rheumatism/American College of Rheumatology classification criteria for systemic lupus erythematosus. Ann Rheum Dis 2019;78(9):1151–9.

2. González-Regueiro JA, Cruz-Contreras M, Merayo-Chalico J, et al. Hepatic manifestations in systemic lupus erythematosus. Lupus 2020;29(8):813–24.

3. Bessone F, Poles N, Roma MG. Challenge of liver disease in systemic lupus erythematosus: Clues for diagnosis and hints for pathogenesis. World J Hepatol 2014;6(6):394–409.

4. Runyon BA, LaBrecque DR, Anuras S. The spectrum of liver disease in systemic lupus erythematosus. Report of 33 histologically-proved cases and review of the literature. Am J Med 1980;69(2): 187–94.

5. Brewer BN, Kamen DL. Gastrointestinal and Hepatic Disease in Systemic Lupus Erythematosus. Rheum Dis Clin North Am 2018;44(1):165–75.

6. Afzal W, Haghi M, Hasni SA, et al. Lupus hepatitis, more than just elevated liver enzymes. Scand J Rheumatol 2020;49(6):427–33.

7. Ebert EC, Hagspiel KD. Gastrointestinal and hepatic manifestations of systemic lupus erythematosus. J Clin Gastroenterol 2011;45(5):436–41.

8. Mustafa M, Bawazir YM. Acute liver failure as the first feature of systemic lupus erythematosus. Rheumatol Int 2021;41(2):469–74.

9. De Santis M, Crotti C, Selmi C. Liver abnormalities in connective tissue diseases. Best Pract Res Clin Gastroenterol 2013;27(4):543–51.

10. Chowdhary VR, Crowson CS, Poterucha JJ, et al. Liver involvement in systemic lupus erythematosus: case review of 40 patients. J Rheumatol 2008; 35(11):2159–64.

11. Li Z, Xu D, Wang Z, et al. Gastrointestinal system involvement in systemic lupus erythematosus. Lupus 2017;26(11):1127–38.

12. Lu MC, Li KJ, Hsieh SC, et al. Lupus-related advanced liver involvement as the initial presentation of systemic lupus erythematosus. J Microbiol Immunol Infect 2006;39(6):471–5.

13. Matsumoto T, Kobayashi S, Shimizu H, et al. The liver in collagen diseases: pathologic study of 160 cases with particular reference to hepatic arteritis, primary biliary cirrhosis, autoimmune hepatitis and nodular regenerative hyperplasia of the liver. Liver 2000;20(5):366–73.

14. Siramolpiwat S, Sakonlaya D. Clinical and histologic features of Azathioprine-induced hepatotoxicity. Scand J Gastroenterol 2017;52(8):876–80.

15. Takahashi A, Abe K, Saito R, et al. Liver dysfunction in patients with systemic lupus erythematosus. Intern Med 2013;52(13):1461–5.

16. Adiga A, Nugent K. Lupus Hepatitis and Autoimmune Hepatitis (Lupoid Hepatitis). Am J Med Sci 2017;353(4):329–35.

17. Miller MH, Urowitz MB, Gladman DD, et al. The liver in systemic lupus erythematosus. Q J Med 1984; 53(211):401–9.

18. Wang CR, Tsai HW. Autoimmune liver diseases in systemic rheumatic diseases. World J Gastroenterol 2022;28(23):2527–45.

19. El-Shabrawi MH, Farrag MI. Hepatic manifestations in juvenile systemic lupus erythematosus. Recent Pat Inflamm Allergy Drug Discov 2014;8(1):36–40.

20. Piga M, Vacca A, Porru G, et al. Liver involvement in systemic lupus erythematosus: incidence, clinical course and outcome of lupus hepatitis. Clin Exp Rheumatol 2010;28(4):504–10.

21. Zheng RH, Wang JH, Wang SB, et al. Clinical and immunopathological features of patients with lupus hepatitis. Chin Med J (Engl) 2013;126(2):260–6.

22. Manderson AP, Botto M, Walport MJ. The role of complement in the development of systemic lupus erythematosus. Annu Rev Immunol 2004;22:431–56.

23. Efe C, Purnak T, Ozaslan E, et al. Autoimmune liver disease in patients with systemic lupus erythematosus: a retrospective analysis of 147 cases. Scand J Gastroenterol 2011;46(6):732–7.

24. Gurung A, Assis DN, McCarty TR, et al. Histologic features of autoimmune hepatitis: a critical appraisal. Hum Pathol 2018;82:51–60.

25. Tiniakos DG, Brain JG, Bury YA. Role of Histopathology in Autoimmune Hepatitis. Dig Dis 2015;33(Suppl 2):53–64.

26. Wang Y, Luo P, Guo T, et al. Study on the correlation between anti-ribosomal P protein antibody and systemic lupus erythematosus. Medicine (Baltim) 2020; 99(20):e20192.

27. Hubscher O, Elsner B. Nodular transformation of the liver in a patient with systemic lupus erythematosus. J Rheumatol 1989;16(3):410–2.

28. Al-Homood IA. Thrombosis in systemic lupus erythematosus: a review article. ISRN Rheumatol 2012; 2012:428269.

29. Sekiya M, Sekigawa I, Hishikawa T, et al. Nodular regenerative hyperplasia of the liver in systemic lupus erythematosus. The relationship with anticardiolipin antibody and lupus anticoagulant. Scand J Rheumatol 1997;26(3):215–7.

30. Leung VK, Ng WL, Luk IS, et al. Unique hepatic imaging features in a patient with nodular regenerative hyperplasia of the liver associating with systemic lupus erythematosus. Lupus 2007;16(3):205–8.

31. Dachman AH, Ros PR, Goodman ZD, et al. Nodular regenerative hyperplasia of the liver: clinical and radiologic observations. AJR Am J Roentgenol 1987;148(4):717–22.

32. Jharap B, van Asseldonk DP, de Boer NK, et al. Diagnosing Nodular Regenerative Hyperplasia of the Liver Is Thwarted by Low Interobserver Agreement. PLoS One 2015;10(6):e0120299.

33. Rubio-Tapia A, Murray JA. The Liver and Celiac Disease. Clin Liver Dis 2019;23(2):167–76.

34. Villavicencio Kim J, Wu GY. Celiac Disease and Elevated Liver Enzymes: A Review. J Clin Transl Hepatol 2021;9(1):116–24.

35. Haggård L, Glimberg I, Lebwohl B, et al. High prevalence of celiac disease in autoimmune hepatitis: Systematic review and meta-analysis. Liver Int 2021;41(11):2693–702.

36. Callichurn K, Cvetkovic L, Therrien A, et al. Prevalence of Celiac Disease in Patients with Primary Biliary Cholangitis. J Can Assoc Gastroenterol 2021;4(1):44–7.

37. Mounajjed T, Oxentenko A, Shmidt E, et al. The liver in celiac disease: clinical manifestations, histologic features, and response to gluten-free diet in 30 patients. Am J Clin Pathol 2011;136(1):128–37.

38. Evans KE, Sanders DS. Celiac disease. Gastroenterol Clin North Am 2012;41(3):639–50.

39. He MM, Lo CH, Wang K, et al. Immune-Mediated Diseases Associated With Cancer Risks. JAMA Oncol 2022;8(2):209–19.

40. Yoosuf S, Singh P, Khaitan A, et al. Prevalence of celiac disease in patients with liver diseases: a systematic review and meta-analyses. Am J Gastroenterol 2023;118(5):820–32.

41. Novacek G, Miehsler W, Wrba F, et al. Prevalence and clinical importance of hypertransaminasaemia in coeliac disease. Eur J Gastroenterol Hepatol 1999;11(3):283–8.

42. Rubio-Tapia A, Murray JA. Liver involvement in celiac disease. Minerva Med 2008;99(6):595–604.

43. Majumdar K, Sakhuja P, Puri AS, et al. Coeliac disease and the liver: spectrum of liver histology, serology and treatment response at a tertiary referral centre. J Clin Pathol 2018;71(5):412–9.

44. Garrido I, Liberal R, Peixoto A, et al. Long-term follow-up and prognosis of celiac hepatitis. Eur J Gastroenterol Hepatol 2022;34(12):1255–60.

45. Roderburg C, Loosen S, Kostev K, et al. Nonalcoholic fatty liver disease is associated with a higher incidence of coeliac disease. Eur J Gastroenterol Hepatol 2022;34(3):328–31.

46. Turesson C, Matteson EL. Genetics of rheumatoid arthritis. Mayo Clin Proc 2006;81(1):94–101.

47. Feuchtenberger M, Kraus L, Nigg A, et al. Methotrexate does not increase the risk of liver fibrosis in patients with rheumatoid arthritis: assessment by ultrasound elastography (ARFI-MetRA study). Rheumatol Int 2021;41(6):1079–87.

48. Gelfand JM, Wan J, Zhang H, et al. Risk of liver disease in patients with psoriasis, psoriatic arthritis, and rheumatoid arthritis receiving methotrexate: A population-based study. J Am Acad Dermatol 2021;84(6):1636–43.

49. Aithal GP. Hepatotoxicity related to antirheumatic drugs. Nat Rev Rheumatol 2011;7(3):139–50.

50. Olsson-White DA, Olynyk JK, Ayonrinde OT, et al. Assessment of liver fibrosis markers in people with rheumatoid arthritis on methotrexate. Intern Med J 2022;52(4):566–73.

51. Hilal G, Akasbi N, Boudouaya H, et al. Liver Fibrosis in Rheumatoid Arthritis Patients Treated with Methotrexate. Curr Rheumatol Rev 2020;16(4):293–7.

52. Craig E, Cappelli LC. Gastrointestinal and Hepatic Disease in Rheumatoid Arthritis. Rheum Dis Clin North Am 2018;44(1):89–111.

53. Wong GW, Heneghan MA. Association of Extrahepatic Manifestations with Autoimmune Hepatitis. Dig Dis 2015;33(Suppl 2):25–35.

54. Sema K, Takei M, Uenogawa K, et al. Felty's syndrome with chronic hepatitis and compatible autoimmune hepatitis: a case presentation. Intern Med 2005;44(4):335–41.

55. Ruderman EM, Crawford JM, Maier A, et al. Histologic liver abnormalities in an autopsy series of patients with rheumatoid arthritis. Br J Rheumatol 1997;36(2):210–3.

56. Ahern MJ, Kevat S, Hill W, et al. Hepatic methotrexate content and progression of hepatic fibrosis: preliminary findings. Ann Rheum Dis 1991;50(7):477–80.

57. Kevat S, Ahern M, Hall P. Hepatotoxicity of methotrexate in rheumatic diseases. Med Toxicol Adverse Drug Exp 1988;3(3):197–208.

58. Langman G, Hall PM, Todd G. Role of non-alcoholic steatohepatitis in methotrexate-induced liver injury. J Gastroenterol Hepatol 2001;16(12):1395–401.

59. Mori S, Arima N, Ito M, et al. Non-alcoholic steatohepatitis-like pattern in liver biopsy of rheumatoid arthritis patients with persistent transaminitis during low-dose methotrexate treatment. PLoS One 2018;13(8):e0203084.

60. Wanless IR. Micronodular transformation (nodular regenerative hyperplasia) of the liver: a report of 64 cases among 2,500 autopsies and a new classification of benign hepatocellular nodules. Hepatology 1990;11(5):787–97.

61. Goritsas C, Roussos A, Ferti A, et al. Nodular regenerative hyperplasia in a rheumatoid arthritis patient without felty's syndrome. J Clin Gastroenterol 2002;35(4):363–4.

62. Cohen ML, Manier JW, Bredfeldt JE. Sinusoidal lymphocytosis of the liver in Felty's syndrome with

a review of the liver involvement in Felty's syndrome. J Clin Gastroenterol 1989;11(1):92–4.

63. Osuga T, Ikura Y, Kadota C, et al. Significance of liver biopsy for the evaluation of methotrexate-induced liver damage in patients with rheumatoid arthritis. Int J Clin Exp Pathol 2015;8(2):1961–6.

64. Zhang C, Shi L, Wang FS. Liver injury in COVID-19: management and challenges. Lancet Gastroenterol Hepatol 2020;5(5):428–30.

65. Xu Z, Shi L, Wang Y, et al. Pathological findings of COVID-19 associated with acute respiratory distress syndrome. Lancet Respir Med 2020;8(4): 420–2.

66. Mokhtari T, Hassani F, Ghaffari N, et al. COVID-19 and multiorgan failure: A narrative review on potential mechanisms. J Mol Histol 2020;51(6):613–28.

67. Fiel MI, El Jamal SM, Paniz-Mondolfi A, et al. Findings of Hepatic Severe Acute Respiratory Syndrome Coronavirus-2 Infection. Cell Mol Gastroenterol Hepatol 2021;11(3):763–70.

68. Luo M, Ballester MP, Soffientini U, et al. SARS-CoV-2 infection and liver involvement. Hepatol Int 2022; 16(4):755–74.

69. Kunutsor SK, Laukkanen JA. Hepatic manifestations and complications of COVID-19: A systematic review and meta-analysis. J Infect 2020; 81(3):e72–4.

70. Bryce C, Grimes Z, Pujadas E, et al. Pathophysiology of SARS-CoV-2: the Mount Sinai COVID-19 autopsy experience. Mod Pathol 2021;34(8):1456–67.

71. Peiris S, Mesa H, Aysola A, et al. Pathological findings in organs and tissues of patients with COVID-19: A systematic review. PLoS One 2021;16(4): e0250708.

72. Wang Y, Liu S, Liu H, et al. SARS-CoV-2 infection of the liver directly contributes to hepatic impairment in patients with COVID-19. J Hepatol 2020;73(4): 807–16.

73. Bongiovanni M, Zago T. Acute hepatitis caused by asymptomatic COVID-19 infection. J Infect 2021; 82(1):e25–6.

74. Chu H, Peng L, Hu L, et al. Liver Histopathological Analysis of 24 Postmortem Findings of Patients With COVID-19 in China. Front Med 2021;8:749318.

75. Haji Esmaeil Memar E, Mamishi S, Sharifzadeh Ekbatani M, et al. Fulminant hepatic failure: A rare and devastating manifestation of Coronavirus disease 2019 in an 11-year-old boy. Arch Pediatr 2020;27(8):502–5.

76. McConnell MJ, Kawaguchi N, Kondo R, et al. Liver injury in COVID-19 and IL-6 trans-signaling-induced endotheliopathy. J Hepatol 2021;75(3):647–58.

77. Sarin SK, Choudhury A, Lau GK, et al. Pre-existing liver disease is associated with poor outcome in patients with SARS CoV2 infection; The APCOLIS Study (APASL COVID-19 Liver Injury Spectrum Study). Hepatol Int 2020;14(5):690–700.

78. Iavarone M, D'Ambrosio R, Soria A, et al. High rates of 30-day mortality in patients with cirrhosis and COVID-19. J Hepatol 2020;73(5): 1063–71.

79. Bartoli A, Cursaro C, Andreone P. Severe acute respiratory syndrome coronavirus-2-associated cholangiopathies. Curr Opin Gastroenterol 2022;38(2): 89–97.

80. Roth NC, Kim A, Vitkovski T, et al. Post-COVID-19 Cholangiopathy: A Novel Entity. Am J Gastroenterol 2021;116(5):1077–82.

81. Faruqui S, Okoli FC, Olsen SK, et al. Cholangiopathy After Severe COVID-19: Clinical Features and Prognostic Implications. Am J Gastroenterol 2021;116(7): 1414–25.

82. Shih AR, Hatipoglu D, Wilechansky R, et al. Persistent Cholestatic Injury and Secondary Sclerosing Cholangitis in COVID-19 Patients. Arch Pathol Lab Med 2022;146(10):1184–93.

83. Hartl L, Haslinger K, Angerer M, et al. Progressive cholestasis and associated sclerosing cholangitis are frequent complications of COVID-19 in patients with chronic liver disease. Hepatology 2022;76(6): 1563–75.

84. Heucke N, Keitel V. COVID-19-associated cholangiopathy: What is left after the virus has gone? Hepatology 2022;76(6):1560–2.

85. Durazo FA, Nicholas AA, Mahaffey JJ, et al. Post-Covid-19 Cholangiopathy-A New Indication for Liver Transplantation: A Case Report. Transplant Proc 2021;53(4):1132–7.

86. Bütikofer S, Lenggenhager D, Wendel Garcia PD, et al. Secondary sclerosing cholangitis as cause of persistent jaundice in patients with severe COVID-19. Liver Int 2021;41(10):2404–17.

87. Garrido I, Lopes S, Simões MS, et al. Autoimmune hepatitis after COVID-19 vaccine - more than a coincidence. J Autoimmun 2021;125: 102741.

88. Marjot T, Moon AM, Cook JA, et al. Outcomes following SARS-CoV-2 infection in patients with chronic liver disease: An international registry study. J Hepatol 2021;74(3):567–77.

89. Mahamid M, Nseir W, Khoury T, et al. Nonalcoholic fatty liver disease is associated with COVID-19 severity independently of metabolic syndrome: a retrospective case-control study. Eur J Gastroenterol Hepatol 2021;33(12):1578–81.

90. Mushtaq K, Khan MU, Iqbal F, et al. NAFLD is a predictor of liver injury in COVID-19 hospitalized patients but not of mortality, disease severity on the presentation or progression - The debate continues. J Hepatol 2021;74(2):482–4.

91. Karlafti E, Paramythiotis D, Pantazi K, et al. Drug-Induced Liver Injury in Hospitalized Patients during SARS-CoV-2 Infection. Medicina (Kaunas) 2022; 58(12).

92. Guardiola J, Lammert C, Teal E, et al. Unexplained liver test elevations after SARS-CoV-2 vaccination. J Hepatol 2022;77(1):251–3.

93. Codoni G, Kirchner T, Engel B, et al. Histological and serological features of acute liver injury after SARS-CoV-2 vaccination. JHEP Rep 2023;5(1):100605.

94. Boettler T, Csernalabics B, Salié H, et al. SARS-CoV-2 vaccination can elicit a CD8 T-cell dominant hepatitis. J Hepatol 2022;77(3):653–9.

95. Vuille-Lessard É, Montani M, Bosch J, et al. Autoimmune hepatitis triggered by SARS-CoV-2 vaccination. J Autoimmun 2021;123:102710.

Systemic Disease and the Liver Part 2

Pregnancy-Related Liver Injury, Sepsis/Critical Illness, Hypoxia, Psoriasis, Scleroderma/Sjogren's Syndrome, Sarcoidosis, Common Variable Immune Deficiency, Cystic Fibrosis, Inflammatory Bowel Disease, and Hematologic Disorders

Maria Isabel Fiel, MD, FAASLD[a],*, Thomas D. Schiano, MD, FAASLD[b]

KEYWORDS

- Liver biopsy • Combined variable immunodeficiency • Pregnancy • Sarcoidosis • Cystic fibrosis
- Nodular regenerative hyperplasia • Granuloma • Sepsis

Key Points

- Nodular regenerative hyperplasia (NRH) and obliterative portal venopathy (OPV) occur commonly in the setting of systemic disease and are associated with non-cirrhotic portal hypertension. Liver biopsy may be the only way to confidently rule out cirrhosis.

- Nonalcoholic fatty liver disease is a frequent liver biopsy finding in the setting of systemic inflammatory states, such as psoriasis, some collagen vascular diseases, and inflammatory bowel disease.

- Liver disease is extremely common in common variable immune deficiency with NRH being the most frequent histological finding.

- The differential diagnosis for abnormal liver chemistry test in myeloproliferative neoplasms, such as polycythemia vera, is broad. Liver biopsy may show extramedullary hematopoiesis, OPV and NRH, sinusoidal dilatation, portal biliopathy, or nonspecific findings.

- Patients surviving protracted critical illness with need for intensive care monitoring, use of mechanical ventilation, and vasopressor support may develop a secondary sclerosing cholangitis, which is now being increasing identified.

ABSTRACT

The liver is involved in many multisystem diseases and commonly may manifest with abnormal liver chemistry tests. The liver test perturbations may be multifactorial in nature, however, as patients are receiving many different medications and can also have intrinsic liver disease that may be exacerbated by the systemic disorder. Some disorders have typical histologic findings that can be diagnosed on liver biopsy, whereas others will show a more nonspecific histology. Clinicians should be aware of these conditions so as to consider the performance of a liver biopsy at the most opportune time and setting to help establish the diagnosis of acute or chronic liver disease.

---

[a] Department of Pathology, Molecular and Cell-Based Medicine, Icahn School of Medicine at Mount Sinai, One Gustave Levy Place, New York, NY 10029, USA; [b] Division of Liver Diseases, Recanati-Miller Transplantation Institute, Icahn School of Medicine at Mount Sinai, One Gustave Levy Place-Box 1104, New York, NY 10029, USA
* Corresponding author.
E-mail address: mariaisabel.fiel@mountsinai.org

Surgical Pathology 16 (2023) 485–498
https://doi.org/10.1016/j.path.2023.04.005
1875-9181/23/© 2023 Elsevier Inc. All rights reserved.

OVERVIEW

In Part 1, the liver histopathology occurring in four diverse systemic diseases was presented—systemic lupus erythematosus, rheumatoid arthritis, celiac disease, and COVID-19, exemplifying the varied clinical conditions that are associated with liver abnormalities. In Part 2 of this review, the authors summarize many other diseases that have liver involvement, often with representative photomicrographs. These include thrombophilia and other hematological conditions, disorders of immunity such as common variable immunodeficiency (CVID), and rheumatological conditions such as systemic sclerosis and psoriasis. Also presented are abnormal liver histological findings occurring in pregnancy, sepsis, and with critical illness.

This review is not meant to be an exhaustive summary of all systemic diseases involving the liver. Infiltrative diseases such as amyloidosis and genetic/metabolic conditions such as Gaucher's disease and lysosomal acid lipase deficiency will not be covered. In reviewing the liver involvement associated with systemic diseases, the authors hope to highlight the disease states when liver biopsy is helpful in establishing a diagnosis, which reinforces the need for close collaboration between the liver pathologist and clinician. Under certain circumstances, liver biopsy may show only nonspecific findings, whereas at other times, pathognomonic or typical histological features will enable timely diagnosis and treatment.

PREGNANCY-RELATED LIVER DISEASES

Liver disorders in pregnancy are infrequent despite pregnant women generally having abnormal liver biochemistries. Up to 3% of all pregnancies are complicated by liver.[1,2] Unique liver diseases occur in pregnancy and will be discussed below.

Hyperemesis Gravidarum

Hyperemesis gravidarum is characterized by intractable vomiting resulting in dehydration and other metabolic abnormalities.[3] Approximately 50% of patients suffering from hyperemesis gravidarum have liver dysfunction.[4] Serum aminotransferases may be elevated up to 20 times the upper limit of normal along with other biochemical abnormalities, which resolve when vomiting resolves.[5] Liver biopsy is not indicated. If a liver biopsy is available, the parenchyma may appear normal or may exhibit mild steatosis.[2] Rarely, cholestasis and scattered necrotic hepatocytes may be seen.[6]

Intrahepatic Cholestasis of Pregnancy

Pregnant women who suffer from intrahepatic cholestasis experience pruritus.[2,7] The underlying pathophysiology is believed to be due to female sex hormones, which induce cholestasis and inhibit the bile salt export pump.[7] Elevated serum bile acids and aminotransferases can be elevated up to 20 times the upper limit of normal. Liver biopsy is not necessary but if done, the findings are those of nonspecific perivenular cholestasis mostly with bile plugs in the canaliculi. Necrosis and lobular and portal inflammation are absent.[6,8]

Preeclampsia and Eclampsia

Approximately 5% of all pregnancies may be complicated by preeclampsia. It is a multisystemic disease and can involve the kidneys, the central nervous system, and the liver. It is characterized by hypertension and proteinuria and if seizures occur, it is then defined to be eclampsia.[2] Abnormal liver biochemistry tests particularly aminotransferases, which can be elevated up to 10 times the upper limit of normal, are characteristic.[7,9] Liver biopsy is not indicated to make a definitive diagnosis, however, if a liver biopsy is available, findings are most prominent in periportal zones such as the presence of fibrin thrombi in the sinusoids, hemorrhage, and hepatocyte necrosis. Thrombi may also be seen in other vessels such as the capillaries in portal tracts as well as hepatic arterioles and portal veins.[6,8]

HELLP syndrome

HELLP syndrome is a combination of hemolysis, elevated liver enzymes, and low platelets. Patients with HELLP syndrome may be asymptomatic or clinically present with abdominal pain, nausea, vomiting, and malaise.[4] Approximately 5% to 10% of patients with preeclampsia develop HELLP.[9] HELLP may show symptoms similar to preeclampsia but it may also develop in women who might not have signs or symptoms of preeclampsia.[2] Liver injury is secondary to intravascular fibrin deposition, hypovolemia, and increased sinusoidal pressure. Raised aminotransferases and mild elevation of bilirubin are typical. The performance of a liver biopsy is a high-risk procedure due to increased risk for bleeding. If histology is available, the changes are similar to those of preeclampsia and can include fibrin deposition in vessels and sinusoids and periportal hepatocyte necrosis and hemorrhage.[8]

Liver Rupture, Infarction, Hematoma

Hepatic rupture, infarction, and hematoma rarely occur in women with preeclampsia or HELLP syndrome.[10] Hepatocellular adenoma, hepatocellular carcinoma, and hemangiomas may also rupture during pregnancy.[11] CT scan (CT) or MRI of the liver may be diagnostic of rupture, hematoma, or infarction.[11]

Acute Fatty Liver of Pregnancy

Acute fatty liver of pregnancy is rare and affects one in 16000 to one in 20,000 pregnancies.[12,13] Clinical presentations include vomiting, abdominal pain, and even hepatic encephalopathy and jaundice.[2,4,7,8,13] Patients may have hypoglycemia, lactic acidosis, hyperammonemia, and microvesicular fat deposition in multiple organs.[2,7,12] The gold standard for diagnosis is a liver biopsy but is not necessary as liver biopsy is rarely performed due to the urgent need to stabilize and deliver the baby.[7,9] Histologically, there is panlobular involvement by small droplet steatosis that expands the cytoplasm of hepatocytes and frequently gives a foamy appearance of the cytoplasm giving a ballooning change similar to what is seen in other liver diseases; distinct small droplets may not be discernible (**Fig. 1**A). Sometimes periportal hepatocytes may be spared.[6] Before the development of clinical criteria, a fat stain such as Oil-red-O or Sudan Black was performed to highlight the presence of microvesicular steatosis, which required frozen tissue (**Fig. 1**B).

SEPSIS/CRITICAL ILLNESS

Liver dysfunction is commonly seen in critically ill patients and clinically may present in different ways.[14–16] Hyperbilirubinemia developing in an intensive care unit patient may be seen as part of the cholestasis of sepsis.[15,17] Cholestasis of sepsis is a complex physiologic process involving Kupffer cell and endothelial cell dysfunction and

Fig. 1. Acute fatty liver of pregnancy. (*A*) Microvesicular steatosis may not be apparent, but instead the hepatocyte cytoplasm looks foamy and may have characteristic features of ballooned hepatocytes. Also seen may be mild cholestasis. The portal tracts show a mild nonspecific inflammation. H&E, original magnification x40. (*B*) The presence of fat droplets within the hepatocyte cytoplasm is highlighted by an Oil-red-O stain. Original magnification x20.

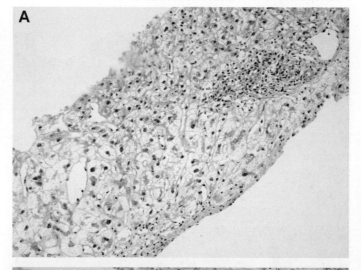
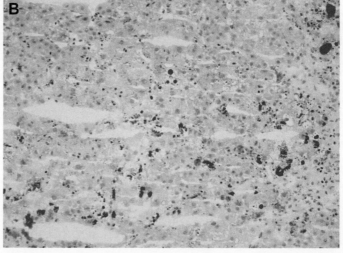

impairment of bile transport but can also be multi-factorial in nature related to drug-induced liver injury (DILI), concurrent acute kidney injury, hemolysis, use of total parenteral nutrition, hypotension, multiple transfusions, and acute-on-chronic liver failure for patients having intrinsic liver disease.[16,18] Patients can develop acalculous cholecystitis or ischemic hepatitis which can further confound the clinical and biochemical presentation.[14,19]

Histology

Liver biopsy performed in this setting may not be helpful as it often shows nonspecific findings such as microthrombi, scattered areas of necrosis and cholangitis lenta.[15,20] Nonspecific changes include focal hepatocyte necrosis, Kupffer cell hyperplasia, and portal inflammation. Sinusoidal congestion, steatosis, and intrahepatic cholestasis ranging from moderate to severe are also seen. The cholestasis is mainly centrilobular and may be seen as intrahepatocytic cholestasis as well as canalicular

bile concretions.[21] Cholangitis lenta shows prominent ductular cholestasis with dilated ductules containing thick inspissated bile[21,22] (Fig. 2A). Two types of liver injury have been described in critically ill patients, the "hepatitic" type that shows portal and lobular inflammation with or without centrilobular necrosis and the second type designated as "mixed" as having both biliary lesions, cholestasis, portal and lobular inflammation, and centrilobular necrosis.[21] Critically ill patients may also develop an often gradual but sometimes a rapid development of cholestasis with high levels of serum alkaline phosphatase and direct bilirubin that may persist, even after their recovery. Cross-sectional imaging may or may not show biliary abnormalities, but a liver biopsy can demonstrate chronic biliary changes such as prominent ductular reaction, portal fibrous expansion and progressive changes of biliary fibrosis, and features that are characteristic of secondary sclerosing cholangitis or critical illness cholangiopathy[23,24] (Fig. 2B).

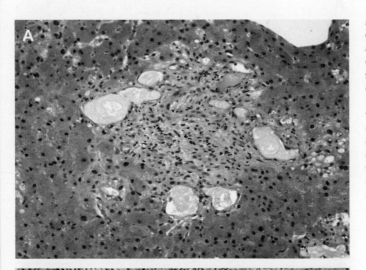

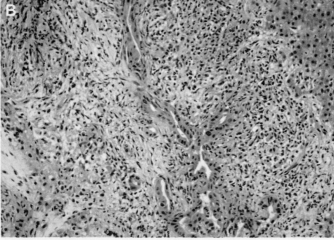

Fig. 2. Sepsis (A). A portal tract is expanded by mild fibrosis. The proliferating bile ductules at the periphery are dilated and contain bile (ductular cholestasis). The lobule also demonstrates cholestasis. This finding is often termed "cholangitis lenta." H&E, original magnification x20. (B) A portal tract is markedly expanded by edema, inflammation, and ductular reaction. Note that the bile ducts are irregular in shape and appear slightly damaged. The latter may be secondary to low-flow state. This finding is also known as "critical illness cholangiopathy." H&E, original magnification x40.

The etiology of this entity is a presumed low flow state within the portal venous/hepatic arterial vascular axis, which similarly occurs post-liver transplantation with interruption of hepatic artery flow to the biliary plexus resulting in ischemic cholangiopathy.[25]

HYPOXIC LIVER INJURY

Hypoxic liver injury (HLI), also known as hypoxic hepatitis, ischemic hepatitis or shock liver, occurs because of insufficient liver perfusion.[26,27] Associated conditions are right- or left-sided heart failure, constrictive cardiomyopathy, and chronic respiratory failure with cor pulmonale.[27] It is estimated to occur in 2.5%–10% of all admissions to the intensive care unit (ICU) with 10% to 50% in-hospital mortality.[26,28] As centrilobular zones are prone to hypoxic damage, liver biopsy shows centrilobular necrosis; very little inflammatory infiltrates are noted (Fig. 3A). Chronic hepatic venous congestion

may lead to dilatation of the sinusoids and hepatocyte atrophy.[14,29] Multiple episodes of HLI will lead to cardiac sclerosis characterized by centrilobular fibrosis with progression to bridging fibrous septa that link central to central zones and eventually cirrhosis (congestive hepatopathy)[29] (Fig. 3B). A heterogeneous distribution of liver involvement by congestion and fibrosis is typical and is secondary to heterogeneous thrombus formation in hepatic and portal vessels. Because of this geographic heterogeneity, typical findings may be missed on liver biopsy. Portal areas are relatively spared.[30]

PSORIASIS

Psoriasis is a common chronic inflammatory skin disease that is being increasingly recognized as a systemic inflammatory disorder and has been shown to have associations with arthritis, inflammatory bowel disease (IBD), cardiometabolic disease, and other conditions. It affects 7.5 million

Fig. 3. Hypoxic liver injury. (*A*) Extensive coagulative-type necrosis involving centrilobular (zone 3) and mid-zones (zone 2) is demonstrated in this photomicrograph. Note the mummified appearance of the necrotic hepatocytes. A mild mononuclear infiltrate is present. There is relative sparing of periportal (zone 1) hepatocytes. H&E, original magnification x20. (*B*) A patient with chronic ischemic hepatopathy may develop extensive fibrosis, which may be heterogeneously distributed. Note the patchy atrophy of hepatocyte plates. Masson trichrome, original magnification x20.

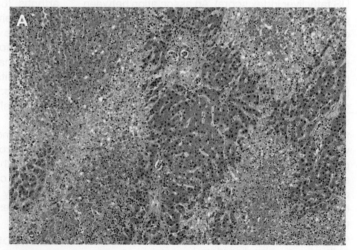

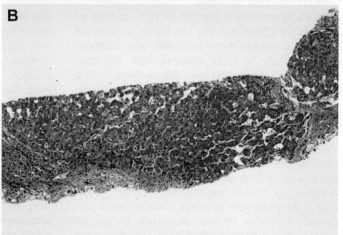

persons in the United States and approximately 125 million worldwide.[31] Psoriasis, especially severe disease, is associated with increased mortality and comorbid disease burden, hypothesized to be the result of chronic inflammation. It may be an independent risk factor for diabetes mellitus and major cardiovascular events with chronic inflammation likely contributing to atherogenesis. There are shared pathophysiologic pathways between psoriasis and cardiovascular disease which include increased oxidative stress, endothelial dysfunction, and chronic T-cell-mediated inflammation. Obesity is an independent risk factor for psoriasis, and the latter is associated with an increased risk of diabetes mellitus and hypertension. Dyslipidemia and the metabolic syndrome may be more prevalent in patients with psoriasis.[31]

Using the National Health and Nutrition Examination Survey, an analysis was performed of 148/5672 (3%) persons with psoriasis and the 1558/5672 (26.8%) respondents meeting criteria for nonalcoholic fatty liver disease (NAFLD) (via the US fatty liver index score). An association between psoriasis and NAFLD was established with an odds ratio of 1.67; 95% CI, 1.03–2.70 with subgroup analysis showing stronger associations in men (OR 2.16), those aged 20 to 39 years old (OR 2.48), and among those without diabetes (OR 1.70). This was a nationally representative cross-sectional study of outpatients; two previous studies examining inpatient populations also found that psoriasis was positively associated with NAFLD.[32,33] Although psoriasis may predispose to comorbidities associated with NAFLD and vice versa, it seems that NAFLD and psoriasis may be directly linked as a consequence of the chronic inflammation seen in the latter.[33] Thus, psoriasis may be a cause for lean NAFLD, as other chronic inflammatory disorders can be, such as collagen vascular disorders.

Psoriatic arthritis is present in 10% to 40% of patients with psoriasis and has higher prevalence in patients having more extensive skin disease. Approximately 15% of patients with psoriasis may have undiagnosed psoriatic arthritis.[34] In a longitudinal cohort study conducted in a psoriatic arthritis clinic, 343/1061 (32%) of patients had liver test abnormalities. The common causes for these abnormalities were DILI and NAFLD with higher body: mass index (BMI), daily alcohol intake, more severe disease, elevated C-reactive protein and use of methotrexate, leflunomide, or biologic therapies (ie, tumor necrosis factor [TNF] inhibitors).[31] Very few liver biopsies however were performed with the clinical diagnosis based on clinical or radiologic (including elastography) criteria. Much of the armamentarium used to treat psoriasis and psoriatic arthritis has potential for causing DILI, which include TNF inhibitors, corticosteroids, nonsteroidal anti-inflammatories, and methotrexate.[34] In the past, azathioprine has also been used which is associated with several different forms of DILI, including a cholestatic hepatitis and nodular regenerative hyperplasia and obliterative portal venopathy (NRH/OPV). Long-term methotrexate use has been less problematic in patients having IBD and rheumatoid arthritis, as compared with those having psoriasis. This was the classic teaching, which recommended the performance of surveillance liver biopsies in patients having psoriasis while receiving methotrexate. In retrospect, this potential for increased fibrosis progression due to methotrexate was probably due to underlying NAFLD and/or diabetes mellitus, both of which are well-established risk factors for accelerated fibrosis progression. Gelfand and colleagues[35] recently published a Danish population-based cohort study of 40,237 persons having psoriatic arthritis (5687), psoriatic arthritis (6520), and rheumatoid arthritis (8030) who received methotrexate between 1997 and 2015. The incidence rate of any liver disease was greatest for patients having psoriasis and lowest for rheumatoid arthritis, which included liver test abnormalities, cirrhosis, or cirrhosis-related hospitalizations. These outcomes were 1.3 to 1.6 times more likely in patients having psoriasis after adjusting for demographics, smoking, alcohol use, comorbidities, and methotrexate dose.[35] Thus, fibrosis progression should be followed at least with elastography in psoriasis patients receiving chronic methotrexate therapy, especially when they have risk factors for having NAFLD and/or diabetes mellitus.

SCLERODERMA/SJOGREN'S

Systemic sclerosis (scleroderma) is a connective tissue disease characterized by fibrosis, vasculopathy of small blood vessels, and immunologic dysfunction associated with specific antibody production.[36] It typically involves the skin, kidneys, lung, heart, and gastrointestinal tract. Its prevalence varies from 30 to 443 per million population. The most common liver disease associated with systemic sclerosis is primary biliary cholangitis (PBC), often as part of the CREST syndrome, which is typified by (+) anti-centromere antibodies.[36] Upwards of 10% of patients with PBC may have CREST syndrome, in which patients may have calcinosis, Raynaud's phenomenon, esophageal dysfunction (often dysmotility and reflux symptoms), sclerodactyly, and telangiectasias.[37] Overlap syndromes with autoimmune hepatitis (AIH) have also been described as well as non-cirrhotic portal hypertension related to NRH, and sclerosing cholangitis. It is important to note that NRH may also occur in the setting of PBC and primary sclerosing cholangitis (PSC).[38,39]

Sjogren syndrome is an autoimmune disorder mainly affecting salivary and lacrimal glands resulting in keratoconjunctivitis sicca which leads to ophthalmologic problems, gastrointestinal reflux disease, dental caries and less frequently lymphoma, peripheral neuropathy, and mononeuritis multiplex. Aminotransferases and alkaline phosphatase may be elevated and can rise and fall in parallel with disease activity.[36] In a study of 42 patients having primary Sjogren syndrome 44% had abnormal liver biochemistries, which correlated with the presence of arthritis, vasculitis, Raynaud's phenomenon, and higher percentages of antinuclear and anti-mitochondrial antibodies. Upward of 10% of patients with Sjogren syndrome have (+) anti-mitochondrial antibodies and meet clinical criteria for having PBC; there is also an association with AIH.[40] Another study examined liver stiffness in 101 patients with Sjogren syndrome and found that a minority of patients had substantial liver fibrosis without an obvious cause, although liver biopsy was not performed.[41] NAFLD may develop in the presence of systemic inflammatory disorders, so it is possible that a subset of these patients had fatty liver contributing to the abnormal liver stiffness. Liver biopsy may thus be necessary in certain patients with Sjogren syndrome to help establish the etiology for abnormal liver tests.

SARCOIDOSIS

Sarcoidosis is a multisystem disease that is commonly characterized by noncaseating epithelioid granulomas.[42] Sarcoidosis can involve any organ; however, the lungs and hilar lymph nodes are the most commonly affected with the liver being the third most common organ affected.[43] Clinical presentations can vary depending on the organ affected, making the diagnosis of sarcoidosis difficult at times, especially in detecting the commonly asymptomatic manifestation.[44,45] Hepatic sarcoidosis is an example of one such manifestation. Studies demonstrate varying rates (6% to 80%) of sarcoidosis involving the liver but a recent study involving 1476 patients with sarcoidosis found 4.2% of patients having liver involvement mainly manifesting with an elevated alkaline phosphatase level.[44] Hepatosplenomegaly may be present with related thrombocytopenia making it difficult at times to reliably exclude or confirm cirrhosis. Symptomatic patients often present with abdominal pain, pruritus, hepatosplenomegaly, fever, night sweats, and weight loss.[46] In more advanced cases, patients may present with portal hypertension (non-cirrhotic or due to cirrhosis) and liver failure requiring liver transplantation.[42,47,48] Immunomodulatory treatment is initiated in patients with appreciable cardiopulmonary, renal, or neurologic disease, but there are scant treatment data on medical therapy for hepatic sarcoidosis.[49]

There are few existing criteria to make a precise diagnosis of hepatic sarcoidosis. Diagnosis is based on a combination of clinical, laboratory, and histological manifestations.[43,45] Current clinical markers include assessing for elevated liver chemistry tests (LFTs) and radiographic imaging of the abdomen demonstrating hepatomegaly or hepatic nodules.[48] The most affirmative diagnostic tool is to obtain a liver biopsy in conjunction with radiologic and laboratory data.

Histology

On liver biopsy, sarcoidosis will commonly show large well-formed noncaseating epithelioid granulomas located mainly at the portal tract or periportal zones. They are generally larger than granulomas seen in other liver conditions. Frequently, granulomas may coalesce forming large masses (**Fig. 4**). These granulomas may eventually be replaced by fibrosis over time. The granulomas contain multinucleated giant cells with minimal lymphocytic cuffing and fibrin depositions at the periphery. The differential diagnosis includes other types of granulomatous hepatitis such as PBC, CVID, infections, idiopathic granulomatous hepatitis, and drug-induced liver injury. Rarely, sarcoid granulomas may undergo central necrosis, leading to suspicion of an infectious etiology.[50] Fernandes and colleagues[50] attributed necrosis as secondary to systemic vasculitis, which may coexist with sarcoidosis. Histochemical stains to rule out acid-fast bacilli and fungi are routinely performed.[51] Other histological features may include bile duct damage and loss, biliary cirrhosis, portal inflammation, and changes consistent with AIH and NRH.[42]

COMMON VARIABLE IMMUNODEFICIENCY

CVID is the most common symptomatic primary immunodeficiency in adults (11.7%–36.3%) with an estimated incidence of 2 to 10/100,000 population.[52] Although the circulating B-cell count is normal in patients, the disorder is characterized by defects in B-cell differentiation leading to significant hypogammaglobulinemia and decreased counts of plasma cell and memory B cells.[53,54]

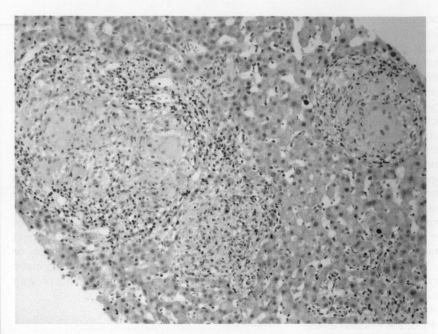

Fig. 4. Hepatic sarcoidosis. Multiple noncaseating coalescent granulomas are seen in this photomicrograph. Most of these granulomas are located adjacent to a portal tract, whereas others may be located in the lobule. Multinucleated giant cells and a mild lymphocytic cuff at the periphery of the granulomas are present. H&E, original magnification x40.

There also seems to be decreased numbers in CD4+ and Treg cells with alteration of T-cell functions. CVID has highly variable and heterogeneous clinical presentations and is typified by decreased plasma cells and globulins leading to infections primarily by bacteria in the sinuses, and respiratory and gastrointestinal tracts as well as autoimmune disorders and risk for malignancies.[52] The hematological system and liver are also commonly involved. The clinical heterogeneity may lead to a delay in formal diagnosis. More than 90% of CVID patients present with various infections such as serial sinusitis, bronchiectasis, pneumonia, or bronchitis, although more severe infections involving the otolaryngeal tract, skin, bone, and urine also occur.[52,55] Interestingly, autoimmunity is a common complication of CVID and may be its initial manifestation. The most frequent autoimmune conditions associated with CVID are cytopenias, such as immune thrombocytopenia and hemolytic anemia, but more systemic disorders can occur such as rheumatoid arthritis, Sjogren disease, systemic lupus erythematosus (SLE), inflammatory bowel-type disease, thyroiditis, and PBC.[52,55] CVID patients also have an increased risk for lymphoproliferation which may be benign causing hepatomegaly, splenomegaly or lymphadenopathy, or lymphoma. The incidence of solid tumors is also increased in CVID, especially that of gastric cancer, with malignancies being a major cause of death in CVID.[52]

Noncaseating granulomatous lesions occur in up to a quarter of CVID patients with the majority affecting the lymph nodes, lungs, and liver. This generally portends a worse overall prognosis. When the lung is involved the patient might initially be misdiagnosed as having sarcoidosis.[52] It is clear that many different types of liver conditions can potentially be associated with CVID and that CVID has features that can occur in patients having liver disease such as hepatosplenomegaly, thrombocytopenia, and granulomas on disease biopsy. At least 10% of patients with CVID present with liver involvement. Liver damage is strongly associated with lymphocytic enteropathy suggesting a pathogenic role of the gut–liver axis. The liver involvement may occur in up to 40% of patients and can range from abnormal liver chemistries (most commonly alkaline phosphatase) to NRH and non-cirrhotic portal hypertension to biliary cirrhosis, finally to reports of hepatocellular carcinoma. Also reported in CVID are chronic hepatitis, sclerosing cholangitis, and AIH. NRH seems to be the most common feature noted on clinically warranted liver biopsy.[52,56,57] The diagnosis of a specific liver disease in CVID can be challenging because serological antibody testing may be unreliable, and thus liver biopsy often becomes necessary. Other features seen on liver biopsy can include nonspecific portal and lobular inflammation, interface hepatitis, lymphocytic infiltration without plasma cells, bile ductular proliferation, and granulomas. A distinct pattern of peri-cellular fibrosis has been noted ranging from focal centrizonal fibrosis to bridging fibrosis at times accompanied by increased sinusoidal lymphocytes.[58]

It is important to survey patients with CVID periodically for the presence of portal hypertension, as once clinical manifestation develop, morbidity and mortality increase. NRH seems to be by far the most common histology seen on liver biopsy and manifests with the radiologic or clinical development of portal hypertension in patients who have CVID for at least a decade. Typically in NRH, liver stiffness is not appreciably elevated and can be a good tool to differentiate non-cirrhotic from cirrhotic portal hypertension. However, NRH in CVID seems to be associated with increased liver stiffness on elastography.[59] DiGiacomo and colleagues[60] compared ultrasound-based transient elastography in 12 CVID patients having biopsy-proven NRH with patients having CVID without NRH and a large cohort of NAFLD patients. Interestingly, elastography results demonstrated a significantly elevated liver stiffness in CVID patients with NRH (mean 13.2 ± 6.2 kPa) as compared with both CVID patients without NRH (mean 4.6 ± 0.9 kPa) and non-CVID patients with NAFLD (mean 6.9 ± 5.5 kPa). No single or composite histopathologic feature of NRH correlated with liver stiffness and stiffness correlated with clinical parameters of portal hypertension.[60] Most patients with NRH already had appreciable portal hypertension in this study so whether elastography can be used early on in CVID as a predictive or prognostic tool for the development of portal hypertension requires further study.

CYSTIC FIBROSIS

Cystic fibrosis (CF) is the most common autosomal recessive genetic disorder in Caucasians. The prevalence of CF liver disease approaches 40% in patients having CF but accounts for only 2% to 5% in overall mortality.[61] CF liver disease is well-described in the pediatric population and is a non-pulmonary cause of morbidity in these patients. As life expectancy has improved, adult-onset CF liver disease is increasingly recognized. Hepatosplenomegaly is extremely common in CF liver disease and from 50% to 90% of patients have abnormal alanine aminotransferase (ALT) or aspartate aminotransferase (AST).[62]

Histology

CF liver disease may present as heterogeneous distribution of biliary-type fibrosis as characterized by periportal fibrosis that can gradually advance to bridging fibrous septa that link portal to portal zones. Along with biliary fibrosis, ductular reaction and dilated ductules that contain inspissated bile may be seen (Fig. 5).[63] These changes are attributed to mutations in the CF transmembrane conduction regulator protein that leads to mucus plugging in cholangiocytes with subsequent periductal inflammation, bile duct damage and proliferation, and periportal fibrosis. Biliary cirrhosis and portal hypertension can result.[64] Some patients with CF develop steatosis which seems multifactorial in nature. Thus, CF is one of the causes (such as celiac disease) of macrovesicular steatosis not due to NAFLD. Whereas hepatic steatosis and focal biliary cirrhosis are more common in pediatric patients with CF, the latter is not as common in adults.[65] In adults, non-cirrhotic

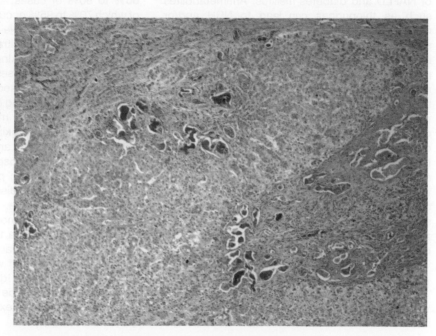

Fig. 5. Cystic fibrosis. Prominent ductules containing thick bile-stained mucoid material are seen at the periphery of portal areas. Note the irregular expansion of the portal tracts secondary to fibrosis (biliary type). The lobules seem light-staining due to involvement by steatosis. H&E, original magnification x20.

portal hypertension may develop due to NRH and OPV.[63] Gallbladder abnormalities and hepatolithiasis may also occur and lead to chronic biliary changes and sclerosing cholangitis type picture.[61] The wide spectrum of histologic liver changes in CF may be patchy in nature and thus may be underrepresented or missed on a liver biopsy sample.

INFLAMMATORY BOWEL DISEASE

Hepatic dysfunction may commonly be seen in patients having IBD.[66,67] PSC is associated much more with ulcerative colitis as compared with Crohn disease and can present with cholestasis at any point throughout the course of the disease.[68] Liver histology may often support the diagnosis of PSC, which is definitively made via cholangiography. Typical PSC may itself have several variant forms such as small duct PSC, an overlap with AIH, and immunoglobulin G4 (IgG4) cholangiopathy, which can only be definitively diagnosed via liver biopsy.[69,70]

Much of the therapeutic armamentarium for IBD has the potential to cause DILI. Many of the biologic agents, especially the anti-TNF agents infliximab and adalimumab, have been associated with causing abnormal aminotransferases with rare reports of acute liver failure and triggering of an AIH.[71] Liver biopsy may or may not assist in the diagnosis as at times there may be nonspecific findings, whereas at others, characteristic findings of AIH and DILI are noted. Methotrexate is associated with the development of progressive liver fibrosis and cirrhosis but more so in the setting of NAFLD and diabetes mellitus. Antimetabolites such as thiopurines can lead to NRH and/or OPV, causes of non-cirrhotic portal hypertension.[72,73] In this case, liver tests may actually be in the normal range but developing thrombocytopenia over time or abnormal liver-spleen imaging may alert the clinician to the possibility of portal hypertension. Thiopurines are also associated with an idiosyncratic DILI typically soon after the onset of treatment.[73] The most common cause of abnormal liver tests in IBD patients is actually NAFLD, which may confound the clinical picture and thus necessitate liver biopsy to help discern the cause of hepatic dysfunction.[74] Much rarer causes of abnormal liver tests in this population, such as granulomatous hepatitis (due to sulfasalazine), portal vein thrombosis, and amyloidosis can only be definitively diagnosed by liver biopsy.[67]

HEMATOLOGIC DISORDERS

Various hematologic conditions may directly involve the liver. Clinical evidence of liver disease may be the first manifestation of these disorders. Leukemias, lymphomas, and multiple myeloma can cause abnormal liver chemistries and in rare cases lead to liver failure. The extent of liver infiltration in relation to abnormal liver enzyme tests is not established. Acute liver failure may occur due to massive infiltration of the liver by leukemia or lymphoma.[75] Acute myelogenous leukemia, acute lymphocytic leukemia (ALL), chronic lymphocytic leukemia (CLL), and chronic myelogenous leukemia (CML) may involve the liver to some degree in half of patients. Non-Hodgkin's lymphoma may frequently involve the liver. The incidence and pattern of liver involvement in hematological malignancies vary. In a study involving 127 patients with hematological malignancies, the investigators found that CML, CLL, and myeloproliferative diseases involved the liver in 80% to 100% of patients while the incidence of liver involvement in ALL, CLL, and non-Hodgkin lymphoma was found in ~50% to 70%. Liver involvement in multiple myeloma was only found in 32% of cases.[76] Barcos and colleagues[77] in a large autopsy study of 1206 cases with acute and chronic leukemia demonstrated liver to be involved by leukemias in 40% to 60% of patients, whereas the liver was involved in 16% to 43% of patients having non-Hodgkin lymphoma.

Primary lymphoma of the liver occurs rarely[78] and is defined as lymphoma without extrahepatic involvement and comprises less than 1% of all lymphomas. Non-Hodgkin lymphoma is the major subtype, particularly diffuse large B-cell lymphoma (DLBCL) being the most common, comprising 60% to 90% of cases.[78] Histologically nodules, of which 70% to 95% occur more frequently as single nodules than multiple or diffuse portal infiltration and sinusoidal infiltration occur in ~5% to 30% of cases.[78] Hodgkin lymphoma may involve the liver in ~15% of cases. Acute liver failure can occur due to ischemia secondary to compression of sinusoids by infiltrating lymphoma cells. Vanishing bile duct syndrome may be a paraneoplastic manifestation of Hodgkin lymphoma and may antedate the diagnosis and may be the cause of an elevated alkaline phosphatase level.[79]

Various characteristic patterns of liver involvement by hematologic disorders may be demonstrated. For example, DLBCL and Burkitt lymphoma occur as tumor nodules, whereas CLL and Hodgkin lymphoma typically occur as portal infiltrates (Fig. 6A). Marginal zone B-cell lymphoma typically present with lymphoepithelial lesions involving the bile ducts.[78] Features of bile duct obstruction may be noted, which is mainly due to compression of extrahepatic bile ducts by lymphadenopathy.

Fig. 6. Liver involvement in hematologic disorders. (*A*) Chronic lymphocytic leukemia (CLL) involving a portal tract. The portal tract is expanded by a monotonous population of lymphoid cells. Immunostains performed on this biopsy-confirmed CLL. H&E, original magnification x20. (*B*) Hemophagocytosis in a patient diagnosed to have CML. Sinusoids are mildly dilated and contain activated histiocytes. Some of these seem to have phagocytosed red blood cells (*arrows*). H&E, original magnification x40.

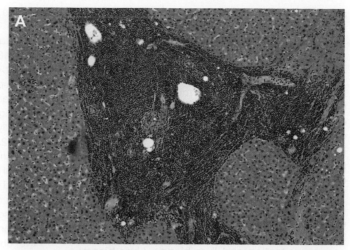

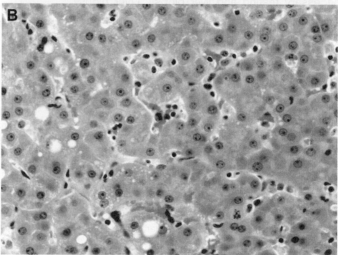

The differential diagnosis of the abnormal liver tests is broad and may also include DILI related to chemotherapy, steatohepatitis due to chemotherapy (CASH), reactivation of viral hepatitis, hematocrit (HCT) induction regimens using total body irradiation and high-dose chemotherapy (sinusoidal obstruction syndrome [SOS]) or HCT induction regimens (SOS) and its complications such as acute and chronic graft vs host disease (GVHD), and opportunistic infections.[75] Hemophagocytosis–lymphohistiocytosis (HLH) may be precipitated by certain viral infections or collagen vascular disease such as Still's disease or may be the first manifestation of hematologic malignancy (**Fig. 6**B). Primary HLH may be due to genetic susceptibility, whereas secondary hemophagocytic syndrome may be triggered by other conditions including hematological disorders. Lymphoma is the most common underlying

condition that may precipitate its development.[80] Aminotransferases 10 to 20 times the upper limit of normal and hyperbilirubinemia may be seen. HLH can lead to liver failure and typically has a poor prognosis. The diagnosis can be made using clinical criteria but liver biopsy is extremely helpful in establishing the diagnosis.

Thrombophilias such as occurring in myeloproliferative neoplasms (ie, polycythemia vera and myelofibrosis) may lead to portal mesenteric vein thrombosis or Budd–Chiari syndrome. In the setting of portal vein thrombosis, liver histology may show changes of NRH or OPV.[81] Portal biliopathy occurs when a long-standing portal vein thrombosis leads to cavernous transformation and a functional obstruction of the biliary system. The presence of significant extramedullary hematopoiesis on liver biopsy may be highly suggestive of an underlying hematologic disorder although lesser degrees may be nonspecific findings.[82]

SUMMARY

In the setting of systemic or multisystem disease, the liver is often involved either primarily by the disease process itself or secondarily with the patient developing abnormal liver chemistry tests. The latter scenario occurs commonly in hospitalized patients and may be multifactorial in nature, related to a combination of medications, infection, transfusions, hypotension, parenteral nutrition, or an exacerbation of underlying chronic liver disease. Understanding what systemic diseases the liver can be involved in is important to avoid unnecessary testing and liver biopsy. Liver biopsy under certain circumstances will help differential diagnose, whereas in others, it may show nonspecific liver histology. Discussion between the pathologist and clinician when both considering the performance of liver biopsy and of its performance is essential.

REFERENCES

1. Ch'ng CL, Morgan M, Hainsworth I, et al. Prospective study of liver dysfunction in pregnancy in Southwest Wales. Gut 2002;51(6):876–80.
2. Joshi D, James A, Quaglia A, et al. Liver disease in pregnancy. Lancet 2010;375(9714):594–605.
3. Goodwin TM. Hyperemesis gravidarum. Obstet Gynecol Clin North Am 2008;35(3):401–17, viii.
4. Hay JE. Liver disease in pregnancy. Hepatology 2008;47(3):1067–76.
5. Conchillo JM, Koek GH. Hyperemesis gravidarum and severe liver enzyme elevation. J Hepatol 2002; 37(1):162–3.
6. Rolfes DB, Ishak KG. Liver disease in pregnancy. Histopathology 1986;10(6):555–70.
7. Westbrook RH, Dusheiko G, Williamson C. Pregnancy and liver disease. J Hepatol 2016;64(4): 933–45.
8. Birkness-Gartman JE, Oshima K. Liver pathology in pregnancy. Pathol Int 2022;72(1):1–13.
9. Sasamori Y, Tanaka A, Ayabe T. Liver disease in pregnancy. Hepatol Res 2020;50(9):1015–23.
10. Pavlis T, Aloizos S, Aravosita P, et al. Diagnosis and surgical management of spontaneous hepatic rupture associated with HELLP syndrome. J Surg Educ 2009;66(3):163–7.
11. Wilson CH, Manas DM, French JJ. Laparoscopic liver resection for hepatic adenoma in pregnancy. J Clin Gastroenterol 2011;45(9):828–33.
12. Castro MA, Fassett MJ, Reynolds TB, et al. Reversible peripartum liver failure: a new perspective on the diagnosis, treatment, and cause of acute fatty liver of pregnancy, based on 28 consecutive cases. Am J Obstet Gynecol 1999;181(2):389–95.
13. Knight M, Nelson-Piercy C, Kurinczuk JJ, et al. A prospective national study of acute fatty liver of pregnancy in the UK. Gut 2008;57(7):951–6.
14. Cheung A, Flamm S. Hepatobiliary complications in critically ill patients. Clin Liver Dis 2019;23(2): 221–32.
15. Vanwijngaerden YM, Wauters J, Langouche L, et al. Critical illness evokes elevated circulating bile acids related to altered hepatic transporter and nuclear receptor expression. Hepatology 2011;54(5):1741–52.
16. Thomson SJ, Cowan ML, Johnston I, et al. 'Liver function tests' on the intensive care unit: a prospective, observational study. Intensive Care Med 2009; 35(8):1406–11.
17. Jenniskens M, Langouche L, Vanwijngaerden YM, et al. Cholestatic liver (dys)function during sepsis and other critical illnesses. Intensive Care Med 2016;42(1):16–27.
18. Strnad P, Tacke F, Koch A, et al. Liver - guardian, modifier and target of sepsis. Nat Rev Gastroenterol Hepatol 2017;14(1):55–66.
19. Huffman JL, Schenker S. Acute acalculous cholecystitis: a review. Clin Gastroenterol Hepatol 2010; 8(1):15–22.
20. Hirata K, Ikeda S, Honma T, et al. Sepsis and cholestasis: basic findings in the sinusoid and bile canaliculus. J Hepatobiliary Pancreat Surg 2001;8(1): 20–6.
21. Garofalo AM, Lorente-Ros M, Goncalvez G, et al. Histopathological changes of organ dysfunction in sepsis. Intensive Care Med Exp 2019;7(Suppl 1):45.
22. Chand N, Sanyal AJ. Sepsis-induced cholestasis. Hepatology 2007;45(1):230–41.
23. Zilkens C, Friese J, Köller M, et al. Hepatic failure after injury - a common pathogenesis with sclerosing cholangitis? Eur J Med Res 2008;13(7):309–13.
24. Engler S, Elsing C, Flechtenmacher C, et al. Progressive sclerosing cholangitis after septic shock: a new variant of vanishing bile duct disorders. Gut 2003;52(5):688–93.
25. Gelbmann CM, Rümmele P, Wimmer M, et al. Ischemic-like cholangiopathy with secondary sclerosing cholangitis in critically ill patients. Am J Gastroenterol 2007;102(6):1221–9.
26. Tapper EB, Sengupta N, Bonder A. The incidence and outcomes of ischemic hepatitis: a systematic review with meta-analysis. Am J Med 2015;128(12): 1314–21.
27. Henrion J, Schapira M, Luwaert R, et al. Hypoxic hepatitis: clinical and hemodynamic study in 142 consecutive cases. Medicine (Baltim) 2003;82(6): 392–406.

28. Trilok G, Qing YC, Li-Jun X. Hypoxic hepatitis: a challenging diagnosis. Hepatol Int 2012;6(4):663–9.

29. Louie CY, Pham MX, Daugherty TJ, et al. The liver in heart failure: a biopsy and explant series of the histopathologic and laboratory findings with a particular focus on pre-cardiac transplant evaluation. Mod Pathol 2015;28(7):932–43.

30. Wanless IR, Liu JJ, Butany J. Role of thrombosis in the pathogenesis of congestive hepatic fibrosis (cardiac cirrhosis). Hepatology 1995;21(5):1232–7.

31. Takeshita J, Grewal S, Langan SM, et al. Psoriasis and comorbid diseases: Epidemiology. J Am Acad Dermatol 2017;76(3):377–90.

32. Ruan Z, Lu T, Chen Y, et al. Association between psoriasis and nonalcoholic fatty liver disease among outpatient US adults. JAMA Dermatol 2022;158(7): 745–53.

33. van der Voort EA, Koehler EM, Dowlatshahi EA, et al. Psoriasis is independently associated with nonalcoholic fatty liver disease in patients 55 years old or older: results from a population-based study. J Am Acad Dermatol 2014;70(3):517–24.

34. Pakchotanon R, Ye JY, Cook RJ, et al. Liver abnormalities in patients with psoriatic arthritis. J Rheumatol 2020;47(6):847–53.

35. Gelfand JM, Wan J, Zhang H, et al. Risk of liver disease in patients with psoriasis, psoriatic arthritis, and rheumatoid arthritis receiving methotrexate: a population-based study. J Am Acad Dermatol 2021;84(6):1636–43.

36. Malnick S, Melzer E, Sokolowski N, et al. The involvement of the liver in systemic diseases. J Clin Gastroenterol 2008;42(1):69–80.

37. Shah AA, Wigley FM. Often forgotten manifestations of systemic sclerosis. Rheum Dis Clin North Am 2008;34(1):221–38, ix.

38. Chapman R, Fevery J, Kalloo A, et al. Diagnosis and management of primary sclerosing cholangitis. Hepatology 2010;51(2):660–78.

39. Colina F, Pinedo F, Solís JA, et al. Nodular regenerative hyperplasia of the liver in early histological stages of primary biliary cirrhosis. Gastroenterology 1992;102(4 Pt 1):1319–24.

40. Montaño-Loza AJ, Crispín-Acuña JC, Remes-Troche JM, et al. Abnormal hepatic biochemistries and clinical liver disease in patients with primary Sjögren's syndrome. Ann Hepatol 2007;6(3):150–5.

41. Lee SW, Kim BK, Park JY, et al. Clinical predictors of silent but substantial liver fibrosis in primary Sjogren's syndrome. Mod Rheumatol 2016;26(4): 576–82.

42. Fauter M, Rossi G, Drissi-Bakhkhat A, et al. Hepatic sarcoidosis with symptomatic portal hypertension: a report of 12 cases with review of the literature. Front Med 2022;9:995042.

43. Syed U, Alkhawam H, Bakhit M, et al. Hepatic sarcoidosis: pathogenesis, clinical context, and treatment options. Scand J Gastroenterol 2016; 51(9):1025–30.

44. Graf C, Arncken J, Lange CM, et al. Hepatic sarcoidosis: clinical characteristics and outcome. JHEP Rep 2021;3(6):100360.

45. Modaresi Esfeh J, Culver D, Plesec T, et al. Clinical presentation and protocol for management of hepatic sarcoidosis. Expet Rev Gastroenterol Hepatol 2015;9(3):349–58.

46. Tadros M, Forouhar F, Wu GY. Hepatic sarcoidosis. J Clin Transl Hepatol 2013;1(2):87–93.

47. Nakanuma Y, Kouda W, Harada K, et al. Hepatic sarcoidosis with vanishing bile duct syndrome, cirrhosis, and portal phlebosclerosis. Report of an autopsy case. J Clin Gastroenterol 2001;32(2): 181–4.

48. Fetzer DT, Rees MA, Dasyam AK, et al. Hepatic sarcoidosis in patients presenting with liver dysfunction: imaging appearance, pathological correlation and disease evolution. Eur Radiol 2016;26(9): 3129–37.

49. Baughman RP, Valeyre D, Korsten P, et al. ERS clinical practice guidelines on treatment of sarcoidosis. Eur Respir J 2021;58(6):2004079.

50. Fernandes SR, Singsen BH, Hoffman GS. Sarcoidosis and systemic vasculitis. Semin Arthritis Rheum 2000;30(1):33–46.

51. Karagiannidis A, Karavalaki M, Koulaouzidis A. Hepatic sarcoidosis. Ann Hepatol 2006;5(4):251–6.

52. Song J, Lleo A, Yang GX, et al. Common variable immunodeficiency and liver involvement. Clin Rev Allergy Immunol 2018;55(3):340–51.

53. Azizi G, Abolhassani H, Asgardoon MH, et al. Autoimmunity in common variable immunodeficiency: epidemiology, pathophysiology and management. Expet Rev Clin Immunol 2017;13(2):101–15.

54. Azizi G, Tavakol M, Rafiemanesh H, et al. Autoimmunity in a cohort of 471 patients with primary antibody deficiencies. Expet Rev Clin Immunol 2017;13(11): 1099–106.

55. Cunningham-Rundles C. The many faces of common variable immunodeficiency. Hematology Am Soc Hematol Educ Program 2012;2012:301–5.

56. Ward C, Lucas M, Piris J, et al. Abnormal liver function in common variable immunodeficiency disorders due to nodular regenerative hyperplasia. Clin Exp Immunol 2008;153(3):331–7.

57. Lima FMS, Toledo-Barros M, Alves VAF, et al. Liver disease accompanied by enteropathy in common variable immunodeficiency: common pathophysiological mechanisms. Front Immunol 2022;13:933463.

58. Crotty R, Taylor MS, Farmer JR, et al. Spectrum of hepatic manifestations of common variable immunodeficiency. Am J Surg Pathol 2020;44(5):617–25.

59. Globig AM, Strohmeier V, Surabattula R, et al. Evaluation of laboratory and sonographic parameters for detection of portal hypertension in patients with

common variable immunodeficiency. J Clin Immunol 2022;42(8):1626–37.

60. DiGiacomo DV, Shay JE, Crotty R, et al. Liver stiffness by transient elastography correlates with degree of portal hypertension in common variable immunodeficiency patients with nodular regenerative hyperplasia. Front Immunol 2022;13:864550.

61. Sakiani S, Kleiner DE, Heller T, et al. Hepatic manifestations of cystic fibrosis. Clin Liver Dis 2019;23(2):263–77.

62. Kamal N, Surana P, Koh C. Liver disease in patients with cystic fibrosis. Curr Opin Gastroenterol 2018;34(3):146–51.

63. Dana J, Debray D, Beaufrère A, et al. Cystic fibrosis-related liver disease: Clinical presentations, diagnostic and monitoring approaches in the era of CFTR modulator therapies. J Hepatol 2022;76(2):420–34.

64. Koh C, Sakiani S, Surana P, et al. Adult-onset cystic fibrosis liver disease: diagnosis and characterization of an underappreciated entity. Hepatology 2017;66(2):591–601.

65. Hillaire S, Cazals-Hatem D, Bruno O, et al. Liver transplantation in adult cystic fibrosis: clinical, imaging, and pathological evidence of obliterative portal venopathy. Liver Transplant 2017;23(10):1342–7.

66. Gaspar R, Branco CC, Macedo G. Liver manifestations and complications in inflammatory bowel disease: a review. World J Hepatol 2021;13(12):1956–67.

67. Mahfouz M, Martin P, Carrion AF. Hepatic complications of inflammatory bowel disease. Clin Liver Dis 2019;23(2):191–208.

68. Ricciuto A, Kamath BM, Griffiths AM. The IBD and PSC Phenotypes of PSC-IBD. Curr Gastroenterol Rep 2018;20(4):16.

69. Lindor KD, Kowdley KV, Harrison ME. ACG clinical guideline: primary sclerosing cholangitis. Am J Gastroenterol 2015;110(5):646–59, [quiz: 60].

70. Björnsson E, Chari ST, Smyrk TC, et al. Immunoglobulin G4 associated cholangitis: description of an emerging clinical entity based on review of the literature. Hepatology 2007;45(6):1547–54.

71. Losurdo G, Brescia IV, Lillo C, et al. Liver involvement in inflammatory bowel disease: what should the clinician know? World J Hepatol 2021;13(11):1534–51.

72. Shaye OA, Yadegari M, Abreu MT, et al. Hepatotoxicity of 6-mercaptopurine (6-MP) and Azathioprine (AZA) in adult IBD patients. Am J Gastroenterol 2007;102(11):2488–94.

73. Musumba CO. Review article: the association between nodular regenerative hyperplasia, inflammatory bowel disease and thiopurine therapy. Aliment Pharmacol Ther 2013;38(9):1025–37.

74. Ritaccio G, Stoleru G, Abutaleb A, et al. Nonalcoholic fatty liver disease is common in IBD patients however progression to hepatic fibrosis by noninvasive markers is rare. Dig Dis Sci 2021;66(9):3186–91.

75. Lettieri CJ, Berg BW. Clinical features of non-Hodgkins lymphoma presenting with acute liver failure: a report of five cases and review of published experience. Am J Gastroenterol 2003;98(7):1641–6.

76. Walz-Mattmüller R, Horny HP, Ruck P, et al. Incidence and pattern of liver involvement in haematological malignancies. Pathol Res Pract 1998;194(11):781–9.

77. Barcos M, Lane W, Gomez GA, et al. An autopsy study of 1206 acute and chronic leukemias (1958 to 1982). Cancer 1987;60(4):827–37.

78. Baumhoer D, Tzankov A, Dirnhofer S, et al. Patterns of liver infiltration in lymphoproliferative disease. Histopathology 2008;53(1):81–90.

79. Pass AK, McLin VA, Rushton JR, et al. Vanishing bile duct syndrome and Hodgkin disease: a case series and review of the literature. J Pediatr Hematol Oncol 2008;30(12):976–80.

80. Zhang L, Zhou J, Sokol L. Hereditary and acquired hemophagocytic lymphohistiocytosis. Cancer Control 2014;21(4):301–12.

81. Mayer JE, Schiano TD, Fiel MI, et al. An association of myeloproliferative neoplasms and obliterative portal venopathy. Dig Dis Sci 2014;59(7):1638–41.

82. Tremblay D, Saberi S, Mascarenhas J, et al. The quantification and significance of extramedullary hematopoiesis seen on liver biopsy specimens. Am J Clin Pathol 2022;158(2):277–82.

Liver Pathology Related to Onco-Therapeutic Agents

Paige H. Parrack, MD[a,b], Stephen D. Zucker, MD[b,c], Lei Zhao, MD, PhD[a,b],*

KEYWORDS

- Checkpoint inhibitor • Protein kinase inhibitor • Tyrosine kinase inhibitor • Monoclonal antibody
- Antibody–drug conjugate • Hormonal therapy • Liver • Hepatotoxicity

Key points

- Immune checkpoint-inhibitor (ICI) hepatitis most often presents histologically as histiocyte-rich, pan-lobular or zone 3 hepatitis with varying frequency of granulomas and endothelialitis. Biliary injury secondary to ICI toxicity has also been described and is often diagnostically challenging due to broader differential diagnosis.

- Hepatic injury associated with protein kinase inhibitors is not uncommon but severe liver toxicity is relatively rare. The injury pattern is diverse and less stereotypical based on limited studies. Hepatic necrosis is the predominant histologic finding reported by most studies.

- A subset of both kinase inhibitors and monoclonal antibodies can lead to reactivation of viral hepatitis.

- Sinusoidal obstruction syndrome and nodular regenerative hyperplasia have been reported in liver injury related to both conventional chemotherapeutic agents and newer oncotherapeutic options.

ABSTRACT

Oncotherapeutic agents can cause a wide range of liver injuries from elevated liver functions tests to fulminant liver failure. In this review, we emphasize a newer generation of drugs including immune checkpoint inhibitors, protein kinase inhibitors, monoclonal antibodies, and hormonal therapy. A few conventional chemotherapy agents are also discussed.

generations of oncotherapeutic agents, including protein kinase inhibitors, monoclonal antibodies, antibody–drug conjugates, hormonal therapies, and immune checkpoint inhibitors (ICIs), are playing increasing roles alongside traditional cytotoxic agents. These newer agents have markedly improved patient outcomes; however, they are not without toxicity, albeit generally less severe than traditional chemotherapy. This review will summarize our current understanding of liver injury caused by oncotherapeutic agents, with an emphasis on novel therapies.

OVERVIEW

ONCOTHERAPEUTIC AGENTS RELATED LIVER INJURY

The landscape of cancer therapeutics has evolved significantly in the last few decades. New

DISCUSSION

IMMUNE CHECKPOINT INHIBITORS

ICIs have had a significant positive impact on the cancer therapy landscape for over a decade. The

---

[a] Department of Pathology, Brigham and Women's Hospital, 75 Francis street, Boston, MA, 02115, USA;
[b] Harvard Medical School; [c] Department of Medicine, Brigham and Women's Hospital, 75 Francis street, Boston, MA, 02115, USA
* Corresponding author.
E-mail address: lzhao19@bwh.harvard.edu

Surgical Pathology 16 (2023) 499–518
https://doi.org/10.1016/j.path.2023.04.006
1875-9181/23/© 2023 Elsevier Inc. All rights reserved.

Abbreviations	
VEGF	vascular endothelial growth factor
CSF	colony stimulating factor
FLT3	FMS-like tyrosine kinase 3
PARP	poly (ADP-ribose) polymerase
PD-1	programmed cell death protein 1
PD-L1	programmed cell death ligand 1
LAG-3	lymphocyte-activation gene 3
CTLA-4	cytotoxic T-lymphocyte associated protein 4

FDA approved the first ICI, ipilimumab, a CTLA-4 inhibitor, for treatment of melanoma in 2011.[1] Subsequently, PD-1 inhibitors (pembrolizumab, nivolumab, cemiplimab), PD-L1 inhibitors (atezolizumab, avelumab, durvalumab), LAG-3 inhibitors (relatlimab) and additional CTLA-4 inhibitors (tremelimumab) were approved for an expanded tumor cohort.[2,3] With the rise of ICI therapy, there has been an emergence of new side effects, immune-related adverse events (irAEs), that present over a broad, systemic spectrum. Patients' symptomatology and organ involvement is dependent on the type and dose of ICI.

All ICIs have been associated with hepatotoxicity, with an incidence that varies from 0.7% to 16%.[4] The single agent with the highest risk of irAEs, including hepatitis, is ipilimumab.[2,5] Combination therapy with anti-CTLA and anti-PD-1 agents confers the greatest incidence and severity of irAEs, including hepatotoxicity,[5,6] and similar rates of ICI hepatitis recently have been described with combination relatlimab and nivolumab.[7] The median time to onset of ICI-induced hepatotoxicity ranges from 0.9 to 3.3 months.[2] Clinically, hepatic irAEs are classified using the Common Terminology Criteria for Adverse Events (CTCAE) grading system, which is defined by the height of elevation in liver enzymes.[8] Based on the patient's presentation and severity of disease, hepatic irAEs are treated by withholding ICIs and administering corticosteroids (with or without additional immunosuppressive agents). In the proper clinical circumstances, liver biopsy is often not necessary for diagnosis and treatment.[4,9]

There are 2 main patterns of ICI injury: hepatocellular and cholangitic. The hepatocellular form typically presents as elevations in alanine transaminase(ALT) and aspartate aminotransferase (AST). The primary histologic feature is lobular inflammation, with 84% of patients manifesting this finding in a review of 95 liver biopsy specimens from patients with high-grade ICI hepatitis.[9] In most of the cases inflammation is panlobular, some with zone 3 accentuation. The inflammation is predominantly lymphocytic and histiocytic, including prominent sinusoidal lymphohistiocytic aggregates, with scattered eosinophils and neutrophils and variable plasma cell density.[10–14] Lobular injury can be associated with centrilobular necrosis, either spotty or confluent.[15] Necrosis is generally associated with anti-CTLA therapy, although at least one case of centrilobular zonal necrosis with anti-PD-1 has been reported.[16] Central vein endothelialitis has been described in a minority of patients[10,15] and can rarely represent the only inflammatory manifestation. Isolated portal inflammation is uncommon, being more often associated with the cholangitic injury pattern (described below), but mild portal inflammation can be seen in cases with lobular predominant injury.[12] Histiocytic aggregates and granulomas are reasonably common in ICI-induced hepatitis.[9,12] Granulomas with epithelioid cells, fibrin ring granulomas, or fibrin deposits are primarily identified in patients receiving anti-CTLA monotherapy or combination therapy, and are less prominent in patients treated with anti-PD-1 or anti-PD-L1 monotherapy.[15] Fibrin ring granulomas are characterized by a central lipid vacuole surrounded by layers of histiocytes and fibrin. They have previously been described in infections (most commonly in *Coxiella burnetti*; Q fever), vascular injury, Hodgkin's disease, and allopurinol hypersensitivity. Everett and colleagues[17] described fibrin ring granulomas in association with steatosis in 2 patients treated with a combination of ipilimumab and nivolumab. Rare reports of sarcoid-like granulomas in the spleen, lung, and skin following ipilimumab therapy[18–20] suggest the possibility of a systemic granulomatous response. Scattered parenchymal microgranulomas were reported in one liver biopsy post-pembrolizumab infusion.[16] Rare cases manifesting with steatosis or a steatohepatitis-like injury pattern have also been described.[10,12,13]

A subset of ICI-induced liver injury manifests as a cholangitic injury pattern, most often reported with nivolumab therapy. Both large and small duct cholangiopathy has been described. On imaging, large duct disease is characterized by diffuse bile duct wall thickening and dilation mimicking primary sclerosing cholangitis or IgG4-related cholangitis.[21] Histologically, large duct disease manifests as fibrotic portal-tract enlargement and ductular reaction. Small duct disease is characterized by variable portal infiltrate. Cohen and colleagues[12] described portal inflammation predominantly composed of neutrophils around ducts and ductules, with a paucity of granulomas. Alternatively, a primary lymphocytic portal infiltrate, with variable eosinophils and plasma cells, has been reported.[22,23] Some cases of acute cholangitis have partial overlap with other patterns including focal lobular inflammation and endotheliitis.[10,12] Bile duct epithelial injury, lymphocytic ductitis/cholangiolitis, ductular reaction, and duct loss have all been reported in biopsies with cholangitic injury pattern.[11,23,24] As a cholangitic pattern is much less common than a hepatocellular injury pattern in ICI-induced liver injury, the former should be diagnosed with caution. Biliary obstruction or biliary tract compression by metastatic tumor, or other causes of cholestasis (eg, sepsis, parenteral nutrition, alternative medications) should be carefully considered.

Rare cases of veno-occlusive disease/sinusoidal obstruction syndrome, graft-versus-host disease after bone marrow transplantation, and allograft rejection after solid organ transplantation have also been reported in the setting of ICI therapy.[25-28]

The histologic patterns of ICI-induced hepatitis have broad morphologic mimics, including other drug-induced liver injury, acute viral hepatitis, and, rarely, hemophagocytic lymphohistiocytosis (in setting of sinusoidal lymphohistiocytic infiltrate). However, the primary diagnostic consideration in the setting of panlobular or zone 3 hepatitis is autoimmune hepatitis, which is characterized by a significant plasma cell infiltrate, necrosis, and severe interface hepatitis.[15] One study[11] directly comparing the histology of ICI-associated liver injury with autoimmune hepatitis found no difference in grading of portal inflammation or lobular injury; however, confluent necrosis and plasmacytosis were significantly more likely to be identified in autoimmune hepatitis. Significant histiocytic inflammation with aggregates

favor ICI-induced hepatitis. Ultimately, a thorough clinical history, including serologic studies for autoantibodies,[29] is helpful in establishing a diagnosis.

In summary, panlobular or zone 3 hepatitis with lymphohistiocytic aggregates (**Fig. 1**A and B) or "microgranulomas" are among the most common findings in ICI-induced liver injury. Granulomatous inflammation (**Fig. 1**C), is more likely to be associated with anti-CTLA therapy, whereas anti-PD-1/anti-PD-L1 therapies manifest milder lobular hepatitis or cholangiopathy (**Fig. 1** D). Along with careful clinical correlation, these histologic patterns can help distinguish ICI-hepatitis from morphologic mimics.

PROTEIN KINASE INHIBITORS

Kinases are enzymes that catalyze the phosphorylation of specific substrates to modulate function. Protein kinases can be classified based on the nature of the substrates, such as tyrosine kinase, serine/threonine kinase, or phosphatidylinositol 3-kinases (PI3K). Tyrosine kinase inhibitors (TKIs) have the broadest range of wild-type and/or mutant kinase targets, such as BCR-ABL, PDGFR, HER2, EGFR, ALK, ROS1, HER2, VEGF, BTK, MET, KIT, RET, and JAKs. Serine/threonine kinase inhibitors include antagonists for wild-type and/or mutant types of TOR, BRAF, MEK1/2, ROCK1/2, and CDK4/CDK6.[30] Dysregulated kinase activity, either through genetic or epigenetic alterations, is often a key driver of tumorigenesis and tumor progression. Kinase inhibition has been achieved with small molecule inhibitors, monoclonal antibodies, and antibody–drug conjugates.[30,31] Since the first tyrosine kinase inhibitor, imatinib, was approved for use in 2001, marked advances have been achieved in the use of kinase inhibitors for targeted cancer therapy. To date, 72 protein kinase inhibitors (PKIs) have been FDA-approved for clinical use.[32]

Although kinase inhibition represents an important breakthrough in cancer therapy, liver-related adverse effects are not uncommon, although still poorly defined, largely due to the rapid development of new drugs and a dearth of systematic studies. It is generally believed that PKI-related liver injury is predominantly idiosyncratic in nature. There appears to be no class effect for PKI-related liver injury, as patients may suffer toxicity from one drug but not another targeting the same kinase pathway, and no direct link between chemical structural properties and hepatotoxicity has been identified.[33,34] *In vitro* studies suggest that inhibition of glycolysis and mitochondrial injury via increased production of reactive oxygen species may be involved in tyrosine kinase inhibitor-

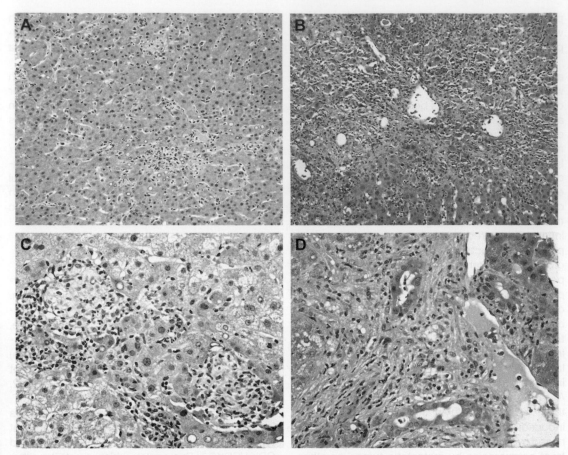

Fig. 1. *Immune checkpoint inhibitors.* (*A*) A 53-year-old woman with metastatic melanoma underwent treatment with concurrent nivolumab and ipilimumab and developed grade 4 liver function test (LFT) elevation. Biopsy showed lobular inflammation composed of a lobular lymphohistiocytic infiltrate. (*B*) A 62-year-old man with a history of metastatic melanoma and treatment with nivolumab monotherapy presented with right upper quadrant pain and elevated LFTs. Biopsy showed extensive centrilobular dropout and mixed inflammatory infiltrate. (*C*) A 69-year-old woman with metastatic melanoma, treated with ipilimumab and nivolumab, presented with elevated LFTs. Biopsy showed non-necrotizing granulomatous inflammation. (*D*) A 76-year-old man with a history of high-grade urothelial carcinoma, treated with pembrolizumab, presented with nausea, acholic stools, jaundice, and elevated LFTs. Biopsy showed periportal edema and bile duct injury with histiocytic and neutrophilic inflammation.

induced liver injury.[35,36] Because most kinase inhibitors are processed through the cytochrome P450 pathway, another hypothesis is that genetic variations or deficiencies in this pathway lead to toxicity from increased levels of reactive metabolites.[37,38] A proportion of patients manifest low level autoantibodies and other features of autoimmunity, and can respond to corticosteroid therapy.[39]

Low-grade hepatotoxicity characterized by transient elevations in ALT and AST is not uncommon; however, high-grade (grades 3–4) hepatotoxicity from PKI is relatively rare, ranging from 0% to 29% in clinical trials.[37] The histologic findings of PKI-related liver injury are not well described. The LiverTox database[40] is a

comprehensive summary of drug-induced liver injury, including liver toxicity related to PKIs documented in clinical trials and postmarketing practice. **Table 1** provides a summary of pathologic findings derived from individual entries in the Liver-Tox database, as well as from additional case reports. It is important to note that toxicity data skews toward agents that have been more widely available, with the most clinical experience. In addition, although case reports typically focus on severe hepatotoxicity, in our experience, most cases of PKI exhibit more mild histologic changes.

Hepatocellular necrosis is the most commonly reported histologic finding (see **Table 1**) and is generally more prominent than what is seen with ICI-related liver injury. The degree of necrosis

Table 1
Summary of drug-induced liver injury related to protein kinase inhibitors[a]

	Generic Name	Brand Name	Kinase Target	Approval	Likelihood Score[b]	Major Uses[c]	Liver Pathology Description
1	Abemaciclib	Verzenio	Cyclin-dependent kinase 4/6	2017	E[a]	Breast cancer	NA
2	Acalabrutinib	Calquence	Bruton kinase	2017	D	Mantle cell lymphoma	NA
3	Afatinib	Gilotrif	EGFR, HER2	2013	D	NSCLC	NA
4	Alectinib	Alecensa	ALK	2015	D	NSCLC	Severe acute hepatitis with ductular proliferation and bridging necrosis[72]
5	Alpelisib	Piqray	PIK3	2019	E[a]	Breast cancer, HR positive, HER2 negative	NA
6	Axitinib	Inlyta	VEGFR 1–3	2012	E[a]	Renal cell cancer	NA
7	Binimetinib	Mektovi	BRAF	2018	E[a]	Melanoma	NA
8	Bortezomib	Velcade	Proteasome	2003	C	Multiple myeloma, Mantle cell lymphoma	Multifocal and confluent hepatocellular necrosis[73], cholestatic pattern of injury with mild portal and lobular inflammation, hepatocellular and canalicular cholestasis[74]
9	Bosutinib	Bosulif	BCR-ABL, scr	2012	D	CML, resistant	NA
10	Brigatinib	Alunbrig	ALK	2017	E[a]	NSCLC	NA
11	Cabozantinib	Cometriq, Cabometyx	MET, VEGFR 2	2012	E[a]	Medullary thyroid cancer, renal cell cancer	NA
12	Carfilzomib	Kyprolis	Proteasome	2012	D	Multiple myeloma, resistant	NA
13	Ceritinib	Zykadia	ALK	2014	D	NSCLC	NA
14	Cobimetinib	Cotellic	MEK	2015	D	Melanoma	NA
15	Copanlisib	Aliqopa	PI3Kα/δ	2017	E[a]	Follicular lymphoma	NA
16	Crizotinib	Xalkori	ALK	2011	C	NSCLC	NA
17	Dabrafenib	Tafinlar	BRAF	2013	E[a]	Melanoma	NA
18	Dacomitinib	Vizimpro	HER1,2,3	2018	E[a]	NSCLC	NA

(continued on next page)

Table 1
(continued)

	Generic Name	Brand Name	Kinase Target	Approval	Likelihood Score[b]	Major Uses[c]	Liver Pathology Description
19	Dasatinib	Sprycel	BCR-ABL, src	2006	D	CML, resistant	Severe hepatitis with widespread necrosis and moderate-to-intense lymphocytic infiltrate[75]
20	Duvelisib	Copiktra	PI3K	2018	E[a]	CLL, small cell lymphoma	NA
21	Enasidenib	IDHIFA	Mutant IDH-2	2017	E[a]	AML	NA
22	Encorafenib	Braftovi	BRAF	2018	E[a]	Melanoma	
23	Entrectinib	Rozlytrek	NTRK, ROS1	2019	E[a]	NSCLC	NA
24	Erdafitinib	Balversa	FGFR	2019	E[a]	Urothelial cancer	NA
25	Erlotinib	Tarceva	EGFR, HER1	2004	B	NSCLC, pancreatic cancer	Submassive necrosis with marked portal inflammation[76]
26	Fedratinib	Inrebic	JAK-2	2019	D	Myelofibrosis	NA
27	Futibatinib	Lytgobi	FGFR	2022	E[a]	Cholangiocarcinoma	NA
28	Gefitinib	Iressa	EGFR	2009	B	NSCLC	Chronic hepatitis, necrosis, and fibrosis[77]
29	Gilteritinib	Xospata	FLT3	2018	E[a]	AML	NA
30	Glasdegib	Daurismo	Hedgehog	2018	E[a]	AML	NA
31	Ibrutinib	Imbruvica	Bruton kinase	2013	D	Mantle cell lymphoma, CLL	A mixed inflammatory cell infiltrate, lobular disarray, hepatocellular ballooning, focal canalicular cholestasis, and necrosis[78]; hepatocellular injury in the centrilobular region, caused by a mixed inflammatory cell infiltrate, and additional canalicular cholestasis[79]; acute hepatitis with mixed acute and chronic inflammation and hepatocellular cholestasis[80]

#	Generic	Brand	Target	Year	Category	Indication	Liver pathology
32	Idelalisib	Zydelig	PI3Kδ	2014	D	CLL, non-Hodgkin lymphoma	In CLL patients, increased infiltrate of CD8+ cytotoxic T cells in the liver[81]
33	Imatinib	Gleevec	BCR-ABL, c-Kit	2001	B	CML, GIST	Massive necrosis[82]; centrilobular necrosis, inflammation and interface hepatitis[83]; cirrhosis with superimposed submassive necrosis, inflammation and cholestasis, HBV reactivation[84], massive necrosis, subsequent cirrhosis[85]; massive necrosis in explant[86]
34	Infigratinib	Truseltiq	FGFR	2021	E[a]	Cholangiocarcinoma	NA
35	Ivosidenib	Tibsovo	Mutant IHD-1	2018	E[a]	AML	NA
36	Ixazomib	Ninlaro	26S Proteasome	2015	E[a]	Multiple myeloma	NA
37	Lapatinib	Tykerb	EGFR, HER2	2007	B	Breast cancer, HER2 positive	Bridging hepatic necrosis and portal inflammation with eosinophils[87]
38	Larotrectinib	Vitrakvi	NTRK	2018	E[a]	Solid tumors	NA
39	Lenvatinib	Lenvima	VEGFR 1–3, FGF 1–4, PDGF, c-Kit, RET	2015/2016/2018	D	Thyroid cancer/renal cell cancer/hepatocellular carcinoma	NA
40	Lorlatinib	Lorbrena	ALK	2018	E[a]	NSCLC	NA
41	Midostaurin	Rydapt	FLT3	2018	E[a]	AML	NA
42	Neratinib	Nerlynx	HER2	2017	E[a]	Breast cancer	NA
43	Nilotinib	Tasigna	BCR-ABL	2007	D	CML, resistant	Severe acute cholestatic hepatitis with bridging necrosis, mixed inflammatory portal infiltrate, cholestasis, and bile ductular proliferation[88]
44	Niraparib	Zejula	PARP	2017	E[a]	Ovarian cancer	NA

(continued on next page)

Table 1
(continued)

	Generic Name	Brand Name	Kinase Target	Approval	Likelihood Score[b]	Major Uses[c]	Liver Pathology Description
45	Olaparib	Lynparza	PARP	2014/2018	E	Ovarian cancer/advanced breast cancer	Submassive necrosis with lobular collapse, moderate-to-severe portal and lobular inflammation with predominantly lymphocytes, cholestasis, acute cholangitis with bile duct injury, and ductal proliferation[89]
46	Osimertinib	Tagrisso	EGFR	2015	E[a]	NSCLC, refractory	Steatohepatitis with macro- and microvesicular steatosis, ballooning degeneration of hepatocytes, periportal lymphocytic infiltration, and canalicular cholestasis[90]; disrupted lobular architecture with pericentral confluent necrosis, parenchymal collapse, mild mixed chronic inflammatory infiltrate predominantly composed of macrophages with rare lymphocytes and plasma cells[91]
47	Palbociclib	Ibrance	ER+, HER2	2015	C	Breast cancer, HER2 negative	"Pseudocirrhosis" due to sinusoidal obstruction syndrome[92]

48	Pazopanib	Votrient	VEGFR 1–3	2009	Renal cell cancer	C	Active cholestatic hepatitis with some degree of bile duct injury and ductular proliferation[93], acute cholestatic hepatitis with spotty necrosis, hepatocellular cholestasis, hepatocyte disarray, and sparse chronic inflammation[94]
49	Pemigatinib	Pemazyre	FGFR	2020	Cholangiocarcinoma, myeloid or lymphoid neoplasms	E[a]	NA
50	Pexidartinib	Turalio	CSF1, FLT3	2019	Tenosynovial giant cell tumor	B	Vanishing bile duct syndrome[95]
51	Ponatinib	Iclusig	BCR-ABL	2013	CML, ALL	E[a]	Mild steatohepatitis[96]
52	Regorafenib	Stivarga	VEGFR 1–3, PDGF	2012	Colorectal cancer, GIST	B	Histopathological liver lesions were different depending on the onset of hepatotoxicity (acute or subacute): acinar zone 3 necrosis in case of acute symptoms, and portal tract inflammation with portocentral bridging and fibrosis in the delayed presentation[97]; severe acute hepatitis in the form of necrotic strands associated with portal necrotic inflammatory activity and lymphocyte infiltration[98]
53	Ribociclib	Kisqali	Cyclin-dependent kinase 4/6	2017	Breast cancer	C	Acute fulminant toxic hepatitis with extensive confluent necrosis and intense inflammation[99], features of autoimmune hepatitis[100]
54	Rucaparib	Rubraca	PARP	2016	Ovarian cancer, advanced	E[a]	NA

(continued on next page)

Table 1
(continued)

	Generic Name	Brand Name	Kinase Target	Approval	Likelihood Score[b]	Major Uses[c]	Liver Pathology Description
55	Ruxolitinib	Jakafi	JAK-1/2	2011/2014/2019	C	Myelofibrosis/polycythemia vera/acute graft-vs-host disease, steroid resistant	Four cases: extramedullary hematopoiesis attributed to the underlying myelofibrosis in 3, and granulomatous hepatitis with loss of bile ducts attributed to drug-induced liver injury in 1, and features suggestive of occlusive portal veinopathy in 1[41]
56	Selumetinib	Koselugo	MEK 1/2	2020	E[a]	Neurofibromatosis type 1	NA
57	Sonidegib	Odomzo	Hedgehog	2015	E[a]	Basal cell skin cancer	NA
58	Sorafenib	Nexavar	VEGFR 1–3	2005/2007/2013	B	Renal cell cancer/hepatocellular cancer/thyroid cancer	Acute hepatitis with parenchymal necrosis, prominent canalicular cholestasis, and lymphocytic infiltrate[101]; intrahepatic cholestasis, parenchymal necrosis, inflammatory infiltrates, as well as significant fibrosis, indicating both acute and chronic liver injury[102]
59	Sunitinib	Sutent	PDGF, c-Kit	2006	B	CML, resistant; GIST, renal cell cancer	Diffuse, severe, centrilobular necrosis with moderate-to-severe steatosis and minimal invasion by the tumor (patient was also treated with acetaminophen)[103]
60	Talazoparib	Talzenna	PARP	2018	E[a]	Breast cancer	NA
61	Trametinib	Mekinist	MEK 1/2	2013	E[a]	Melanoma	NA
62	Vandetanib	Caprelsa	VEGFR 2	2011	E[a]	Medullary thyroid cancer	NA

63	Vemurafenib	Zelboraf	BRAF	2011	E[a]	Melanoma	Cholestatic injury with granulomas, eosinophils, and lymphocytic infiltration of the bile ducts[42]
64	Vismodegib	Erivedge	Hedgehog	2012	C	Basal cell skin cancer	Cholestasis with portal fibrosis[104]
65	Zanubrutinib	Brukinsa	BTK	2019	E[a]	Mantle cell lymphoma	Patchy necrosis, cholestasis, moderate-to-severe lobular and portal inflammation with lymphocytes, plasma cells, neutrophils, and eosinophils, suggestive of drug-induced liver injury[105]

[a] Drug information including name, kinase target, approval, likelihood score, and major use was derived from the LiverTox database.[40]
[b] Likelihood score indicates the likelihood of association with drug induced liver injury, based upon the known potential of the drug to cause such injury (definition provided by the LiverTox database).
[c] Abbreviations: ALL, acute lymphocytic leukemia; AML, acute myeloid leukemia; CLL, chronic lymphocytic leukemia; CML, chronic myelogenous leukemia; GIST, gastrointestinal stromal tumor; NSCLC, non-small cell lung cancer.

ranges from patchy to bridging, confluent, or massive. Centrilobular accentuation has been described in some reports. Centrilobular necrosis is also seen in acetaminophen toxicity; however, unlike acetaminophen toxicity, PKI-induced necrosis is often associated with inflammation, generally lymphocytic predominant or mixed. Granulomatous inflammation and histiocytic infiltrates appear to be uncommon.[41,42] Bile ductular reaction and cholestasis often coexist with necrosis. Bile duct injury, bile ductitis, and duct loss were noted only in single case reports with olaparib (PARP inhibitor), pazopanib (VEGF inhibitor), pexidartinib (CSF and FLT3 inhibitor), ruxolitinib (JAK inhibitor), and vemurafenib (BRAF inhibitor) (see **Table 1**). As with ICI hepatotoxicity, caution should be taken when attributing biliary injury to PKI use, as alternative causes, such as malignant biliary obstruction, should be considered. Hepatitis B reactivation in patients who are HBsAg positive has been documented in multiple reports (**Table 2**). It remains unclear if the reactivation is through kinase inhibition or other immune modulation. Although pseudocirrhosis also has been reported in at least one instance (see **Table 1**), a clear causal link with PKI use remains to be determined.

PKIs have been shown to potentiate the antineoplastic effect of ICI by priming and modulating the tumor microenvironment.[30] In patients receiving sequential or combination PKI and ICI therapy, it can be challenging to delineate the culprit agent responsible for liver injury. A recent analysis of adverse events associated with concurrent ICI and PKI therapy found that toxicity was more commonly related to PKI, although findings were not liver specific.[43] In a case series describing hepatitis associated with combination use of TKI and ICI, in one case where a liver biopsy was obtained, liver histology showed active lobular hepatitis with neutrophilic abscesses and lobular granulomas with central deposits of fibrin.[44]

In summary, hepatic necrosis with variable inflammation appears to be the predominant injury pattern in PKI-related hepatotoxicity. Additionally, cholestasis and ductular reaction also can be present, whereas biliary injury is less common. Hepatitis B reactivation also has been described. **Figs. 2** and **3** highlight histologic changes identified after therapy with PKIs.

ADDITIONAL MONOCLONAL ANTIBODIES AND ANTIBODY–DRUG CONJUGATES

Rituximab, a monoclonal antibody targeting CD20, was approved for treatment of B-cell non-Hodgkin lymphoma in 1997[45] and is still being used today for a broader spectrum of diseases, including autoimmune conditions. Instances of serum aminotransferase elevations and acute liver injury have been reported but, overall, are quite uncommon in adults. A case report of an adult patient with rituximab-associated acute liver injury and an autoimmune hepatitis-like presentation described histologic findings of perivenular and lobular inflammation composed of lymphocytes and plasma cells.[46] Although high-grade hepatitis has been described in pediatric patients treated with rituximab in combination with other chemotherapeutic agents, it is unclear if liver injury is directly attributable to rituximab.[47] With regard to the liver, the most significant adverse effect of rituximab is reactivation of hepatitis B, which can lead to acute hepatitis and liver failure. Reactivation of other viruses, including adenovirus[48] and hepatitis C,[49] has been described. Other monoclonal antibodies (such as anti-TNF therapies infliximab and adalimumab) have also led to reactivation of hepatitis B.[50]

Table 2
Reports of HBV reactivation with protein kinase inhibitor therapy

	Generic Name	Brand Name	Kinase Target	References
1	Acalabrutinib	Calquence	Bruton kinase	Markham & Dhillon,[106] 2018
2	Carfilzomib	Kyprolis	Proteasome	Muchtar et al,[107] 2016
3	Dasatinib	Sprycel	BCR-ABL, src	Ando et al,[108] 2015
4	Ibrutinib	Imbruvica	Bruton kinase	Herishanu et al,[109] 2017
5	Imatinib	Gleevec	BCR-ABL, c-Kit	Kang et al,[84] 2009; Walker et al,[110] 2014
6	Nilotinib	Tasigna	BCR-ABL	Uhm et al,[111] 2018
7	Osimertinib	Tagrisso	EGFR	Kang & Meng,[112] 2022
8	Ruxolitinib	Jakafi	JAK-1/2	Sjoblom et al,[113] 2022

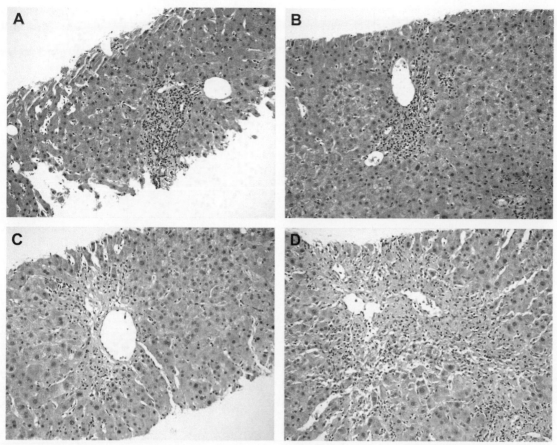

Fig. 2. Kinase inhibitors. (A, B) An 83-year-old man with metastatic clear cell renal cell carcinoma was undergoing treatment with cabozantinib. His clinical course was complicated by transaminitis, and biopsy showed multifocal mild portal inflammation primarily composed of lymphocytes with few admixed plasma cells. *(C, D)* In a separate case, a patient was enrolled in a clinical trial for an experimental kinase inhibitor and developed centrilobular hepatitis.

Trastuzumab is a monoclonal antibody targeting the HER2 receptor. As a single agent, trastuzumab has been tolerated very well with rare cases of serum aminotransferase elevation. Liver biopsies are not usually required since the enzyme elevations are self-limited, but one biopsy revealed mild portal and interface inflammation.[51] Unlike trastuzumab, ado-trastuzumab emtansine (T-DM1), in which trastuzumab is conjugated with emtansine, a cytotoxic anti-microtubule drug,[52] frequently has been associated with liver injury. In a clinical trial of 361 patients, 4.4% and 6.6% developed grade 3 to 4 elevations in AST and ALT, respectively.[53] A cholestatic injury pattern[54] also has rarely been reported. A small cohort of case reports have identified non-cirrhotic portal hypertension due to nodular regenerative hyperplasia (NRH) after T-DM1 therapy (**Fig. 4**). Liver biopsies demonstrated sinusoidal dilation with atrophic foci and alternating thickened and thinned hepatic plates, without inflammation or fibrosis.[55,56] Additionally, there have been case reports of sinusoidal obstruction syndrome developing after several years of treatment with T-DM1. Liver histology is described as showing sinusoidal dilatation and congestion with collagen fiber growth.[57,58]

HORMONAL THERAPY

Tamoxifen is a selective estrogen receptor modulator primarily used for the treatment of breast cancer. Tamoxifen has been associated with hepatotoxicity primarily consisting of steatosis and acute steatohepatitis, with rare cases of progression to cirrhosis.[59] Peliosis hepatis has also been associated with long-term anti-estrogen treatment.[60] With discontinuation of the medication, liver enzymes generally improve. Of note, steatohepatitis also has been reported with other chemotherapeutic agents, including

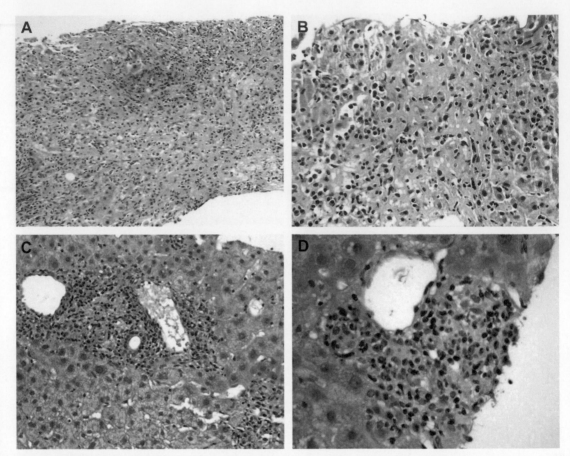

Fig. 3. Additional kinase inhibitors. (*A, B*) A 66-year-old woman with non-small cell lung carcinoma, treated with erlotinib, presents with painless jaundice, elevated liver function tests, elevated bilirubin, and synthetic dysfunction. Biopsy showed submassive necrosis with prominent plasmocytic infiltrates. (*C, D*) A 62-year-old man with metastatic clear cell renal cell carcinoma, treated with pazopanib, presented with grade 3 AST and ALT elevations. Biopsy showed a mixed portal inflammatory infiltrate, cholangiolitis, and portal venulitis (Images for Parts C, D courtesy of Dr Leona Doyle).

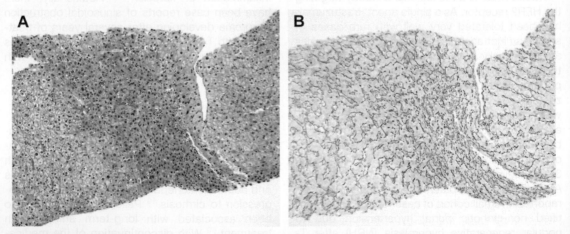

Fig. 4. Ado-trastuzumab emtansine. A 36-year-old woman with invasive ductal carcinoma of the breast was treated with ado-trastuzumab emtansine after bilateral mastectomy. She developed increasing LFTs, and a biopsy showed nodular regenerative hyperplasia characterized by alternating hepatocyte plate hypertrophy and atrophy (*A*), which is best highlighted by reticulin staining (*B*).

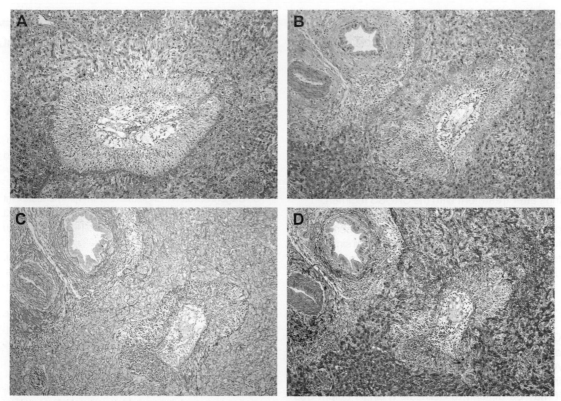

Fig. 5. CROSS regimen effects. A 62-year-old man with lower esophageal/gastro-esophageal junction adenocarcinoma and metastases had neoadjuvant treatment with carboplatin, paclitaxel, and radiation therapy. Multifocal liver hyperpigmentation was noted during the resection; a liver wedge showed sinusoidal dilation, hepatocyte cord atrophy, and venous injury with subepithelial edema (*A, B*). Reticulin (*C*) and trichrome (*D*) stains highlight vein wall fibrosis, suggestive of a sinusoidal obstruction/veno-occlusive injury pattern.

immunotherapy, 5-fluorouracil, irinotecan, methotrexate, and L-asparginase.[61]

CONVENTIONAL ONCOTHERAPEUTIC AGENTS USED FOR GASTROINTESTINAL PRIMARIES

Colorectal Cancer: FOLFOX and FOLFIRI

FOLFOX and FOLFIRI are standard chemotherapy regimens for advanced-stage and metastatic colorectal cancer. FOLFOX includes leucovorin calcium, 5-fluorouracil (5-FU), and oxaliplatin, whereas leucovorin calcium, 5-FU, and irinotecan comprise FOLFIRI. A significant but rare side effect with 5-FU is hyperammonemic encephalopathy where patients manifest high plasma ammonia levels with only mild-to-moderate aminotransferase elevations.[62] The development of hepatic steatosis is estimated to occur in up to 47% of patients treated with 5-FU,[63] but steatohepatitis is uncommon. In contrast, steatohepatitis is more often identified with irinotecan therapy. A unique complication of intra-arterial 5-FU administered for treatment of liver metastases is secondary sclerosing cholangitis.[64] The notable side effect of oxaliplatin is sinusoidal injury, which has been estimated to occur in 19% to 52% of patients.[65] Oxaliplatin-related sinusoid injury may present as a spectrum of sinusoidal dilatation, sinusoidal obstruction syndrome, or NRH. Sinusoidal obstruction syndrome (SOS) has been characterized grossly as blue surface coloration of the liver due to underlying centrilobular congested and distended sinusoids.[63] SOS lesions are typically located in the subcapsular region with disruption of the sinusoidal wall, perisinusoidal hemorrhage, and rare hepatocellular necrosis.[66] NRH is the most severe type of injury with diffuse small regenerative nodules with peripherally atrophic hepatocytes or dilated sinusoids.[66]

Esophageal and Gastric Primaries: CROSS Regimen and FLOT Regimen

The Chemoradiotherapy for Esophageal Cancer followed by Surgery Study (CROSS) trial marked a significant change in treatment strategy for esophageal or esophagogastric junction primaries by incorporating neoadjuvant chemoradiotherapy. The neoadjuvant regimen includes carboplatin, pacli-taxel, and concurrent 41.4 Gy radiotherapy.[67] A small subset of patients who receive high-dose car-boplatin develop transient hyperbilirubinemia and elevated aminotransferase levels[68]; however, acute or severe liver injury is rare. Similar to carboplatin, the most common manifestation of paclitaxel-induced liver injury is serum aminotransferase eleva-tions,[69] although grade 3 or higher liver injury is infre-quent. One case report described a patient who developed fatal acute hepatic necrosis after a com-bined dose of paclitaxel and trastuzumab.[70] A case from our institution (Fig. 5) highlights histologic find-ings after treatment with the CROSS regimen.

The FLOT regimen (fluorouracil, leucovorin, oxali-platin, and docetaxel) is a common treatment option for gastric primaries. Docetaxel causes a similar liver test abnormalities to paclitaxel, with rare reports of cholestatic or mixed patterns of liver injury.[71]

SUMMARY

Oncotherapeutic agent-related liver injury is a feared adverse effect that often impedes cancer treatment. Although some agents produce a stereotypical injury pattern, when multiple agents are combined, it may be difficult to delineate a single culprit due to overlapping histologic features. Even in these scenarios, liver histology can aid in clinical manage-ment, by excluding alternative causes of liver injury (eg, tumor recurrence, infection, vascular obstruc-tion, biliary obstruction, graft vs. host disease, un-derlying chronic liver diseases).

CLINICS CARE POINTS

- Liver injury mediated by immune-checkpoint inhibitors or protein kinase inhibitors has broad clinical and histologic presentations. Close correlation with a patient's history is essential for distinguishing drug-induced hepatitis from morphologic mimics.

- Onco-therapeutic agents have overlapping patterns of injury; however, some patterns may favor different therapies. In ICI-induced toxicity, the predominant injury pattern is panlobular/zone 3 hepatitis with lymphohis-tiocytic aggregates, and in PKI-related hepa-totoxicity, hepatic necrosis with variable inflammation has been reported most often.

- Liver biopsy can facilitate clinical management by narrowing differential diagnosis and excluding alternative causes of liver injury.

DISCLOSURE

The authors do not have any conflicts of interest related to this article.

REFERENCES

1. Ledford H. Melanoma drug wins US approval. Na-ture 2011;471(7340):561.
2. Suzman DL, Pelosof L, Rosenberg A, et al. Hepato-toxicity of immune checkpoint inhibitors: An evolving picture of risk associated with a vital class of immu-notherapy agents. Liver Int 2018;38(6):976–87.
3. Bagchi S, Yuan R, Engleman EG. Immune Checkpoint Inhibitors for the Treatment of Cancer: Clinical Impact and Mechanisms of Response and Resistance. Annu Rev Pathol Mech Dis 2021;16(1):223–49.
4. Peeraphatdit TB, Wang J, Odenwald MA, et al. Hepatotoxicity From Immune Checkpoint Inhibitors: A Systematic Review and Management Recom-mendation. Hepatology 2020;72(1):315–29.
5. Martins F, Sofiya L, Sykiotis GP, et al. Adverse ef-fects of immune-checkpoint inhibitors: epidemi-ology, management and surveillance. Nat Rev Clin Oncol 2019;16(9):563–80.
6. Wolchok JD, Chiarion-Sileni V, Gonzalez R, et al. Overall Survival with Combined Nivolumab and Ipi-limumab in Advanced Melanoma. N Engl J Med 2017;377(14):1345–56.
7. Amaria RN, Postow M, Burton EM, et al. Neoadju-vant relatlimab and nivolumab in resectable mela-noma. Nature 2022;611(7934):155–60.
8. Reynolds K, Thomas M, Dougan M. Diagnosis and Management of Hepatitis in Patients on Checkpoint Blockade. Oncol 2018;23(9):991–7.
9. Li M, Sack JS, Bell P, et al. Utility of Liver Biopsy in Diagnosis and Management of High-grade Immune Checkpoint Inhibitor Hepatitis in Patients With Can-cer. JAMA Oncol 2021;7(11):1711–4.
10. Johncilla M, Misdraji J, Pratt DS, et al. Ipilimumab-associated Hepatitis: Clinicopathologic Character-ization in a Series of 11 Cases. Am J Surg Pathol 2015;39(8):1075–84.
11. Zen Y, Yeh MM. Hepatotoxicity of immune check-point inhibitors: a histology study of seven cases in comparison with autoimmune hepatitis and idio-syncratic drug-induced liver injury. Mod Pathol 2018;31(6):965–73.
12. Cohen JV, Dougan M, Zubiri L, et al. Immune checkpoint inhibitor related liver injury: Histopatho-logic pattern does not correlate with response to immune suppression. Mod Pathol Off J U S Can Acad Pathol Inc 2021;34(2):426–37.
13. Simonelli M, Di Tommaso L, Baretti M, et al. Patho-logical characterization of nivolumab-related liver injury in a patient with glioblastoma. Immuno-therapy 2016;8(12):1363–9.

14. Kleiner DE, Berman D. Pathologic Changes in Ipilimumab-related Hepatitis in Patients with Metastatic Melanoma. Dig Dis Sci 2012;57(8). 2233–40.

15. De Martin E, Michot JM, Papouin B, et al. Characterization of liver injury induced by cancer immunotherapy using immune checkpoint inhibitors. J Hepatol 2018;68(6):1181–90.

16. Aivazian K, Long GV, Sinclair EC, et al. Histopathology of pembrolizumab-induced hepatitis: a case report. Pathology 2017;49(7):789–92.

17. Everett J, Srivastava A, Misdraji J. Fibrin Ring Granulomas in Checkpoint Inhibitor-induced Hepatitis. Am J Surg Pathol 2017;41(1):134–7.

18. Andersen R, Nørgaard P, Al-Jailawi MKM, et al. Late development of splenic sarcoidosis-like lesions in a patient with metastatic melanoma and long-lasting clinical response to ipilimumab. OncoImmunology 2014;3(8):e954506.

19. Reule RB, North JP. Cutaneous and pulmonary sarcoidosis-like reaction associated with ipilimumab. J Am Acad Dermatol 2013;69(5):e272–3.

20. Berthod G, Lazor R, Letovanec I, et al. Pulmonary Sarcoid-Like Granulomatosis Induced by Ipilimumab. J Clin Oncol 2012;30(17):e156–9.

21. Kawakami H, Tanizaki J, Tanaka K, et al. Imaging and clinicopathological features of nivolumab-related cholangitis in patients with non-small cell lung cancer. Invest New Drugs 2017;35(4):529–36.

22. Zen Y, Chen YY, Jong YM, et al. Immune-related adverse reactions in the hepatobiliary system: second-generation check-point inhibitors highlight diverse histological changes. Histopathology 2020;76(3):470–80.

23. Gelsomino F, Vitale G, D'Errico A, et al. Nivolumab-induced cholangitic liver disease: a novel form of serious liver injury. Ann Oncol 2017;28(3):671–2.

24. Doherty GJ, Duckworth AM, Davies SE, et al. Severe steroid-resistant anti-PD1 T-cell checkpoint inhibitor-induced hepatotoxicity driven by biliary injury. ESMO Open 2017;2(4):e000268.

25. Straub BK, Ridder DA, Schad A, et al. [Liver injury induced by immune checkpoint inhibitor-therapy : Example of an immune-mediated drug side effect]. For Pathol 2018;39(6):556–62.

26. Merryman RW, Kim HT, Zinzani PL, et al. Safety and efficacy of allogeneic hematopoietic stem cell transplant after PD-1 blockade in relapsed/refractory lymphoma. Blood 2017;129(10):1380–8.

27. Gassmann D, Weiler S, Mertens JC, et al. Liver Allograft Failure After Nivolumab Treatment-A Case Report With Systematic Literature Research. Transplant Direct 2018;4(8):e376.

28. Dada R, Usman B. Allogeneic hematopoietic stem cell transplantation in r/r Hodgkin lymphoma after treatment with checkpoint inhibitors: Feasibility and safety. Eur J Haematol 2019;102(2):150–6.

29. Karamchandani DM, Chetty R. Immune checkpoint inhibitor-induced gastrointestinal and hepatic injury. pathologists' perspective. J Clin Pathol 2018;71(8):665–71.

30. Cohen P, Cross D, Jänne PA. Kinase drug discovery 20 years after imatinib: progress and future directions. Nat Rev Drug Discov 2021; 20(7):551–69.

31. Lee PY, Yeoh Y, Low TY. A recent update on small-molecule kinase inhibitors for targeted cancer therapy and their therapeutic insights from mass spectrometry-based proteomic analysis. FEBS J 2022. https://doi.org/10.1111/febs.16442.

32. Roskoski R. Properties of FDA-approved small molecule protein kinase inhibitors: A 2023 update. Pharmacol Res 2023;187:106552.

33. Jiang H, Jin Y, Yan H, et al. Hepatotoxicity of FDA-approved small molecule kinase inhibitors. Expert Opin Drug Saf 2021;20(3):335–48.

34. Shah RR, Morganroth J, Shah DR. Hepatotoxicity of Tyrosine Kinase Inhibitors: Clinical and Regulatory Perspectives. Drug Saf 2013;36(7):491–503.

35. Paech F, Bouitbir J, Krähenbühl S. Hepatocellular Toxicity Associated with Tyrosine Kinase Inhibitors: Mitochondrial Damage and Inhibition of Glycolysis. Front Pharmacol 2017;8:367.

36. Mingard C, Paech F, Bouitbir J, et al. Mechanisms of toxicity associated with six tyrosine kinase inhibitors in human hepatocyte cell lines. J Appl Toxicol 2018;38(3):418–31.

37. Houron C, Danielou M, Mir O, et al. Multikinase inhibitor-induced liver injury in patients with cancer: A review for clinicians. Crit Rev Oncol Hematol 2021;157:103127.

38. Shi Q, Yang X, Ren L, et al. Recent advances in understanding the hepatotoxicity associated with protein kinase inhibitors. Expert Opin Drug Metab Toxicol 2020;16(3):217–26.

39. Sobri EA, Zahrani Z, Zevallos E, et al. Imatinib-induced immune hepatitis: Case report and literature review. Hematology 2007;12(1):49–53.

40. LiverTox: Clinical and Research information on drug-induced liver injury. National Institute of Diabetes and Digestive and Kidney Diseases; 2012. Available at: http://www.ncbi.nlm.nih.gov/books/NBK547852/. Accessed February 15, 2023.

41. Tremblay D, Putra J, Vogel A, et al. The Implications of Liver Biopsy Results in Patients with Myeloproliferative Neoplasms Being Treated with Ruxolitinib. Case Rep Hematol 2019;2019:3294046.

42. Spengler EK, Kleiner DE, Fontana RJ. Vemurafenib-induced Granulomatous hepatitis. Hepatol Baltim Md 2017;65(2):745–8.

43. Gao L, Yang X, Yi C, et al. Adverse Events of Concurrent Immune Checkpoint Inhibitors and Antiangiogenic Agents: A Systematic Review. Front Pharmacol 2019;10:1173.

44. Carretero-González A, Salamanca Santamaría J, Castellano D, et al. Three case reports: Temporal association between tyrosine-kinase inhibitor-induced hepatitis and immune checkpoint inhibitors in renal cell carcinoma. Medicine (Baltim) 2019;98(47):e18098.

45. Grillo-Lopez A, White C, Dallaire B, et al. Rituximab The First Monoclonal Antibody Approved for the Treatment of Lymphoma. Curr Pharm Biotechnol 2000;1(1):1–9.

46. Galiatsatos P, Assouline S, Gologan A, et al. Rituximab-induced autoimmune hepatitis: A case study and literature review. Can Liver J 2020;3(4):381–6.

47. Rituxan prescribing information - Genentech. Available at: https://www.gene.com/download/pdf/rituxan_prescribing.pdf. (Accessed: 31st October, 2022). https://www.gene.com/download/pdf/rituxan_prescribing.pdf. Accessed November 1, 2022.

48. Iyer A, Mathur R, Deepak BV, et al. Fatal Adenoviral Hepatitis After Rituximab Therapy. Arch Pathol Lab Med 2006;130(10):1557–60.

49. Torres HA, Hosry J, Mahale P, et al. Hepatitis C virus reactivation in patients receiving cancer treatment: a prospective observational study. Hepatol Baltim Md 2018;67(1):36–47.

50. El Jamaly H, Eslick GD, Weltman M. Meta-analysis: hepatitis B reactivation in patients receiving biological therapy. Aliment Pharmacol Ther 2022;56(7):1104–18.

51. Srinivasan S, Parsa V, Liu CY, et al. Trastuzumab-induced hepatotoxicity. Ann Pharmacother 2008;42(10):1497–501.

52. Barok M, Joensuu H, Isola J. Trastuzumab emtansine: mechanisms of action and drug resistance. Breast Cancer Res 2014;16(2):209.

53. Perez EA, Barrios C, Eiermann W, et al. Trastuzumab Emtansine With or Without Pertuzumab Versus Trastuzumab Plus Taxane for Human Epidermal Growth Factor Receptor 2-Positive, Advanced Breast Cancer: Primary Results From the Phase III MARIANNE Study. J Clin Oncol Off J Am Soc Clin Oncol 2017;35(2):141–8.

54. Garrido I, Magalhães A, Lopes J, et al. Trastuzumab Emtansine-Induced Nodular Regenerative Hyperplasia: Is Dose Reduction Enough as a Preventable Measure? Dig Dis 2022;40(6):787–92.

55. Force J, Saxena R, Schneider BP, et al. Nodular Regenerative Hyperplasia After Treatment With Trastuzumab Emtansine. J Clin Oncol 2016;34(3):e9–12.

56. Lepelley M, Allouchery M, Long J, et al. Nodular Regenerative Hyperplasia Induced by Trastuzumab Emtansine: Role of Emtansine? Ann Hepatol 2018;17(6):1067–71.

57. Fujii Y, Doi M, Tsukiyama N, et al. Sinusoidal obstruction syndrome post-treatment with trastuzumab emtansine (T-DM1) in advanced breast cancer. Int Cancer Conf J 2019;9(1):18–23.

58. Duret-Aupy N, Lagarce L, Blouet A, et al. Liver sinusoidal obstruction syndrome associated with trastuzumab emtansine treatment for breast cancer. Therapie 2019;74(6):675–7.

59. Saphner T, Triest-Robertson S, Li H, et al. The association of nonalcoholic steatohepatitis and tamoxifen in patients with breast cancer. Cancer 2009;115(14):3189–95.

60. van Erpecum KJ, Janssens AR, Kreuning J, et al. Generalized peliosis hepatis and cirrhosis after long-term use of oral contraceptives. Am J Gastroenterol 1988;83(5):572–5.

61. Meunier L, Larrey D. Chemotherapy-associated steatohepatitis. Ann Hepatol 2020;19(6):597–601.

62. Advani PP, Fakih MG. 5-FU-induced Hyperammonemic Encephalopathy in a Case of Metastatic Rectal Adenocarcinoid Successfully Rechallenged with the Fluoropyrimidine Analog, Capecitabine. Anticancer Res 2011;31(1):335–8.

63. Zorzi D, Laurent A, Pawlik TM, et al. Chemotherapy-associated hepatotoxicity and surgery for colorectal liver metastases. Br J Surg 2007;94(3):274–86.

64. Hohn D, Melnick J, Stagg R, et al. Biliary sclerosis in patients receiving hepatic arterial infusions of floxuridine. J Clin Oncol 1985;3(1):98–102.

65. Chun YS, Laurent A, Maru D, et al. Management of chemotherapy-associated hepatotoxicity in colorectal liver metastases. Lancet Oncol 2009;10(3):278–86.

66. Rubbia-Brandt L, Lauwers GY, Wang H, et al. Sinusoidal obstruction syndrome and nodular regenerative hyperplasia are frequent oxaliplatin-associated liver lesions and partially prevented by bevacizumab in patients with hepatic colorectal metastasis. Histopathology 2010;56(4):430–9.

67. van Hagen P, Hulshof MCCM, van Lanschot JJB, et al. Preoperative Chemoradiotherapy for Esophageal or Junctional Cancer. N Engl J Med 2012;366(22):2074–84.

68. Canetta R, Bragman K, Smaldone L, et al. Carboplatin: current status and future prospects. Cancer Treat Rev 1988;15:17–32.

69. Kümmel S, Paepke S, Huober J, et al. Randomised, open-label, phase II study comparing the efficacy and the safety of cabazitaxel versus weekly paclitaxel given as neoadjuvant treatment in patients with operable triple-negative or luminal B/HER2-negative breast cancer (GENEVIEVE). Eur J Cancer 2017;84:1–8.

70. Mandaliya H, Baghi P, Prawira A, et al. A Rare Case of Paclitaxel and/or Trastuzumab Induced Acute Hepatic Necrosis. Case Rep Oncol Med 2015;2015:825603.

71. Wang Z, Liang X, Yu J, et al. Non-genetic risk factors and predicting efficacy for docetaxel–drug-induced liver injury among metastatic breast cancer patients. J Gastroenterol Hepatol 2012;27(8):1348–52.

72. Zhu VW, Lu Y, Ou SHI. Severe Acute Hepatitis in a Patient Receiving Alectinib for ALK-Positive Non–Small-Cell Lung Cancer: Histologic Analysis. Clin Lung Cancer 2019;20(1):e77–80.

73. Kim Y, Kim KY, Lee SH, et al. A Case of Drug-Induced Hepatitis due to Bortezomib in Multiple Myeloma. Immune Netw 2012;12(3):126–8.

74. Jain A, Malhotra P, Suri V, et al. Cholestasis in a Patient of Multiple Myeloma: A Rare Occurrence of Bortezomib Induced Liver Injury. Indian J Hematol Blood Transfus 2016;32(Suppl 1):181–3.

75. Clément M, Cervoni JP, Renosi F, et al. Acute fulminant hepatitis related to the use of dasatinib: First case report. Clin Res Hepatol Gastroenterol 2022; 46(8):102004.

76. Liu W, Makrauer FL, Qamar AA, et al. Fulminant Hepatic Failure Secondary to Erlotinib. Clin Gastroenterol Hepatol 2007;5(8):917–20.

77. Ho C, Davis J, Anderson F, et al. Side effects related to cancer treatment: CASE 1. Hepatitis following treatment with gefitinib. J Clin Oncol Off J Am Soc Clin Oncol 2005;23(33):8531–3.

78. Tafesh ZH, Coleman M, Fulmer C, et al. Severe Hepatotoxicity due to Ibrutinib with a Review of Published Cases. Case Rep Gastroenterol 2019; 13(2):357–63.

79. Nandikolla AG, Derman O, Nautsch D, et al. Ibrutinib-induced severe liver injury. Clin Case Rep 2017;5(6):735–8.

80. Kahn A, Horsley-Silva JL, Lam-Himlin DM, et al. Ibrutinib-induced acute liver failure. Leuk Lymphoma 2018;59(2):512–4.

81. Lampson BL, Kasar SN, Matos TR, et al. Idelalisib given front-line for treatment of chronic lymphocytic leukemia causes frequent immune-mediated hepatotoxicity. Blood 2016;128(2): 195–203.

82. Lin NU, Sarantopoulos S, Stone JR, et al. Fatal hepatic necrosis following imatinib mesylate therapy. Blood 2003;102(9):3455–6.

83. Tonyali O, Coskun U, Yildiz R, et al. Imatinib mesylate-induced acute liver failure in a patient with gastrointestinal stromal tumors. Med Oncol 2010;27(3):768–73.

84. Kang BW, Lee SJ, Moon JH, et al. Chronic myeloid leukemia patient manifesting fatal hepatitis B virus reactivation during treatment with imatinib rescued by liver transplantation: case report and literature review. Int J Hematol 2009;90(3):383–7.

85. Spataro V. Nilotinib in a patient with postnecrotic liver cirrhosis related to imatinib. J Clin Oncol Off J Am Soc Clin Oncol 2011;29(3):e50–2.

86. Martínez Pascual C, Valdés Mas M, de la Peña Moral JM, et al. [Fulminating hepatitis for imatinib in a patient with chronic myeloid leukaemia]. Med Clin 2011;137(7):329–30.

87. Peroukides S, Makatsoris T, Koutras A, et al. Lapatinib-induced hepatitis: a case report. World J Gastroenterol 2011;17(18):2349–52.

88. Belopolsky Y, Grinblatt DL, Dunnenberger HM, et al. A Case of Severe, Nilotinib-Induced Liver Injury. ACG Case Rep J 2019;6(2):e00003.

89. Alshelleh M, Park J, John V, et al. Olaparib-Induced Immune-Mediated Liver Injury. ACG Case Rep J 2022;9(1):e00735.

90. Cheng Y, Chang W, Yen H, et al. Osimertinib-related liver injury with successful osimertinib rechallenge: A case report. Thorac Cancer 2022; 13(15):2271–4.

91. González I, Chatterjee D. Histopathological Features of Drug-Induced Liver Injury Secondary to Osimertinib. ACG Case Rep J 2019;6(2): e00011.

92. Vuppalanchi R, Saxena R, Storniolo AMV, et al. Pseudocirrhosis and liver failure in patients with metastatic breast cancer after treatment with palbociclib. Hepatology 2017;65(5):1762–4.

93. Klempner SJ, Choueiri TK, Yee E, et al. Severe pazopanib-induced hepatotoxicity: clinical and histologic course in two patients. J Clin Oncol Off J Am Soc Clin Oncol 2012;30(27):e264–8.

94. Choi JW, Yoo JJ, Kim SG, et al. Pazopanib-induced severe acute liver injury. Medicine (Baltim) 2021; 100(46):e27731.

95. Piawah S, Hyland C, Umetsu SE, et al. A case report of vanishing bile duct syndrome after exposure to pexidartinib (PLX3397) and paclitaxel. NPJ Breast Cancer 2019;5:17.

96. Department of Haematology, Hospital Sultanah Aminah, Johor Bahru, Malaysia, Boo Y, Liam CC, Toh S, et al. Rechallenge of ponatinib in chronic myeloid leukaemia after hepatotoxicity. Hong Kong Med J 2019;162–3.

97. Sacré A, Lanthier N, Dano H, et al. Regorafenib induced severe toxic hepatitis: characterization and discussion. Liver Int Off J Int Assoc Study Liver 2016;36(11):1590–4.

98. Béchade D, Desjardin M, Castain C, et al. Fatal Acute Liver Failure as a Consequence of Regorafenib Treatment in a Metastatic Colon Cancer. Case Rep Oncol 2017;10(2):790–4.

99. Topcu A, Yasin AI, Shbair AT, et al. A case report of fulminant hepatitis due to ribociclib with confirmed by liver biopsy in breast cancer. J Oncol Pharm Pract Off Publ Int Soc Oncol Pharm Pract 2022; 28(1):242–6.

100. 209092ORIG1S000 - Food and Drug Administration. Available at: https://www.accessdata.fda.gov/drugsatfda_docs/nda/2017/209092Orig1s000-MultidisciplineR.pdf. Accessed October 27, 2022.

101. Murad W, Rabinowitz I, Lee FC. Sorafenib-Induced Grade Four Hepatotoxicity in a Patient with Recurrent Gastrointestinal Stromal Tumor (GIST): A

Case Report and Review of Literature. ACG Case Rep J 2014;1(2):115–7.

102. Wang QL, Li XJ, Yao ZC, et al. Sorafenib-induced acute-on-chronic liver failure in a patient with hepatocellular carcinoma after transarterial chemoembolization and radiofrequency ablation: A case report. Mol Clin Oncol 2017;7(4):693–5.

103. Weise AM, Liu CY, Shields AF. Fatal liver failure in a patient on acetaminophen treated with sunitinib malate and levothyroxine. Ann Pharmacother 2009;43(4):761–6.

104. Sanchez BE, Hajjafar L. Severe Hepatotoxicity in a Patient Treated With Hedgehog Inhibitor: First Case Report. Gastroenterology 2011;5(Supplement 1):140.

105. Atallah E, Wijayasiri P, Cianci N, et al. Zanubrutinib-induced liver injury: a case report and literature review. BMC Gastroenterol 2021;21:244.

106. Markham A, Dhillon S. Acalabrutinib: First Global Approval. Drugs 2018;78(1):139–45.

107. Muchtar E, Gatt ME, Rouvio O, et al. Efficacy and safety of salvage therapy using Carfilzomib for relapsed or refractory multiple myeloma patients: a multicentre retrospective observational study. Br J Haematol 2016;172(1):89–96.

108. Ando T, Kojima K, Isoda H, et al. Reactivation of resolved infection with the hepatitis B virus immune escape mutant G145R during dasatinib treatment for chronic myeloid leukemia. Int J Hematol 2015; 102(3):379–82.

109. Herishanu Y, Katchman H, Polliack A. Severe hepatitis B virus reactivation related to ibrutinib monotherapy. Ann Hematol 2017;96(4):689–90.

110. Walker EJ, Simko JP, Ko AH. Hepatitis B Viral Reactivation Secondary to Imatinib Treatment in a Patient with Gastrointestinal Stromal Tumor. Anticancer Res 2014;34(7):3629–34.

111. Uhm J, Kim SH, Oh S, et al. High Incidence of Hepatitis B Viral Reactivation in Chronic Myeloid Leukemia Patients Treated with Tyrosine Kinase Inhibitors. Blood 2018;132(Supplement 1):3010.

112. Kang Y, Meng F. Acute fulminant hepatitis associated with osimertinib administration in a lung cancer patient with chronic hepatitis B: The first mortality case report. Thorac Cancer 2022;13(7): 1091–4.

113. Sjoblom M, Chtioui H, Fraga M, et al. Hepatitis B reactivation during ruxolitinib treatment. Ann Hematol 2022;101(9):2081–6.

Liver Pathology After Hematopoietic Stem Cell Transplantation

Ragini Phansalkar, PhD[a], Neeraja Kambham, MD[a],
Vivek Charu, MD, PhD[a,b],*

KEYWORDS

- Liver • Stem cell transplant • Sinusoidal obstruction syndrome • Veno-occlusive disease
- Graft-versus-host disease • Iron overload • Infection

Key points

- Liver injury is a common complication of hematopoietic stem cell transplant.

- Medications taken before or after stem cell transplant can cause endothelial cell injury leading to sinusoidal obstruction syndrome.

- Classic hepatic graft-versus-host disease usually occurs concurrently with graft-versus-host disease in other organs, but the hepatitic variant can occur in isolation.

- Iron overload in the setting of hematopoietic stem cell transplant typically occurs as a result of repeated transfusions.

- Stem cell transplant patients are at risk for a number of systemic opportunistic viral infections.

ABSTRACT

Hematopoietic stem cell transplantation is used to treat a variety of hematologic malignancies and autoimmune conditions. The immunosuppressive medications as well as other therapies used both before and after transplantation leave patients susceptible to a wide spectrum of complications, including liver injury. Causes for liver damage associated with stem cell transplantation include sinusoidal obstruction syndrome, graft-versus-host disease, iron overload, and opportunistic infection. Here, the authors review the clinical and pathological findings of these etiologies of liver injury and provide a framework for diagnosis.

OVERVIEW

Hematopoietic stem cell transplant (HSCT) is a lifesaving treatment for hematologic malignancies and severe autoimmune conditions, in which diseased blood and immune cells are replaced with transplanted healthy progenitors.[1] In allogeneic HSCT, the newly grafted progenitor cells come from a donor, whereas in autologous HSCT, they come from the recipient themselves. HSCT is a complex and lengthy process, involving donor–recipient human leukocyte antigen matching, pretransplant conditioning with myeloablative (or non-myeloablative) chemotherapy or radiation, and numerous posttransplant maintenance medications including immunosuppressive drugs and antimicrobial prophylaxis. Liver injury is a common and often serious complication of HSCT that can occur at any point during the HSCT process.[2,3] The liver biopsy remains essential to establish the etiology of liver injury in HSCT patients and guide treatment decisions. Arriving at an accurate, clinically useful diagnosis from liver biopsy specimens can be challenging for the practicing pathologist, in part due to the careful clinicopathologic

[a] Department of Pathology, Lane Building, L235, 300 Pasteur Drive, Stanford, CA 94305, USA; [b] Department of Medicine, Quantitative Sciences Unit, Stanford, CA, USA
* Corresponding author. 300 Pasteur Drive, Edwards R248B, Stanford, CA 94305.
E-mail address: vcharu@stanford.edu

Surgical Pathology 16 (2023) 519–532
https://doi.org/10.1016/j.path.2023.04.007

correlation required in these cases. Here, the authors detail the spectrum of liver pathology that can occur following HSCT, focusing on drug-induced liver injury (DILI) (including sinusoidal obstruction syndrome), graft-versus-host disease (GVHD), iron overload, and opportunistic infections.

DRUG-INDUCED LIVER INJURY

SINUSOIDAL OBSTRUCTION SYNDROME/ VENO-OCCLUSIVE DISEASE

Pathogenesis

Sinusoidal obstruction syndrome (SOS) occurs due to damage of sinusoidal and central venular endothelial cells. The inciting endothelial cell injury can come from multiple sources related to HSCT, including chemotherapy or radiation-based conditioning regimens and agents for GVHD prophylaxis.[4] Injury to endothelial cells leads to breaks in the sinusoidal barrier and allowing for extravasation of red blood cells (RBCs), fluid, and other debris into the space of Disse.[4–6] The expansion of the space of Disse causes narrowing of the sinusoids.[4–6] Additional sloughing of endothelial cells can build up in the sinusoids, eventually causing venous obstruction and portal hypertension.[4]

Risk Factors

The risk of SOS varies based on patient and treatment characteristics. In adults undergoing allogeneic HSCT with traditional myeloablative conditioning regimens, the incidence is between 10% and 15%.[4] In contrast, adults undergoing autologous HSCT or allogeneic transplant with a reduced-intensity conditioning regimen have an incidence of less than 10%.[4,7–9] Conditioning regimens most likely to cause SOS include high-dose or unfractionated radiation, and cyclophosphamide, especially when given in combination with treatments that reduce the capacity of the liver to neutralize its toxic metabolite, such as busulfan, carmustine, and total body irradiation.[6,8,10] Similarly, drugs used after transplantation for GVHD prophylaxis can also lead to SOS, particularly the combination of tacrolimus with sirolimus or methotrexate.[6] Although sirolimus use has not been definitively linked to SOS, its combination with a cyclophosphamide-based conditioning or methotrexate has.[11] Finally, certain targeted leukemia therapies including gemtuzumab ozogamicin and inotuzumab ozogamicin are also associated with an increased risk of SOS.[8]

Patient factors are also a significant contributor to risk for SOS. There is a 3 to 10 times greater risk in patients with preexisting liver disease before transplantation, indicated by elevated aspartate aminotransferase (AST) or bilirubin.[6] In addition, iron overload and increased ferritin level are also independent risk factors for SOS.[6,12] Preexisting systemic damage to endothelial cells may also contribute to SOS, as indicated by a study showing increased odds for developing severe SOS in patients with reduced lung diffusion capacity.[13] Genetic factors may also contribute the GSTM1-null genotype, and the HFE C282Y allele has been associated with an increased risk of SOS.[8] Finally, children undergoing allogeneic stem cell transplant have a greater risk of SOS compared with adults, approximately 20%.[14] This is thought to be due to a reduced capacity of the pediatric liver to neutralize toxic metabolites.[5] Thus, in children a young age (<2) is associated with a higher risk of SOS as well.[8,14,15]

Clinical Presentation and Diagnosis

SOS often manifests within 30 days of transplant with early signs being visible within one day of transplant.[8] The classic clinical presentation of SOS stems from the effects of portal hypertension and includes rapid weight gain, ascites, hepatomegaly, and jaundice as well as right upper quadrant pain.[5,10] There can be a difference in clinical presentation of SOS between children and adults with children being less likely to present with jaundice.[7]

In 2016, the European Society for Blood and Marrow Transplantation released a new set of diagnostic criteria for SOS in adults.[6] The new criteria differentiate between classical (within 21 days of transplant) and late-onset SOS (more than 21 days after transplant).[6] Classical SOS requires hyperbilirubinemia as well as at least two features of portal hypertension (painful hepatomegaly, weight gain >5%, and ascites).[6] The late-onset criteria are more flexible, still allowing for the classical presentation but also allowing cases without this presentation if they have biopsy-proven SOS, or if they have hemodynamic or ultrasound evidence of SOS with two additional features (hyperbilirubinemia, weight gain >5%, painful hepatomegaly, or ascites).[6]

New diagnostic criteria for pediatric SOS have also recently been adopted.[14] Similar to the adult late-onset criteria, hyperbilirubinemia is not a strict requirement, and the presence of two or more of the following signs is sufficient to make the diagnosis: transfusion-refractory thrombocytopenia, weight gain greater than 5%, hepatomegaly, ascites, and hyperbilirubinemia.[14]

The noninvasive diagnosis of SOS is an area of active research with proteomics-based biomarkers[16] and advances in transient elastography showing promise.[17]

Microscopic Features

The endothelial cell injury and subsequent sinusoidal blockage underlying SOS are reflected in the microscopic findings on liver biopsy. SOS is characterized by central vein and/or sinusoidal changes; the distribution of histopathologic findings can be heterogenous and can depend on the severity of disease. Classic findings include (1) central venous subendothelial edema, RBC extravasation, and fibrin deposition (Fig. 1A–C); (2) zone 3 sinusoidal dilation and congestion with RBCs with extravasated RBCs within the space of Disse (the space between the damaged endothelial lining and the hepatocyte) and hepatic plate atrophy (Fig. 1D). In some cases, histologic evidence of endothelial damage, such as endothelial nuclear swelling, can be appreciated. In cases with severe endothelial injury, hemorrhagic necrosis can be seen, often in a perivenular distribution (Fig. 1E–F); in mild cases, only sinusoidal congestion and zone 3 cholestasis may be visible. Over time, venular obliteration and perivenular fibrosis can occur, as well as sinusoidal fibrosis.[4,18,19] In many cases, trichrome-stained sections help visualize the histopathologic changes better than hematoxylin & eosin (H&E) stained sections alone.

Differential Diagnosis

Congestion of the sinusoids and features of venous outflow obstruction raise a differential diagnosis that includes Budd–Chiari syndrome and congestive hepatopathy. These conditions are often easy to exclude with pertinent clinical information. Mild cases of SOS (eg, those with pericentral cholestasis and mild sinusoidal congestion alone) can be subtle, and the differential diagnosis would include ischemic injury to the liver. Often, GVHD is in the clinical differential diagnosis; severe bile duct epithelial changes are uncommon in the setting of isolated SOS, and we note that patients can have concurrent SOS and GVHD. Clinical correlation is imperative in these cases, and the presence of extrahepatic GVHD may be helpful. Caution is warranted to avoid overinterpretation of biliary changes as several studies have demonstrated that liver biopsies in patients with venous outflow obstruction can have portal findings mimicking chronic biliary tract disease (eg, portal inflammation, portal-based fibrosis, mild bile ductular proliferation).[20]

Treatment

Timely identification and management of SOS is essential, as severe SOS has a mortality rate greater than 80%.[4] Treatment for SOS is largely supportive including diuretics, paracentesis, and avoidance of hepatotoxic medications.[7] Defibrotide, an oligonucleotide-based medication with protective effects on endothelial cells, is the only medication with food and drug administration (FDA)-approval for SOS after bone marrow transplant and has been shown to be effective for both adult and pediatric patients.[7,8]

OTHER CAUSES OF DRUG-INDUCED LIVER INJURY AFTER HEMATOPOIETIC STEM CELL TRANSPLANT

Although DILI is a common cause of liver complications after HSCT,[21] it is difficult to definitively identify and diagnose because numerous agents used in the transplantation process are hepatotoxic, and DILI can manifest in a variety of ways. Drugs that have been implicated in liver injury include conditioning regimen drugs (eg, busulfan and cyclophosphamide), GVHD prophylaxis medications (eg, cyclosporine and methotrexate), and antibacterial and antifungal prophylaxis (eg, trimethoprim–sulfamethoxazole, and azole antifungal drugs). Although some drugs cause dose-dependent intrinsic liver injury (eg, cyclosporine), others cause idiosyncratic injury (eg, sulfonamides, azoles).[22] Pathways involved in the development of DILI include oxidative stress, activated mitogen activated protein (MAP) kinases, mitochondrial stress, and immune responses.[22] Specific risk factors for DILI depend on the medication but can include age, female sex, and combination with other medications.[22]

DILI as a histopathologic diagnosis remains a diagnosis of exclusion. Histopathologic findings in DILI are heterogeneous, and a pattern-based approach has been advocated to improve diagnostic accuracy. Histopathologic patterns of DILI have been well-reviewed elsewhere and are out of scope for this review.[23–25]

GRAFT-VERSUS-HOST DISEASE

Pathogenesis

The liver is one of the primary targets of GVHD, in addition to the skin and the tubular gastrointestinal (GI) tract.[21,26] Liver damage in acute GVHD is mediated primarily by cytotoxic T and natural killer (NK) cells derived from donor bone marrow, which identify the host tissue as foreign.[21,27,28] The initial activation of graft-derived immune cells is in part secondary to cytokines and other inflammatory factors released in response to conditioning regimens used in the HSCT process.[21,28,29] When

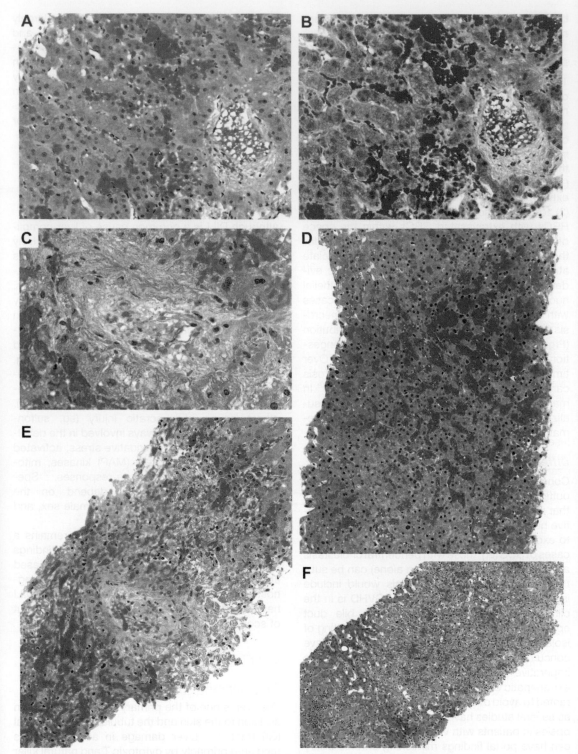

Fig. 1. Histologic findings in sinusoidal obstruction syndrome. Central vein subendothelial edema with entrapped red blood cells (RBCs) and pericentral sinusoidal congestion, seen by H&E (*A, C*) and trichrome stain (*B*). Low-power view of sinusoidal congestion (*D*). In severe cases, pericentral hemorrhagic necrosis can be seen (*E, F*).

the activated donor cells interact with major histocompatibility complex (MHC) antigens on recipient antigen presenting cells, this leads to spropagation of the immune response.[29] Other immune components including T follicular helper cells, B cells, and autoantibodies have been implicated in chronic GVHD.[21,28,29]

Risk Factors

Major histocompatibility complex and minor histocompatibility antigen mismatch are a major risk factor for the development of acute GVHD.[30] Although acute GVHD does not necessarily precede chronic GVHD and can in fact occur concurrently with it, it can be a risk factor.[29] Male gender and the presence of HCV have also been shown to be associated with chronic GVHD.[30,31]

Clinical Presentation and Diagnosis

Cholestasis is a key manifestation of GVHD in the liver, and the clinical presentation is defined by signs and symptoms of cholestasis including progressive jaundice, hyperbilirubinemia, and elevated alkaline phosphatase.[27,28,32] Common bile duct dilation can be seen in conjunction with elevated bilirubin.[33] Typical presentation of GVHD is mild elevations of AST and alanine transaminase (ALT) and elevated alkaline phosphatase.[21] The timing of the initial presentation can be highly variable due to the wide spectrum of posttransplant drug regimens. There is also a less common hepatitic variant of GVHD, which presents with markedly elevated AST and ALT, which can be over 10 times the normal limit[21,27,28] and a smaller increase in alkaline phosphatase.[34] The hepatitic GVHD typically follows a reduction in immunosuppression[21] and is reported to occur on average 9 months after transplant.[34] Although typical liver GVHD often happens concurrently with GVHD in other organs (especially skin and tubular GI tract), the hepatitic variant is known to occur in isolation.[21,28,34] A similar hepatitic GVHD reaction can also occur following donor lymphocyte infusion.[21,32]

The most recent national institutes of health (NIH) consensus regarding the clinical diagnosis of GVHD was published in 2014 and defines two forms of GVHD: acute and chronic.[35] Classic acute GVHD is diagnosed when symptoms of GVHD (cholestasis, in addition to other systemic manifestations such as diarrhea and maculopapular rash) occur within 100 days of transplant.[35] Late-onset or persistent GVHD is diagnosed when these symptoms occur more than 100 days after transplant, as long as the patient does not meet clinical criteria for chronic

GVHD.[35] The 2014 consensus report does not identify any liver-specific features as criteria for chronic GVHD, but there are manifestations in other organ systems that are unique to chronic GVHD, including sclerosis in the skin, esophageal webs, and bronchiolitis obliterans syndrome.[35] When these features are present, GVHD can either be diagnosed independently, or as part of an "overlap" syndrome, if the patient also has manifestations of acute GVHD.[35] Liver biopsy should be considered to confirm the hepatic features of GVHD. Importantly, however, a diagnosis of acute versus chronic GVHD usually cannot be determined based on liver findings alone, so clinical correlation is especially important to make this distinction. Further, other causes of liver damage and cholestasis should be considered and excluded before making a diagnosis of hepatic GVHD, and hepatic GVHD should not be definitively diagnosed in the absence of other systemic manifestations.[21]

Microscopic Features

Damage to bile ducts is the primary histologic feature of hepatic GVHD and underlies the cholestatic pattern of liver injury seen clinically.[27,28] Injured bile ducts can have epithelial nuclear abnormalities such as pleomorphism, overlap, and loss of polarity, as well as vacuoles in epithelial cell cytoplasm without prominent bile ductular reaction (Fig. 2A–D).[21,27,30] Inflammatory infiltrate with lymphocytes in the bile duct epithelium can also be seen and is often mild due to immunosuppressive medications.[27] In pronounced cases, lobular canalicular cholestasis can be seen (Fig. 2E). As GVHD is a common complication of HSCT, it should not be excluded based only on a negative biopsy, especially early in the disease course (within 35 days of transplant), or if the specimen is inadequate.[21,27,28] Later in the disease course (eg, after 90 days following transplant), bile duct injury can lead to bile duct loss and portal fibrosis (Fig. 2F).[27,28] With disease progression, bile ducts can be difficult to identify on H&E alone. In these cases, cytokeratin 7 or cytokeratin 19 staining can be used to identify bile ducts or to demonstrate bile duct loss (Fig. 2G).[30] Chronic GVHD cannot be diagnosed based on liver biopsy alone, as acute and chronic hepatic GVHD have similar manifestations, including bile duct loss and portal fibrosis.[28] Histologic changes in other organs, including sclerosis, can support a diagnosis of chronic GVHD.[29]

In the hepatitic variant of GVHD, microscopic examination shows more extensive lobular

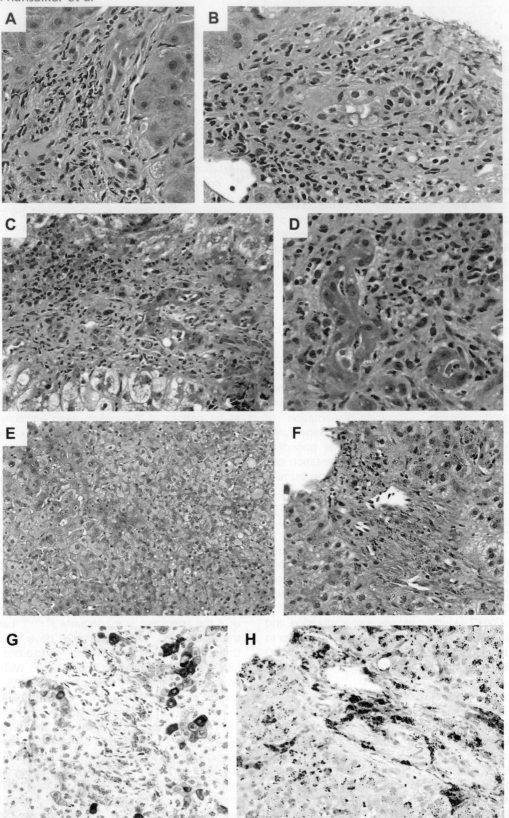

Fig. 2. Histologic findings in hepatic graft-versus-host disease (GVHD). The hallmark finding in acute GVHD is bile duct injury, characterized by cytoplasmic attenuation, uneven cellular spacing and loss of polarity (*A*), cytoplasmic vacuolization (*B*), nuclear pleomorphism and apoptosis (*C*, *D*). In severe cases, lobular canalicular cholestasis can be seen (*E*). In progression to chronic disease, duct loss can be seen (*F*), confirmed by CK7 immunohistochemistry (*G*). Severe hemosiderosis may be an incidental finding in patients with GVHD or may be a direct contributor to bile duct injury (*H*).

inflammatory infiltrate with lymphocytes, plasma cells, and macrophages; foci of necrosis[21] and acidophil bodies[34] may be seen. Bile duct injury is a less prominent feature of this variant.[21]

Differential Diagnosis

Several other possibilities must be excluded before making a diagnosis of GVHD. DILI can sometimes present with bile duct injury and cholestasis.[28] Parenteral nutrition-associated liver disease can also present with cholestatic injury, especially in infants.[36,37] Hepatotropic infections may also present with bile duct injury, but usually also other features of infection, including neutrophilic cholangitis, hepatocyte necrosis, and/or lobular inflammation.[21,28] Obstructive causes of cholestasis also present with robust bile ductular reaction and neutrophilic infiltrate in contrast to GVHD.[21]

The hepatitic variant of GVHD, due to more extensive inflammatory infiltrate, can also have histologic overlap with hepatotropic infections and DILI.[27,34] This less common variant is a diagnosis of exclusion.

Treatment

GVHD is typically treated with immunosuppressive therapy including steroids[28] as well as janus kinase (JAK) inhibitors (ruxolitinib and itacitinib), Bruton tyrosine kinase inhibitor (ibrutinib), and proteasome inhibitors (bortezomib and carfilzomib).[26]

IRON OVERLOAD

Pathogenesis

Iron is an essential metal for cellular metabolism, but there are no physiologically regulated means of iron excretion. Four major cell types determine body iron content and distribution: (1) duodenal enterocytes, responsible for dietary iron absorption; (2) erythroid precursors, responsible for iron utilization; (3) reticuloendothelial macrophages, responsible for iron storage and recycling; and (4) hepatocytes, responsible for iron storage and endocrine regulation.[38] Iron overload in the setting of HSCT occurs primarily as a result of multiple transfusions and ineffective erythropoiesis, resulting in increased intestinal absorption of iron, as contributing factors. Untreated transfusional iron overload can result in damage to the liver, endocrine organs (eg, pancreatic beta cells), and the heart.

Circulating iron (eg, iron released from enterocytes and reticuloendothelial macrophages) binds to free sites on the plasma iron-transport protein, transferrin. In normal conditions, transferrin-binding capacity of iron exceeds plasma iron concentrations, but in the setting of iron overload, transferrin becomes saturated with iron and the excess iron in circulation binds to low-molecular-weight compounds (eg, citrate). This non-transferrin bound iron (NTBI) is readily taken up by certain cell types, including hepatocytes and cardiomyocytes; excess iron is primarily stored in the form of hemosiderin.[38,39] The excess uptake of iron as NTBI can cause cellular damage via free radical generation. The liver is the most important organ for iron storage as it has the largest capacity to sequester excess iron. Although our focus is on iron-mediated liver injury, cardiac toxicity is often more clinically important as patients with transfusional iron overload are at risk of sudden death due to cardiac failure.[40]

Clinical Presentation and Diagnosis

Liver dysfunction in the setting of transfusional iron overload can be insidious, presenting with only moderate elevations in serum transaminases, with otherwise normal liver function tests. Laboratory and radiologic assessment of iron overload status can be helpful.[41,42] Calculation of iron intake by simply recording the number of units of blood transfused is cost-effective and generally predictive of total iron accumulation in the body. Serum ferritin and transferrin levels are an inaccurate measure of total body iron accumulation but are often used due to widespread availability. Liver iron concentration (LIC) largely reflects total body iron accumulation, and the best noninvasive measure of LIC is via MRI (both ferritin and hemosiderin are paramagnetic and can be identified by MRI).[42–44] Importantly, LIC may not reflect iron toxicity in other organs, particularly, the heart, and cardiac-specific measures of iron overload are important in assessing cardiac toxicity.[42]

Microscopic Features

The main two compartments of the liver affected by iron overload are the hepatocytes and the Kupffer cells. Hepatic iron is stored mainly as ferritin and hemosiderin with hemosiderin being the predominant form of *stainable iron*. On routine H&E stain, hemosiderin deposits are golden-brown refractile granules (**Fig.** 3A, B). Small amounts of hemosiderin can be difficult to visualize on H&E stained sections; histochemical stains, particularly Perls' Prussian blue stain, highlights hemosiderin granules in blue. The normal liver has no stainable iron, and as such, any stainable iron deserves mention.

Transfusional iron overload initially results in iron accumulation in Kupffer cells ("mesenchymal

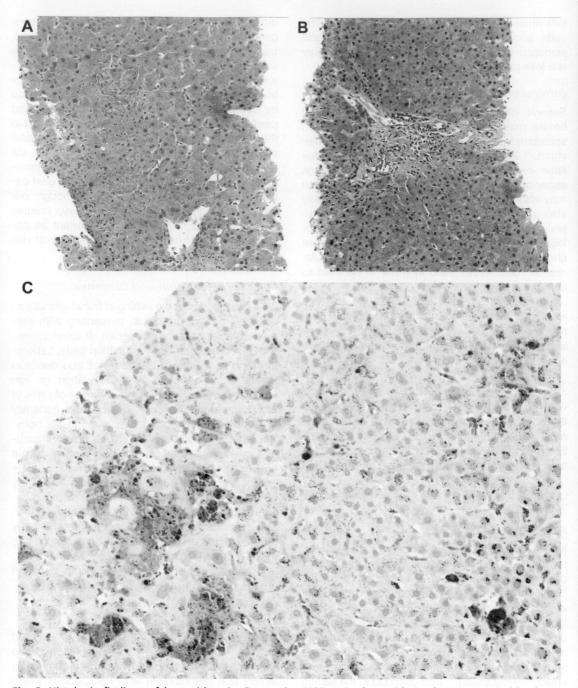

Fig. 3. Histologic findings of hemosiderosis. On routine H&E stain, hemosiderin deposits are golden-brown refractile granules, here seen in the lobule and lobular macrophages (*A*) and the portal tract (*B*). In the setting of HSCT, patients often have long-standing iron overload, resulting in a mixed parenchymal and mesenchymal pattern of hemosiderosis, in which coarse hemosiderin granules are dispersed within hepatocytes and Kupffer cells, highlighted by Perls' Prussian blue stain (*C*).

pattern of hemosiderosis"). In the setting of HSCT, patients often have long-standing iron overload, resulting in a mixed parenchymal and mesenchymal pattern of hemosiderosis, in which coarse hemosiderin granules are dispersed within

hepatocytes and Kupffer cells (**Fig.** 3C). In more severe cases, hemosiderin may be present within the bile duct epithelium as well. Cellular injury from iron overload can progress to bridging fibrosis and cirrhosis.

Although several grading systems for hepatic iron deposition have been developed, they suffer from poor intraobserver and interobserver repeatability. Semiquantification of iron deposition in hepatocytes and Kupffer cells are often presented separately in cases where the cause of iron overload is unclear; this is not commonly an issue in the setting of HSCT.[45]

Differential Diagnosis

Although hemosiderosis of the liver is largely a straightforward histological diagnosis, it may accompany other causes of liver disease. For example, hepatic iron overload is a risk factor for SOS as well as opportunistic infections, and these etiologies should be carefully evaluated for in the biopsied material.[46,47] The relationship between hepatic iron overload and GVHD is unclear.[48,49] Some studies have suggested that hepatic hemosiderosis can exacerbate hepatic GVHD (Fig. 2H).[50] Others have suggested that enzyme abnormalities in patients with hepatic iron overload can mimic GVHD, and patients thought to have both GVHD and iron overload based on liver biopsy may show normalization of their liver enzymes with phlebotomy/iron chelation despite failure to do so after immunosuppression.[51] In severe cases of hepatic iron overload, hemosiderin deposition in the bile duct epithelium may be associated with bile duct injury; distinguishing these cases from GVHD (with background hepatic hemosiderosis) can be challenging, and clinical correlation for other signs of GVHD is often helpful to clarify the differential diagnosis.

Treatment

The mainstay of treatment of iron overload after HSCT is iron chelation therapy. Phlebotomy may be considered in patients without significant anemia.[40]

OPPORTUNISTIC INFECTIONS

Patients undergoing HSCT are at an increased risk of infections due to a variety of interacting factors, including (1) the underlying hematologic disease; (2) the conditioning regimen used and the associated duration of neutropenia and mucosal injury; (3) the degree of histocompatibility mismatch between donor and recipient (for allogeneic HSCT recipients); (4) the presence of latent donor/recipient infections (eg, Epstein–Barr virus [EBV], cytomegalovirus [CMV]) (5) the immunosuppressive regimen used to prevent and/or treat GVHD; and (6) environmental exposures.

In addition, transplant recipients experience a prolonged period of high infection risk due to certain components of immunity, in particular CD4 T-cells and CD4-supported humoral immunity, not returning to normal levels for years following transplant.[52]

The specific combination of donor and recipient latent infection status also affects the likelihood of reactivated infections. For instance, transplant recipients with latent CMV are less likely to experience reactivation with a CMV-infected donor than with a CMV-naïve donor, because in the former case the donor graft will already contain CMV-primed memory T cells.[53]

The range of systemic infections (bacterial, viral, and fungal) affecting patients undergoing HSCT is broad. Here, the authors focus on four hepatotropic herpesvirus infections that can be seen in the post-HSCT setting primarily as a result of reactivation: EBV, CMV, adenovirus, and herpes simplex virus (HSV).

EPSTEIN–BARR VIRUS HEPATITIS AND POSTTRANSPLANT LYMPHOPROLIFERATIVE DISORDERS

EBV reactivation can present in the liver as active infection, EBV hepatitis, with flu-like symptoms, or in the form of EBV-related posttransplant lymphoproliferative disorders (PTLDs). PTLDs after HSCT have a reported incidence of between 1.2% and 12.9%,[52,54] though PTLD in the liver is especially rare. In one study, the highest rate of EBV reactivation occurred within 2 months of transplant.[54] The key laboratory findings in EBV hepatitis include leukocytosis with atypical lymphocytes.[55] The detection of heterophile antibodies can also support the diagnosis, though the test does not have a very high sensitivity or specificity.[55] On histology, a lobular hepatitis pattern is seen with atypical lymphocytes in sinusoids and portal tracts, but without significant hepatocellular damage or acidophil bodies.[56] The lymphocytes can be seen lining up side-by-side in the sinusoids, assuming a "string of beads" pattern that is a characteristic finding for EBV hepatitis (Fig. 4A).[55,56] Noncaseating granulomas consisting of epithelioid histiocytes admixed with small lymphocytes or fibrin rings may also be present.[55,56] The extent of portal inflammation can be variable. In situ hybridization (ISH) for EBV-encoded RNA (EBER) may be positive in scattered cells, but due to the scarcity of these positive cells, especially in a small core biopsy, a negative EBER-ISH does not rule out EBV hepatitis.[55,57]

EBV-associated PTLD is characterized by varying degrees of lymphocytic infiltration of the liver

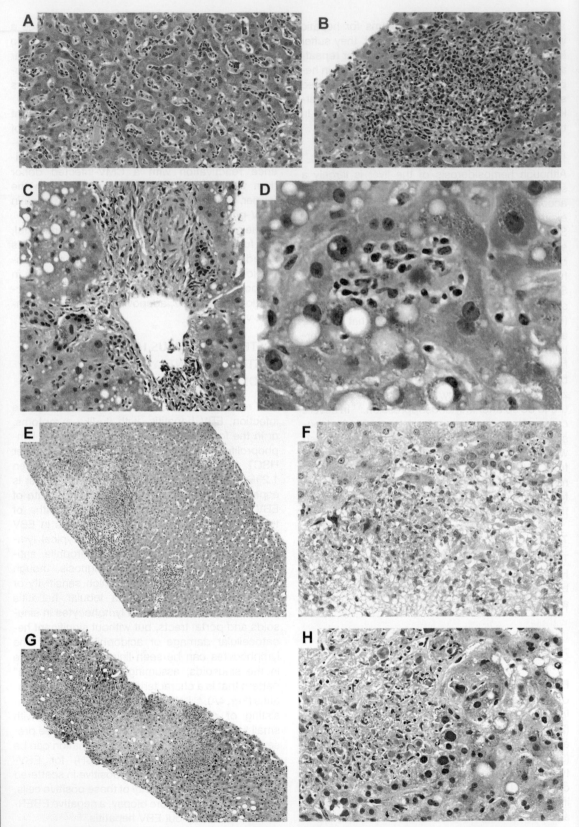

Fig. 4. Histologic findings of selected viral infections in the liver. In EBV hepatitis, lymphocytes can be seen expanding sinusoids (*A*). EBV-positive polymorphic posttransplant lymphoproliferative disorder demonstrates mixed lymphoplasmacytic inflammation composed of polyclonal B cells in portal areas, effacing portal

and is divided into four categories: (1) early lesions demonstrate mixed lymphoplasmacytic inflammation composed of polyclonal B cells in portal areas with preserved architecture; (2) polymorphic PTLD demonstrates similar findings as in early lesions, effacing portal architecture, and a subset of which demonstrate monoclonal kappa- or lambda-light chain restriction (Fig. 4B); (3) monomorphic PTLD is characterized by a mass-forming monoclonal proliferation of typically B cells (though rarely T cell or T/NK-monomorphic PTLD can occur), meeting criteria for a diagnosis of lymphoma, with destruction of the hepatic architecture; and (4) classic Hodgkin lymphoma.[58–60] Although EBER-ISH may be positive in a variable number of cells, (between 1% and 40% in one study[61,62]), by definition, it is detectable in EBV-associated PTLD.

CYTOMEGALOVIRUS HEPATITIS

The risk of CMV reactivation is significant, occurring in over 50% of seropositive allogenic transplant recipients in one study.[63] Historically, CMV infection was seen in the early post-engraftment period of depressed T-cell immunity; however, infections are now emerging later in the engraftment process due to effective antiviral prophylaxis and the longer period of recipient immunosuppression used to prevent GVHD.[52] CMV most commonly causes pneumonia, gastrointestinal disease, and retinitis,[52] but in rare cases can also cause hepatitis. A key, though nonspecific, histologic finding for CMV hepatitis that may prompt a CMV immunostain is the presence of lobular "mini-microabscesses" composed of neutrophils.[56,64] Although not always present, amphophilic nuclear inclusions can be diagnostic (Fig. 4C, D).[64] Other histologic findings are also nonspecific including portal and lobular chronic inflammation.[56] In one study of CMV hepatitis after bone marrow transplantation, hepatocellular damage on histology was limited, without significant necrosis, cholestasis or bile duct injury, and notable primarily for the inflammatory aggregates.[64]

ADENOVIRUS HEPATITIS

Adenovirus hepatitis, though less common than other viral hepatitis or other forms of adenovirus infection after bone marrow transplant, has a high mortality rate, up to 88% in one study.[65]

Adenovirus infection can be a result of reactivation (usually over 90 days after transplant), or post-transplant exposure (usually within 90 days of transplant).[65] In one study, the incidence of adenovirus infection after transplant in children was over twice that in adults.[66] Similar to other viruses, an extended period of T-cell depletion increases the risk of adenovirus infection,[67] as does GVHD.[65,66] It is common for adenovirus to affect the gastrointestinal tract with diarrhea being a presenting symptom.[66] Histologic findings in the liver are notable for hepatocyte necrosis without a specific zonal pattern which ranges from small and well circumscribed to more expansive (Fig. 4E).[56,68] Lymphocytic inflammation is usually present but mild in comparison to the degree of necrosis.[56,68] The hepatocytes surrounding the necrosis can have enlarged atypical nuclei and fat droplets (Fig. 4F).[56] In some cases, bile duct epithelial cells may be infected as well. Another histologic pattern is that of "pox-like" granulomas with collections of histiocytes/macrophages associated with hepatic necrosis in a non-zonal distribution.

HERPES SIMPLEX VIRUS HEPATITIS

HSV hepatitis occurs in the setting of reactivation post-HSCT, and seropositive patients typically receive prophylaxis, which has been shown to reduce the incidence of HSV reactivation. HSV hepatitis is rare but can be life-threatening. Most of the patients with HSV hepatitis also have oropharyngeal or genital manifestations.[69,70] On biopsy, classic HSV hepatitis is characterized by well-circumscribed areas of coagulative necrosis (so-called "punched-out" lesions) with minimal inflammation (Fig. 4G). These areas of necrosis are non-zonal, and in severe cases, massive necrosis can be seen. Viral inclusions may be seen in hepatocyte nuclei at the margins of necrotic areas (Fig. 4H). Classic inclusions are ground-glass or smudged nuclei with margination of chromatin; multinucleated cells are less common in the liver, compared with mucocutaneous lesions. IHC against HSV1/2 is confirmatory.

SUMMARY

The liver is susceptible to multiple forms of injury in the setting of HSCT, including drug-induced injury,

---

architecture (*B*). In CMV hepatitis, although not always present, amphophilic nuclear inclusions can be diagnostic (*C, D*). Adenovirus hepatitis is characterized by non-zonal coagulative necrosis (*E*), with characteristic intranuclear inclusions seen at the periphery of necrotic areas (*F*). HSV hepatitis can also demonstrate well-circumscribed areas of coagulative necrosis (*G*), and characteristic intranuclear inclusions seen at the periphery of necrotic areas (*H*).

GVHD, iatrogenic iron overload, and opportunistic infections in the context of immunosuppression. The extent of histologic overlap between etiologically distinct forms of liver injury, and the heterogeneity in the severity of liver injury make interpretation of liver biopsies after HSCT challenging. Integration of the histologic findings with the clinical history and impression is often essential to arrive at the correct diagnosis.

CLINICS CARE POINTS

- Interpretation of liver biopsies after HSCT require careful correlation with the patient's clinical history and laboratory data.

- The most common etiologies of liver injury after HSCT are: (i) sinusoidal obstruction syndrome; (ii) other forms of drug-induced liver injury; (iii) acute and chronic graft-versus-host disease; (iv) iron overload; and (v) infections.

- Multiple contributing etiologies to liver injury may be present in the same biopsy.

FUNDING

VC is supported by the National Center for Advancing Translational Sciences of the National Institutes of Health under Award Number KL2TR003143.

DISCLOSURE

The authors have nothing to disclose.

REFERENCES

1. Bazinet A, Popradi G. A general practitioner's guide to hematopoietic stem-cell transplantation. Curr Oncol 2019;26(3):187–91.
2. Hogan WJ, Maris M, Storer B, et al. Hepatic injury after nonmyeloablative conditioning followed by allogeneic hematopoietic cell transplantation: a study of 193 patients. Blood 2004;103(1):78–84.
3. Sakai M, Strasser SI, Shulman HM, et al. Severe hepatocellular injury after hematopoietic cell transplant: incidence, etiology and outcome. Bone Marrow Transplant 2009;44(7):441–7.
4. Mohty M, Malard F, Abecassis M, et al. Sinusoidal obstruction syndrome/veno-occlusive disease: current situation and perspectives-a position statement from the European Society for Blood and Marrow Transplantation (EBMT). Bone Marrow Transplant 2015;50(6):781–9.
5. Bonifazi F, Barbato F, Ravaioli F, et al. Diagnosis and treatment of VOD/SOS after allogeneic hematopoietic stem cell transplantation. Front Immunol 2020;11:489.
6. Mohty M, Malard F, Abecassis M, et al. Revised diagnosis and severity criteria for sinusoidal obstruction syndrome/veno-occlusive disease in adult patients: a new classification from the European Society for Blood and Marrow Transplantation. Bone Marrow Transplant 2016;51(7):906–12.
7. Corbacioglu S, Richardson PG. Defibrotide for children and adults with hepatic veno-occlusive disease post hematopoietic cell transplantation. Expet Rev Gastroenterol Hepatol 2017;11(10):885–98.
8. Dalle J-H, Giralt SA. Hepatic veno-occlusive disease after hematopoietic stem cell transplantation: risk factors and stratification, prophylaxis, and treatment. Biol Blood Marrow Transplant 2016;22(3):400–9.
9. Lewis C, Kim HT, Roeker LE, et al. Incidence, predictors, and outcomes of veno-occlusive disease/sinusoidal obstruction syndrome after reduced-intensity allogeneic hematopoietic cell transplantation. Biol Blood Marrow Transplant 2020;26(3):529–39.
10. Bayraktar UD, Seren S, Bayraktar Y. Hepatic venous outflow obstruction: three similar syndromes. World J Gastroenterol 2007;13(13):1912–27.
11. Cutler C, Stevenson K, Kim HT, et al. Sirolimus is associated with veno-occlusive disease of the liver after myeloablative allogeneic stem cell transplantation. Blood 2008;112(12):4425–31.
12. Maradei SC, Maiolino A, de Azevedo AM, et al. Serum ferritin as risk factor for sinusoidal obstruction syndrome of the liver in patients undergoing hematopoietic stem cell transplantation. Blood 2009;114(6):1270–5.
13. Matute-Bello G, McDonald GD, Hinds MS, et al. Association of pulmonary function testing abnormalities and severe veno-occlusive disease of the liver after marrow transplantation. Bone Marrow Transplant 1998;21(11):1125–30.
14. Corbacioglu S, Carreras E, Ansari M, et al. Diagnosis and severity criteria for sinusoidal obstruction syndrome/veno-occlusive disease in pediatric patients: a new classification from the European society for blood and marrow transplantation. Bone Marrow Transplant 2018;53(2):138–45.
15. Corbacioglu S, Jabbour EJ, Mohty M. Risk factors for development of and progression of hepatic veno-occlusive disease/sinusoidal obstruction syndrome. Biol Blood Marrow Transplant 2019;25(7):1271–80.
16. Akil A, Zhang Q, Mumaw CL, et al. Biomarkers for diagnosis and prognosis of sinusoidal obstruction syndrome after hematopoietic cell transplantation. Biol Blood Marrow Transplant 2015;21(10):1739–45.

17. Colecchia A, Ravaioli F, Sessa M, et al. Liver stiffness measurement allows early diagnosis of veno-occlusive disease/sinusoidal obstruction syndrome in adult patients who undergo hematopoietic stem cell transplantation: results from a monocentric prospective study. Biol Blood Marrow Transplant 2019; 25(5):995–1003.

18. Carreras E, Diaz-Ricart M. The role of the endothelium in the short-term complications of hematopoietic SCT. Bone Marrow Transplant 2011;46(12): 1495–502.

19. Richardson P, Guinan E. The pathology, diagnosis, and treatment of hepatic veno-occlusive disease: current status and novel approaches. Br J Haematol 1999;107(3):485–93.

20. Kakar S, Batts KP, Poterucha JJ, et al. Histologic changes mimicking biliary disease in liver biopsies with venous outflow impairment. Mod Pathol 2004; 17(7):874–8.

21. Matsukuma KE, Wei D, Sun K, et al. Diagnosis and differential diagnosis of hepatic graft versus host disease (GVHD). J Gastrointest Oncol 2016; 7(Suppl 1):S21–31.

22. Andrade RJ, Aithal GP, Björnsson ES, et al. EASL clinical practice guidelines: drug-induced liver injury. J Hepatol 2019;70(6):1222–61.

23. Kleiner DE, Chalasani NP, Lee WM, et al. Hepatic histological findings in suspected drug-induced liver injury: systematic evaluation and clinical associations. Hepatology 2014;59(2):661–70.

24. Kleiner DE. The histopathological evaluation of drug-induced liver injury. Histopathology 2017;70(1):81–93.

25. Kleiner DE. Liver histology in the diagnosis and prognosis of drug-induced liver injury. Clin Liver Dis 2014;4(1):12–6.

26. Kurya AU, Aliyu U, Tudu AI, et al. Graft-versus-host disease: therapeutic prospects of improving the long-term post-transplant outcomes. Transplantation Reports 2022;7(4):100107.

27. Mourad N, Michel RP, Marcus VA. Pathology of gastrointestinal and liver complications of hematopoietic stem cell transplantation. Arch Pathol Lab Med 2019;143(9):1131–43.

28. Kambham N, Higgins JP, Sundram U, et al. Hematopoietic stem cell transplantation: graft versus host disease and pathology of gastrointestinal tract, liver, and lung. Adv Anat Pathol 2014;21(5):301–20.

29. Ghimire S, Weber D, Mavin E, et al. Pathophysiology of GvHD and other HSCT-related major complications. Front Immunol 2017;8:79.

30. Salomao M, Dorritie K, Mapara MY, et al. Histopathology of graft-vs-host disease of gastrointestinal tract and liver: an update. Am J Clin Pathol 2016; 145(5):591–603.

31. Chen C-T, Liu C-Y, Yu Y-B, et al. Characteristics and risk of chronic graft-versus-host disease of liver in allogeneic hematopoietic stem cell transplant recipients. PLoS One 2017;12(9):e0185210.

32. Akpek G., Boitnott JK., Lee LA., et al. Hepatitic variant of graft-versus-host disease after donor lymphocyte infusion: presented in the poster session at the 2002 Tandem BMT Meeting, February 21-26, 2002; Orlando, FL. Blood 2002;100(12): 3903–3907. .

33. Ketelsen D, Vogel W, Bethge W, et al. Enlargement of the common bile duct in patients with acute graft-versus-host disease: what does it mean? Am J Roentgenol 2009;193(3):W181–5.

34. Ma SY, Au WY, Ng IOL, et al. Hepatitic graft-versus-host disease after hematopoietic stem cell transplantation: clinicopathologic features and prognostic implication. Transplantation 2004;77(8):1252–9.

35. Jagasia MH, Greinix HT, Arora M, et al. National institutes of health consensus development project on criteria for clinical trials in chronic graft-versus-host disease: I. The 2014 diagnosis and staging working group report. Biol Blood Marrow Transplant 2015;21(3):389–401.

36. Żalikowska-Gardocka M, Przybyłkowski A. Review of parenteral nutrition-associated liver disease. Clin Exp Hepatol 2020;6(2):65–73.

37. Dahms BB, Halpin TC. Serial liver biopsies in parenteral nutrition-associated cholestasis of early infancy. Gastroenterology 1981;81(1):136–44.

38. Fleming RE, Ponka P. Iron overload in human disease. N Engl J Med 2012;366(4):348–59.

39. Kohgo Y, Ikuta K, Ohtake T, et al. Body iron metabolism and pathophysiology of iron overload. Int J Hematol 2008;88(1):7–15.

40. Hoffbrand AV, Taher A, Cappellini MD. How I treat transfusional iron overload. Blood 2012;120(18): 3657–69.

41. Au WY, Lam WM, Chu WC, et al. A magnetic resonance imaging study of iron overload in hemopoietic stem cell transplant recipients with increased ferritin levels. Transplant Proc 2007;39(10):3369–74.

42. Wood JC. Guidelines for quantifying iron overload. Hematology 2014;2014(1):210–5.

43. Maximova N, Gregori M, Boz G, et al. MRI-based evaluation of multiorgan iron overload is a predictor of adverse outcomes in pediatric patients undergoing allogeneic hematopoietic stem cell transplantation. Oncotarget 2017;8(45):79650–61.

44. Wurschi GW, Mentzel H-J, Herrmann K-H, et al. MRI as an alternative to serum ferritin for diagnosis of iron overload in children in the context of immune response after stem cell transplantation. Pediatr Transplant 2019;23(8):e13583.

45. Batts KP. Iron overload syndromes and the liver. Mod Pathol 2007;20(Suppl 1):S31–9.

46. Lai X, Liu L, Zhang Z, et al. Hepatic veno-occlusive disease/sinusoidal obstruction syndrome after hematopoietic stem cell transplantation for thalassemia

major: incidence, management, and outcome. Bone Marrow Transplant 2021;56(7):1635–41.

47. Marty FM, Baden LR. Infection in the hematopoietic stem cell transplant recipient. Hematopoietic Stem Cell Transplantation 2008;421–48. https://doi.org/10.1007/978-1-59745-438-4_19.

48. Trottier BJ, Burns LJ, DeFor TE, et al. Association of iron overload with allogeneic hematopoietic cell transplantation outcomes: a prospective cohort study using R2-MRI-measured liver iron content. Blood 2013;122(9):1678–84.

49. Armand P, Sainvil M-M, Kim HT, et al. Does iron overload really matter in stem cell transplantation? Am J Hematol 2012;87(6):569–72.

50. Deeg HJ, Spaulding E, Shulman HM. Iron overload, hematopoietic cell transplantation, and graft-versus-host disease. Leuk Lymphoma 2009;50(10):1566–72.

51. Kamble RT, Selby GB, Mims M, et al. Iron overload manifesting as apparent exacerbation of hepatic graft-versus-host disease after allogeneic hematopoietic stem cell transplantation. Biol Blood Marrow Transplant 2006;12(5):506–10.

52. Ramaprasad C, Pursell KJ. Infectious complications of stem cell transplantation. In: Stosor V, Zembower TR, editors. Infectious complications in cancer patients. Cham: Springer International Publishing; 2014. p. 351–70.

53. Stern L, Withers B, Avdic S, et al. Human cytomegalovirus latency and reactivation in allogeneic hematopoietic stem cell transplant recipients. Front Microbiol 2019;10:1186.

54. Ru Y, Zhang X, Song T, et al. Epstein–Barr virus reactivation after allogeneic hematopoietic stem cell transplantation: multifactorial impact on transplant outcomes. Bone Marrow Transplant 2020;55(9):1754–62.

55. Schechter S, Lamps L. Epstein-Barr virus hepatitis: a review of clinicopathologic features and differential diagnosis. Arch Pathol Lab Med 2018;142(10):1191–5.

56. Torbenson MS, Moreira RK, Zhang L. Surgical pathology of the liver. Philadelphia, PA: lippincott williams & wilkins; 2017.

57. Suh N, Liapis H, Misdraji J, et al. Epstein-Barr virus hepatitis: diagnostic value of in situ hybridization, polymerase chain reaction, and immunohistochemistry on liver biopsy from immunocompetent patients. Am J Surg Pathol 2007;31(9):1403–9.

58. Randhawa PS, Markin RS, Starzl TE, et al. Epstein-Barr virus-associated syndromes in immunosuppressed liver transplant recipients. Clinical profile and recognition on routine allograft biopsy. Am J Surg Pathol 1990;14(6):538–47.

59. Taylor AL, Marcus R, Bradley JA. Post-transplant lymphoproliferative disorders (PTLD) after solid organ transplantation. Crit Rev Oncol Hematol 2005;56(1):155–67.

60. Quintanilla-Martinez L, Swerdlow SH, Tousseyn T, et al. New concepts in EBV-associated B, T, and NK cell lymphoproliferative disorders. Virchows Arch 2023;482(1):227–44.

61. Randhawa PS, Jaffe R, Demetris AJ, et al. Expression of Epstein-Barr virus-encoded small RNA (by the EBER-1 gene) in liver specimens from transplant recipients with post-transplantation lymphoproliferative disease. N Engl J Med 1992;327(24):1710–4.

62. Nelson BP, Wolniak KL, Evens A, et al. Early posttransplant lymphoproliferative disease: clinicopathologic features and correlation with mTOR signaling pathway activation. Am J Clin Pathol 2012;138(4):568–78.

63. George B, Pati N, Gilroy N, et al. Pre-transplant cytomegalovirus (CMV) serostatus remains the most important determinant of CMV reactivation after allogeneic hematopoietic stem cell transplantation in the era of surveillance and preemptive therapy. Transpl Infect Dis 2010;12(4):322–9.

64. McDonald GB, Sarmiento JI, Rees-Lui G, et al. Cytomegalovirus hepatitis after bone marrow transplantation: an autopsy study with clinical, histologic and laboratory correlates. J Viral Hepat 2019; 26(11):1344–50.

65. Keramari S, Poutoglidou F, Poutoglidis A, et al. Adenoviral infections in bone marrow transplanted adult patients: a review of the 44 cases reported in the last 25 years. Cureus. 13(11), 2021, e19865.

66. Baldwin A, Kingman H, Darville M, et al. Outcome and clinical course of 100 patients with adenovirus infection following bone marrow transplantation. Bone Marrow Transplant 2000;26(12):1333–8.

67. Chakrabarti S, Mautner V, Osman H, et al. Adenovirus infections following allogeneic stem cell transplantation: incidence and outcome in relation to graft manipulation, immunosuppression, and immune recovery. Blood 2002;100(5):1619–27.

68. Schaberg KB, Kambham N, Sibley RK, et al. Adenovirus hepatitis: clinicopathologic analysis of 12 consecutive cases from a single institution. Am J Surg Pathol 2017;41(6):810.

69. Uhlin M, Stikvoort A, Sundin M, et al. Risk factors and clinical outcome for herpes simplex virus reactivation in patients after allogeneic hematopoietic stem cell transplantation. Biol Blood Marrow Transplant 2015;21(2):S170.

70. Norvell JP, Blei AT, Jovanovic BD, et al. Herpes simplex virus hepatitis: an analysis of the published literature and institutional cases. Liver Transpl 2007; 13(10):1428–34.

Primary Sclerosing Cholangitis, Small Duct Primary Sclerosing Cholangitis, IgG4-Related Sclerosing Cholangitis, and Ischemic Cholangiopathy

Diagnostic Challenges on Biopsy

Katy L. Lawson, MD, Hanlin L. Wang, MD, PhD*

KEYWORDS

- Primary sclerosing cholangitis • Small duct primary sclerosing cholangitis
- IgG4-related sclerosing cholangitis • Ischemic cholangiopathy • Bile duct • Liver • Biopsy

Key Points

- Sclerosing bile duct injury and clinical cholestasis are nonspecific findings seen in many entities. On biopsy, pathologists are often forced to issue descriptive sign outs that require careful clinical correlation; however, certain clinical, radiologic, and pathologic features may help narrow the differential.

- Primary sclerosing cholangitis (PSC) is a diagnosis of exclusion that is strongly associated with inflammatory bowel disease (IBD), shows cholangiographic "beading" of the biliary tree, lacks effective treatment, and harbors an increased risk of malignancy, particularly cholangiocarcinoma.

- Small duct primary sclerosing cholangitis (sd-PSC) is a rare variant of PSC with normal cholangiography due to the pathologic stricturing of intrahepatic microscopic bile ducts. Despite its better prognosis, sd-PSC is a progressive disease that requires liver biopsy for diagnosis.

- IgG4-related sclerosing cholangitis (IgG4-SC) is often associated with other IgG4-related fibrosclerosing diseases, particularly autoimmune pancreatitis, and is remarkably steroid-responsive.

- Ischemic cholangiopathy results from impaired blood supply to the biliary tree, most often due to surgery, hepatic artery thrombosis/stenosis, or therapeutic infusion.

ABSTRACT

Pathologists face many challenges when diagnosing sclerosing biliary lesions on liver biopsy. First, histologic findings tend to be nonspecific with similar to identical features seen in numerous conditions, from benign to outright malignant. In addition, the patchy nature of many of these entities amplifies the inherent limitations of biopsy sampling. The end result often forces pathologists to issue descriptive sign outs that require careful clinical correlation; however, certain clinical, radiologic, and histologic features may be of diagnostic assistance. In this article, we review key elements of four sclerosing biliary processes whose proper identification has significant prognostic and therapeutic implications.

Department of Pathology and Laboratory Medicine, David Geffen School of Medicine, Ronald Reagan UCLA Medical Center, University of California Los Angeles, 10833 Le Conte Avenue, Los Angeles, CA 90095, USA
* Corresponding author.
E-mail address: hanlinwang@mednet.ucla.edu

Surgical Pathology 16 (2023) 533–548
https://doi.org/10.1016/j.path.2023.04.008
1875-9181/23/© 2023 Elsevier Inc. All rights reserved.

surgpath.theclinics.com

OVERVIEW

Primary sclerosing cholangitis (PSC), small duct primary sclerosing cholangitis (sd-PSC), IgG4-related sclerosing cholangitis (IgG4-SC), and ischemic cholangiopathy are distinct entities that share clinical and pathologic overlap and have major prognostic and therapeutic implications. Each may present with varying degrees of clinical cholestasis, ranging from asymptomatic elevations of serum alkaline phosphatase (ALP) to full stigmata of biliary cirrhosis. Their unifying histologic feature is biliary sclerosis, a nonspecific pathologic finding that likely represents a common final pathway for chronic bile duct injury of many causes. Distinction between these entities on biopsy is challenging; however, certain clinical, radiologic, and histologic findings may help narrow the differential. Here we review the clinicopathologic features and current literature of these sclerosing biliary processes to assist in diagnosis on biopsy.

PRIMARY SCLEROSING CHOLANGITIS

OVERVIEW OF PRIMARY SCLEROSING CHOLANGITIS

Primary sclerosing cholangitis is a rare, idiopathic, progressive biliary disease characterized by multifocal inflammation, fibrosis, and destruction of intra- and/or extrahepatic bile ducts, leading to biliary cirrhosis. PSC exhibits a highly variable clinical course; however, lack of effective treatment eventually necessitates liver transplantation. While definitive pathogenesis remains elusive, PSC is considered a heterogeneous disease with genetic, autoimmune, and inflammatory underpinnings. PSC is strongly associated with inflammatory bowel disease (IBD) and patients are at increased risk of associated malignancy, particularly cholangiocarcinoma. Diagnosis is based on characteristic cholangiographic findings in the proper clinical context. Liver biopsy is seldom indicated, but performed in patients with atypical clinical and/or radiological findings.

CLINICAL FEATURES OF PRIMARY SCLEROSING CHOLANGITIS

While epidemiologic statistics vary widely, PSC is a rare disease that affects less than 200,000 individuals in the US and less than 250,000 in the EU, with an estimated prevalence of 1 per 10,000.[1,2] Several studies indicate the incidence of PSC, like many other autoimmune and idiopathic inflammatory conditions, is inexplicably on the rise.[3,4]

Approximately 60% to 70% of PSC patients are male and the peak age at diagnosis is between 30 and 40 years.[5] Up to 80% of patients with PSC are diagnosed with IBD, most commonly ulcerative colitis.[6,7] Since the diagnosis of IBD may precede, follow, or occur concurrently with that of PSC, full staging intestinal biopsies at diagnosis and close clinicopathologic surveillance throughout the disease course are highly recommended.[8] Interestingly, patients with PSC-IBD appear to have a unique phenotype of IBD marked by earlier-in-life presentation and more extensive but less active, even asymptomatic, disease.[9] Recent genome-wide association studies (GWAS) further reveal genetic differences in IBD with and without PSC.[10] Up to 25% of patients with PSC harbor other autoimmune diseases, as well.[11]

The majority of patients with PSC present with indolent, asymptomatic disease; however, clinical courses are highly variable, ranging from years-long asymptomatic periods to a highly aggressive process with complications ranging from benign to malignant. Regardless of course, nearly all patients eventually progress to biliary cirrhosis. Factors such as patient age, sex, and type of associated IBD may affect prognosis.[12]

PSC is associated with a considerable risk for malignancies, which account for nearly half of PSC-related deaths.[13] The most notable is cholangiocarcinoma, where the risk is up to 1000 times higher than in the general population and 30% to 50% of cases occur within the first year following PSC diagnosis.[14] In patients with PSC-IBD, the risk of colorectal carcinoma is 10-fold higher and lifetime risk approaches 30%.[15] Increased frequencies of benign and malignant gallbladder abnormalities are also reported.[16] As such, current PSC recommendations advocate for serial imaging every 6 to 12 months and regular assessment of serum CA19-9 levels.[17]

Imaging plays an essential role in PSC diagnosis. Endoscopic retrograde cholangiopancreatography (ERCP), magnetic resonance cholangiopancreatography (MRCP), and direct cholangiography all yield the characteristic PSC findings: focal or multifocal stricturing with associated saccular dilation of intra- and extrahepatic bile ducts, lending a so-called "beads-on-a-string" appearance.[6] Pathologic sclerosis in PSC is patchy but may develop at all levels of the biliary tree. Given its favorable sensitivity, specificity, and cost-effectiveness, MRCP is the current modality of choice.[18]

Biochemical tests usually indicate a cholestatic profile with elevations of ALP and γ-glutamyl transferase (GGT; typically 2–3 times the upper limits of normal).[6] These enzymes may fluctuate due to the naturally waxing-waning course of the disease; thus, normal ALP and/or GGT levels do not necessarily exclude PSC diagnosis. Aminotransferase and bilirubin levels are often normal upon diagnosis, but may increase with disease progression. A wide range of nonspecific autoantibodies may be detected at relatively low titers, likely indicating general immune dysregulation. A small proportion of patients with PSC show elevated serum IgG4 concentrations, which seemingly portends a worse prognosis;[19] but otherwise fail to meet the diagnostic criteria for IgG4-SC (discussed later in discussion).

At this time, no effective medical treatments exist for PSC. Surgical management remains the mainstay of therapy. Biliary obstruction managed with ERCP stenting is performed only in patients with significant stricturing of extrahepatic and large intrahepatic bile ducts, so-called "dominant strictures," which affect 36% to 50% of patients and are associated with significantly worse outcomes.[8] Smaller bile duct radiological interventions are not yet feasible. Liver transplantation is the only curative therapy, with a median time of 10 to 12 years from diagnosis until transplantation[8] and 5-year survival rates of 80% to 85%.[20] Recurrence of PSC post-transplantation occurs in ~20% of patients.[21]

Lastly, PSC falls under a spectrum that includes two rare variants: sd-PSC (discussed later in discussion) and overlap syndrome with autoimmune hepatitis (PSC-AIH), which is outside the scope of this article but reviewed elsewhere.[22] Unlike PSC, both variants require tissue confirmation for diagnosis.

PATHOGENESIS OF PRIMARY SCLEROSING CHOLANGITIS

While considerable advances in understanding the pathogenesis of PSC have been made in recent years, a definitive etiology remains elusive. PSC's strong association with IBD and recent genetic studies point toward a component of autoimmunity, with over 20 associated genes currently identified that predominantly localize to the HLA complex or other loci related to adaptive immune function.[5,23] However, genetic determinants are seen in less than 10% of patients with PSC, clearly emphasizing a predominant role of environmental factors on ultimate disease susceptibility.[23] Disordered gut microbiota resulting in inflammatory "leakage" into portal circulation is another postulated etiology for bile duct damage.[24] So too is the inherent toxicity of bile, as well as the host protective mechanisms keeping bile in check.[25]

Unfortunately, pathogenic hypotheses run contradictory to therapy. The ineffectiveness of immunosuppressive or immunomodulatory drugs, the progression of PSC after colectomy (ie, in the absence of a "leaky gut"), and the little benefit derived from bile toxin-reducing agents all conspire to confound potential etiologies. Thus, PSC is currently considered a heterogeneous disease wherein immunologic priming in a genetically predisposed individual meets other possible confounding host or exogenous factors in a yet-unclear pathologic progression.

MICROSCOPIC FEATURES OF PRIMARY SCLEROSING CHOLANGITIS

Histologically, the classically-described "onion-skin" concentric bile duct fibrous obliteration is infrequently seen on tissue sampling, estimated to be found in less than 25% of needle biopsies, due to such fibrosis mainly involving medium-sized (septal) ducts that aren't routinely sampled by liver biopsy (**Fig. 1**).[26] More often, biopsy-based histologic findings are nonspecific and vary according to disease stage. In early or minimally-active stages, minimal to mild portal and periportal inflammation, predominantly lymphocytic, is seen. Bile ducts may show features of injury and degeneration characterized by nuclear disarray and cytoplasmic vacuolization and eosinophilia. Over time, there is progressive atrophy, narrowing, and eventual loss (ductopenia) of small and medium-sized bile ducts,[26] which may or may not leave a round fibroobliterative scar in portal tracts (**Fig. 2**). Chronic biliary injury and resultant cholestasis often lead to ductular reaction, accumulation of copper binding protein in periportal hepatocytes, and progressive periportal fibrosis, which ultimately leads to bridging fibrosis and biliary cirrhosis.[26] Extravasated bile may also elicit a granulomatous or xanthomatous response. A novel histologic classification system recently exhibited the most significant predictive value for PSC prognosis.[27]

DIAGNOSIS AND DIFFERENTIAL DIAGNOSIS OF PRIMARY SCLEROSING CHOLANGITIS

PSC is diagnosed on clinical and biochemical findings of cholestasis in conjunction with characteristic multifocal strictures of the intra- and/or extrahepatic bile ducts that lend a so-called "beads-on-a-string" appearance on cholangiography (**Fig. 3**). It is a diagnosis of exclusion that requires clinical exclusion of secondary sclerosing cholangitis. Rather uniquely, invasive liver biopsy is not a diagnostic requirement and may indeed

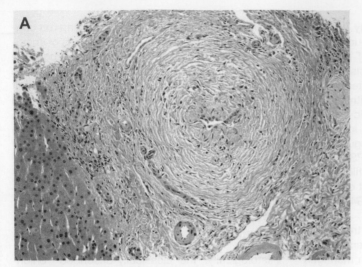

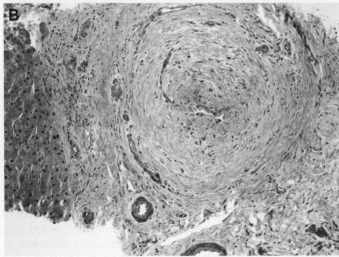

Fig. 1. The classic "onion-skin" lesion of PSC characterized by concentric fibrosis around a bile duct. There is marked luminal narrowing with epithelial degeneration and atrophy. Minimal lymphocytic infiltrates and mild ductular reaction are noted in the portal tract (A; original magnification x200). "Onion-skin" fibrosis is better demonstrated on trichrome stain (B; original magnification x200).

fail to capture pathologic findings given the patchy nature of stricturing disease.[28] Liver biopsy may be performed to assess disease severity or to rule out PSC variants, comorbidities, or malignancy. Because PSC is a diagnosis of exclusion and histologic findings are nonspecific, pathologists often resort to descriptive sign outs with findings "compatible with PSC in the correct clinical setting."

Differential diagnoses of PSC include sd-PSC, IgG4-SC, and ischemic cholangiopathy (Table 1), each discussed later in discussion; in addition to many other disorders that lead to biliary strictures (so-called "secondary sclerosing cholangitis"), such as longstanding mechanical biliary obstruction, infectious cholangitis including AIDS-related cholangiopathy, prior biliary surgery, and drug-induced bile duct injury, among others (Table 2). Complete biochemical testing and extensive clinical history are critical for excluding other diagnoses and detecting overlap/variant conditions.

Pitfalls
IN DIAGNOSING PRIMARY SCLEROSING CHOLANGITIS

!PSC is a radiological and clinical diagnosis of exclusion. When performed, liver biopsy may show nonspecific portal inflammation, features of bile duct injury and degeneration, ductopenia, "onion-skin" periduct concentric fibrosis, and varying degrees of fibrosis.

!Cholangiocarcinoma must be considered in every PSC biopsy and explant given the increased risk.

!Elevated IgG4 levels (often 1.5x normal) are seen in a subset of patients with PSC and should be interpreted alongside the diagnostic criteria of IgG4-SC to avoid this pitfall.

Fig. 2. Ductopenia seen in a PSC case. The hepatic artery and portal vein branches are present. Cholestasis is noted in liver parenchyma (*A*; original magnification x200). The bile duct is entirely replaced by a round fibroobliterative scar (*arrow*) in another PSC case (*B*; original magnification x200).

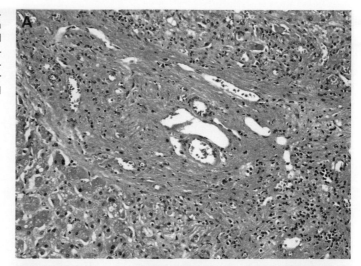

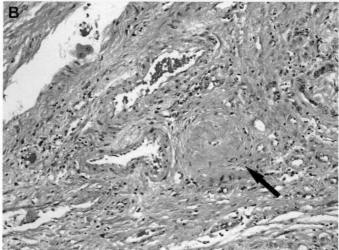

SMALL DUCT PRIMARY SCLEROSING CHOLANGITIS

OVERVIEW OF SMALL DUCT PRIMARY SCLEROSING CHOLANGITIS

The sd-PSC variant is clinically and histologically identical to its large duct ("classic") counterpart, but is uniquely undetectable on cholangiography due to stricuting of intrahepatic microscopic bile ducts and thus requires histologic evaluation for diagnosis. While sd-PSC portends a better prognosis than classic PSC, it is considered a progressive disease that may result in biliary cirrhosis independently or through progression to large duct PSC. Transplantation is the only cure, and post-transplant recurrence has been reported.

CLINICAL FEATURES OF SMALL DUCT PRIMARY SCLEROSING CHOLANGITIS

sd-PSC is very rare, occurring in estimated 0.15 per 100,000 individuals and accounts for ∼6% of the entire PSC spectrum.[29] There are no specific clinical or biochemical features that distinguish small duct from large duct PSC, although sd-PSC may be more likely to be associated with Crohn disease.[30] Thus, suspicion for sd-PSC arises only when cholangiography fails to detect the characteristic "beading" in a patient otherwise suspected to have PSC.[31]

Despite sd-PSC's variable clinical course, multiple studies demonstrate a more favorable long-term prognosis marked by overall- and liver-related morbidity and mortality compared to

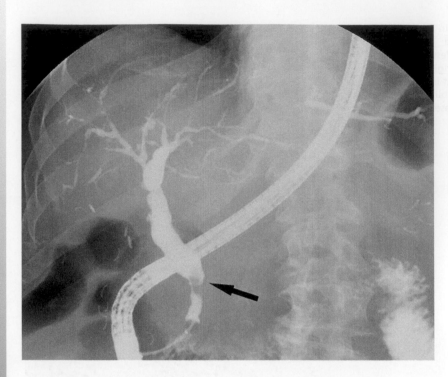

Fig. 3. ERCP showing multiple segmental strictures of the biliary tree in a PSC patient. A dominant stricture with upstream dilation is seen in the distal common bile duct (*arrow*).

classic PSC.[31–34] Further, sd-PSC is not at increased risk for cholangiocarcinoma.[31] However, sd-PSC is considered a progressive disease that may independently result in death or end-stage liver disease requiring transplantation.[31] Interestingly, approximately 25% of patients progress to large duct PSC, with its attendant cholangiographic features, associated malignancy risk, and potential for biliary cirrhosis.[31,33] This progression has led some to conclude that sd-PSC is a precursor to large duct disease, although sd-PSC's ability to independently progress to end-stage liver disease hints at more complex biologic interplay.

MICROSCOPIC FEATURES OF SMALL DUCT PRIMARY SCLEROSING CHOLANGITIS

Liver biopsy is necessary to diagnose sd-PSC, whose histologic features are indistinguishable from those of large duct PSC (detailed above). The patchy nature of the disease and inherent sampling bias are major limitations of biopsy. Like classic PSC, histologic features of sd-PSC can be nonspecific and pathologists often resort to descriptive sign outs requiring clinical correlation.

DIAGNOSIS AND DIFFERENTIAL DIAGNOSIS OF SMALL DUCT PRIMARY SCLEROSING CHOLANGITIS

sd-PSC is a diagnosis of exclusion in patients with clinical and biochemical cholestasis, normal cholangiogram, and liver biopsy findings compatible with PSC histology. Differential diagnoses include those for large duct PSC (detailed above), and adult-onset bile acid transport disorders, which may be similar or identical to all aspects of sd-PSC diagnosis but require heightened clinical awareness, strong family history documentation, and genetic testing to confirm.[35]

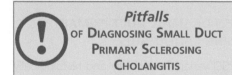

> ### Pitfalls
> OF DIAGNOSING SMALL DUCT PRIMARY SCLEROSING CHOLANGITIS
>
> !A negative cholangiogram does not rule out the PSC spectrum. In patients highly suspicious for PSC, a liver biopsy is necessary to exclude sd-PSC.
>
> !Like large duct PSC, the histologic features of sd-PSC are often nonspecific and require clinical correlation.
>
> !Adult-onset bile acid transport disorders are underrecognized differential diagnoses that must be considered in patients with family histories of cholestatic liver disease and/or lack of the common PSC association with IBD.

Table 1
Histologic features of sclerosing cholangitides that may help guide differential on biopsy

Nonspecific features that may be shared by all entities	Fibrous bile duct obliteration
	Portal and periportal inflammation
	Progressive atrophy, narrowing, and eventual loss of bile ducts
	Cholestasis
	Ductular reaction
	Accumulation of copper binding protein in periportal hepatocytes
	Progressive portal-based fibrosis, which ultimately leads to biliary cirrhosis
	Granulomatous or xanthomatous response due to extravasated bile
IgG4-SC	Denser inflammatory cell infiltrates rich in plasma cells
	Increased IgG4+ cells by immunohistochemistry
	Storiform fibrosis
	Portal-based fibroinflammatory nodules
Ischemic cholangiopathy	Bile casts
	Bilomas

Table 2
Etiologies of sclerosing cholangitides with overlapping histologic features to classic PSC

Immunologic	Primary sclerosing cholangitis
	Small duct primary sclerosing cholangitis
	IgG4-related sclerosing cholangitis
	Eosinophilic cholangitis
	Mast cell cholangiopathy
	Langerhans cell histiocytosis
	Systemic vasculitis
	Primary biliary cholangitis
	Sarcoidosis
	Amyloidosis
Infectious	AIDS cholangiopathy (Cryptosporidium parvum, CMV, Microsporidia, and so forth)
	Helminth infection (Clonorchis, Opisthorchis, Ascaris, and so forth)
	Bacterial cholangitis (Escherichia coli, Klebsiella, Pseudomonas, Proteus sp., and so forth)
	Ascending cholangitis
Congenital	Caroli disease
	Cystic fibrosis
Neoplasm-associated	Masses of extrahepatic bile duct, pancreatic head, and ampulla
	Intraductal papillary neoplasms of bile duct
	Diffuse intrahepatic malignancies (primary and metastatic)
	Hodgkin lymphoma
Iatrogenic and therapy-related	Hepatic transplantation (due to ischemia, allograft rejection, or infection)
	Postoperative stricturing
	Intra-arterial chemotherapy infusion (fluoropyrimidines)
	Radiation therapy
	Drugs (amoxicillin-clavulanic acid, ketamine, and so forth)
Miscellaneous	Ischemic cholangiopathy
	Cholangiolithiasis

Abbreviations: AIDS, acquired immunodeficiency syndrome; CMV, cytomegalovirus; PSC, primary sclerosing cholangitis.

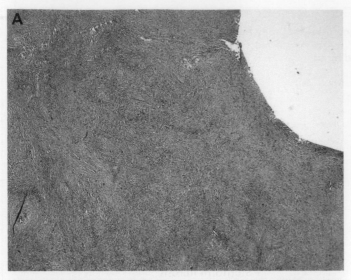

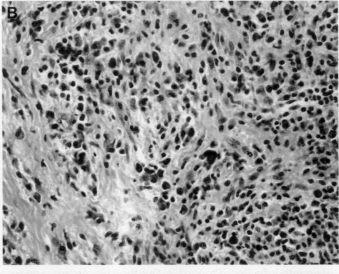

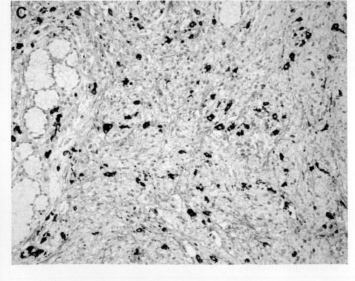

Fig. 4. IgG4-SC showing transmural inflammatory cell infiltrates in a fibrotic background with a storiform appearance seen in a common bile duct resection (*A*; original magnification x20). The inflammatory infiltrates consist of plasma cells and lymphocytes with scattered eosinophils (*B*; original magnification x400). Numerous IgG4+ plasma cells are demonstrated by immunohistochemistry (*C*; original magnification x200).

Fig. 5. A biopsy of strictured left hepatic duct from a patient with clinically suspected IgG4-SC showing dense inflammatory cell infiltrates in a fibrotic background with no storiform pattern. The mucosal surface is eroded and denuded due to prior stent placement (A; original magnification x100). Higher power view showing prominent plasma cells with scattered lymphocytes and neutrophils (B; original magnification x400). Numerous IgG4+ plasma cells are demonstrated by immunohistochemistry (C; original magnification x400).

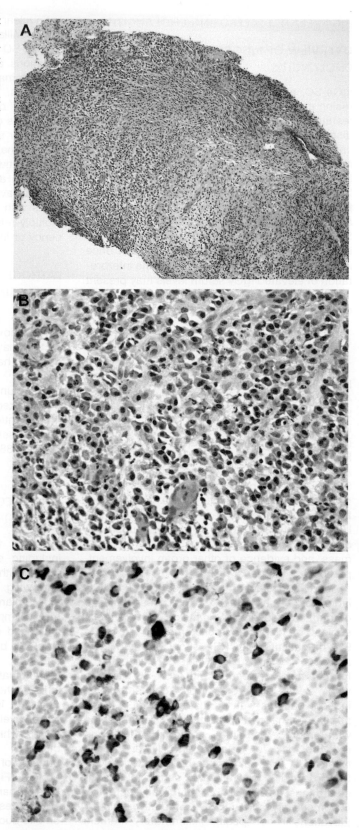

IgG4-RELATED SCLEROSING CHOLANGITIS

OVERVIEW OF IgG4-RELATED SCLEROSING CHOLANGITIS

IgG4-SC, also known as IgG4-associated sclerosing cholangitis (IAC), is a hepatobiliary manifestation of IgG4-related fibroinflammatory diseases that frequently co-presents with autoimmune pancreatitis (AIP), but may otherwise mimic PSC clinically, radiologically, and histologically. Distinction between the 2 is crucial as IgG4-SC may completely resolve with steroid therapy and has a more favorable prognosis if appropriately managed. So important is IgG4-SC diagnosis that current recommendations include testing serum IgG4 levels at least once in all patients with PSC.[20] However, the interpretation of elevated IgG4 serum levels may present its own challenges and appropriate diagnosis requires careful clinicopathologic correlation.

CLINICAL FEATURES OF IgG4-RELATED SCLEROSING CHOLANGITIS

IgG4-SC is rare, with an estimated prevalence of 4.6 per 100,000 individuals.[36] Like PSC, IgG4-SC is male-predominant and presents with clinical cholestasis; though patients tend to be older (mean age: 63 years, compared to 44 years for PSC) and have a high coexistence of AIP.[37,38] AIP is seen in over 90% of patients with IgG4-SC at presentation and may serve as its first clue.[37,38] Radiologic features are variable, but frequently include long and multifocal strictures involving any part of the biliary tree, upstream dilatation, thickened bile duct walls, a liver/hilar mass, and evidence of other organ involvement, particularly the pancreas.[39]

Apart from biochemical cholestasis, IgG4-SC laboratory results range from nonspecific to outright troublesome. Serum IgG4 levels are a subject of diagnostic consternation, as up to 9% of patients with PSC show elevated IgG4 and no specific cut-off value is delineated.[19] Further, not every patient with IgG4-SC presents with elevated serum IgG4 concentrations; indeed, patients with normal serum IgG4 levels appear to have a distinct clinical phenotype with more favorable prognosis, including reduced risk for relapse and fewer organs involved.[40] That said, when patients with IgG4-SC do present with elevated serum IgG4 concentrations, a value of $\geq$2.8 g/L greatly increases the specificity and negative predictive value.[40] Elevations in nonspecific inflammatory markers and IgE may be seen, along with positive antinuclear antibody titers and peripheral eosinophilia.[41]

IgG4-SC diagnosis has major therapeutic implications as immediate treatment, even when asymptomatic, may prevent hepatobiliary complications. Systemic corticosteroids are the mainstay of therapy and induce remission in two-thirds of patients; however, relapse is common after steroid withdrawal.[28,42] The presence of proximal extrahepatic/intrahepatic strictures is predictive of relapse.[38] Rituximab, a CD20-depletion agent, and other immunosuppressive agents have found success in a subset of patients with IgG4-SC with incomplete remission, multiply-relapsed disease, or steroid dependency or intolerance.[43]

PATHOGENESIS OF IgG4-RELATED SCLEROSING CHOLANGITIS

Definitive pathogenesis of IgG4-SC remains elusive, however autoimmune and environmental factors may play a role. A history of allergy and/or atopy has been described in 40% to 60% of patients.[41] Up to 10% of patients have other autoimmune conditions.[42] IgG4-SC has also been linked with chronic exposure to occupational antigens (such as solvents, industrial dusts, pesticides, industrial oils or polymers) in 52% to 88% of patients in the UK and Dutch cohorts.[44]

MICROSCOPIC FEATURES OF IgG4-RELATED SCLEROSING CHOLANGITIS

IgG4-SC typically affects large bile ducts, including extrahepatic, hilar and perihilar bile ducts, with marked wall thickening and luminal narrowing. Histologically, it shows significantly more inflammation than PSC, with dense transmural lymphoplasmacytic infiltrates, often with increased eosinophils.[37] Neutrophils are inconspicuous but can be prominent in the area of ulceration. Lymphoid aggregates and focal granulomatous inflammation can be seen. The inflammation may surround bile ducts but usually does not involve biliary epithelium and instead targets veins (so-called "perivenular accentuation"), which may result in obliterative phlebitis.[45,46] The background shows varying degrees of fibrosis that may assume a storiform pattern (**Fig. 4**). It should be emphasized that these characteristic features readily recognizable on resection specimens may not be evident on bile duct biopsies due to the small size of the specimens, crushing artifact, and compounding inflammation/ulceration associated with stent placement (**Fig. 5**).

When intrahepatic small bile ducts are involved, the typical features of IgG4-SC described above may not be prominent. A liver biopsy may show nonspecific portal and lobular inflammation, cholestasis, bile duct injury, and varying degrees of portal-based fibrosis. A rather unique feature seen in ~50% of cases is the presence of portal-based fibroinflammatory nodules composed of lymphocytes, plasma cells, eosinophils, fibroblasts, and myofibroblasts (**Fig. 6**).[37] The typical changes of other chronic biliary diseases, such as florid ductal lesion in primary biliary cholangitis or "onion-skin" fibrosis in PSC, are not seen.[46] Liver biopsy for diagnosis of IgG4-SC is seldom made given its notoriously low sensitivity.

DIAGNOSIS AND DIFFERENTIAL DIAGNOSIS OF IgG4-RELATED SCLEROSING CHOLANGITIS

IgG4-SC is diagnosed using an adaption of the HISORt (Histology, Imaging, Serology, Other organ involvement, and Response to therapy) criteria for AIP, on the basis of two or more main manifestations.[38] These include elevated serum IgG4 levels, suggestive pancreatic imaging findings, other organ involvement, and biopsy or resection specimens showing increased IgG4+ plasma cells, combined with a significant response to corticosteroid treatment (**Table 3**).[47] Greater than 10 IgG4+ cells per high-power field (HPF) in a biopsy or greater than 50 in a resection specimen, along with an IgG4/IgG ratio greater than 40% are considered diagnostic.[48] Importantly, an abundance of IgG4+ cells alone is not sufficient for diagnosis as these cells may be seen in PSC and other conditions.[49] Differential diagnoses are similar to those for PSC, with particular attention to inflammatory cell-rich conditions like infectious cholangitides and lymphomas.

Pitfalls
OF DIAGNOSING
IgG4-RELATED
SCLEROSING CHOLANGITIS

!Not every patient with IgG4-SC presents with elevated serum IgG4 concentrations, and low levels may be seen in many other conditions including PSC.

!Increased IgG4+ plasma cells on biopsy may be seen in other conditions such as PSC and cholangiocarcinoma.

!The presence of concomitant AIP combined with histologic features of dense lymphoplasmacytic infiltrates, storiform fibrosis, obliterative phlebitis, and increased IgG4+ cells greatly raises suspicion for IgG4-SC.

!Interpretation of IgG4 and IgG immunostains may be troublesome due to high background staining (particularly IgG).

ISCHEMIC CHOLANGIOPATHY

OVERVIEW OF ISCHEMIC CHOLANGIOPATHY

Ischemic cholangiopathy, also known as ischemic cholangitis, results in focal to extensive bile duct damage due to the impairment of the peribiliary vascular plexus (PVP), which is supplied exclusively by the hepatic arteries (HA). Most biliary ischemic events are iatrogenic; however, a host of systemic diseases and inflammatory states may also induce ischemia. Depending on the extent and velocity of the arterial obstructive process, ischemic cholangiopathy may present acutely with necrosis and biliary casts, or chronically with sclerosing histologic findings resembling PSC.

CLINICAL FEATURES OF ISCHEMIC CHOLANGIOPATHY

Patients with ischemic cholangiopathy classically present with a range of clinical findings, from asymptomatic elevations in ALP to end-stage liver disease with its attendant stigmata. Since blood is supplied to the intra- and extrahepatic bile ducts solely via the HAs, disruptions tend to proportionally affect the biliary system they supply.

The predominant site of ischemic injury is the middle third of the common bile duct, followed by the hepatic duct confluence, with intrahepatic involvement being the least common.[50] Radiologic features correspond to the stage of ischemic injury, ranging from intraductal filling defects in the early stages to collections of bile-stained necrosum (so-called "bilomas") seen in severe manifestations.[51]

PATHOGENESIS OF ISCHEMIC CHOLANGIOPATHY

Proximal blockade of large HAs is mostly seen in the transplant setting with HA thrombosis. Distal blockade of small hepatic arterioles and the PVP is most often attributed to HA infusion with chemotherapeutic agents, advanced AIDS, hereditary

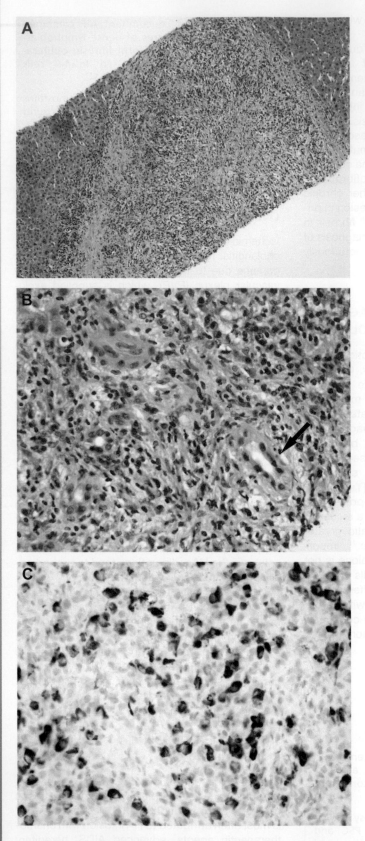

Fig. 6. A liver biopsy from a patient with elevated serum IgG4 levels and abnormal MRCP findings similar to those of PSC showing a portal-based fibroinflammatory nodule (*A*; original magnification x100). Features of bile duct injury are noted (*arrow*) but "onion-skin" fibrosis is not evident (*B*; original magnification x400). Numerous IgG4+ plasma cells are demonstrated by immunohistochemistry (*C*; original magnification x400).

Table 3
HISORt diagnostic criteria for IgG4-SC diagnosis[a]

Histology of biopsy	>10 IgG4+ plasma cells/HPF Plus features described in **Table 1**
Imaging	One or more strictures involving intrapancreatic, intrahepatic or extrahepatic bile ducts Strictures may migrate over time
Serology	Increased serum IgG4 concentration
Other organ involvement	Pancreatic lesions including: classic features of AIP on imaging or histology (seen in >90% of patients with IgG4-SC), enlargement, mass lesion, focal pancreatic duct structuring, and atrophy Retroperitoneal fibrosis Renal lesions Salivary or lacrimal gland enlargement
Response to steroid therapy	Normalization of liver enzymes within 4–6 wk with or without complete resolution of stricturing on imaging

Abbreviations: AIP, autoimmune pancreatitis; HISORt, Histology, Imaging, Serology, Other organ involvement, and Response to therapy; HPF, high power field; IgG4-SC, IgG4-related sclerosing cholangitis.
[a] Adapted and modified for diagnosis of IgG4-SC from Ghazale A, et al. Gastroenterology. 2008; 134 (3):706-715 (ref.[38]).

hemorrhagic telangiectasia, polyarteritis nodosa, atherosclerosis, radiation therapy, and various insults from liver transplantation, including reperfusion injury, ABO incompatibility, rejection, and CMV infection.[50]

MICROSCOPIC FEATURES OF ISCHEMIC CHOLANGIOPATHY

Ischemic biliary injury shows variable histologic findings, likely depending on the acuity and extent of hepatic arterial interruption and the underlying condition. Early stages of ischemia may result in biliary epithelial injury leading to nuclear pyknosis, cytoplasmic eosinophilia and vacuolization, necrosis, sloughing, and bile casts (a mixture of desquamated biliary epithelium and bile), which may in turn obstruct and/or dilate the bile ducts.[51] Full thickness biliary necrosis is usually the result of acute and complete blockage of arterial blood supply, typically seen in liver transplantation complicated by HA thrombosis. Bilomas are another finding of severe ischemia resulting from bile constituent spill-over first into the portal tract then parenchyma, causing necrosis and formation of intrahepatic collections of bile-stained necrosum. Bile duct stenosis with periductal fibrosis, epithelial atrophy, and eventually ductopenia similar to that seen in PSC is often seen in response to prior acute injury or as part of a more insidious or chronic arterial impairment.[51] In severe cases, the liver parenchyma may also show features of ischemic injury such as zone 3 necrosis, hepatocyte ballooning, and cholestasis.

Ischemic cholangiopathy is challenging to demonstrate on liver biopsy since intrahepatic biliary involvement is the least common site of involvement. In these instances, rather than commenting directly on biliary pathology, pathologists are often forced to rely on surrogate parenchymal changes and write descriptive sign outs requiring clinical correlation.

DIAGNOSIS AND DIFFERENTIAL DIAGNOSIS OF ISCHEMIC CHOLANGIOPATHY

Ischemic cholangiopathy is usually diagnosed by MR cholangiography showing compromised arterial blood supply. If biopsy is performed and captures an affected region, bile casts and bilomas are relatively specific for ischemic injury. Sclerosis and bile duct loss are seen in the later phase of the diseases (**Fig. 7**). Differential diagnoses primarily include PSC, infectious cholangitis, and chronic ductopenic rejection in liver transplant.

DISCLOSURE

The authors have no commercial or financial conflicts of interest to disclose.

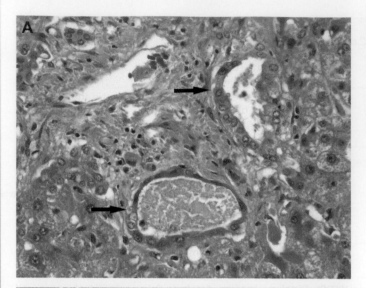

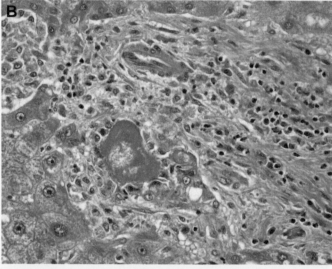

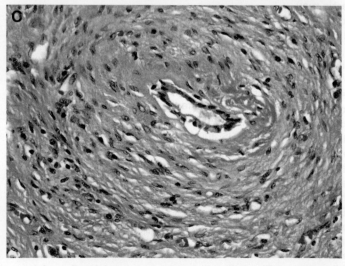

Fig. 7. Ischemic cholangiopathy showing features of biliary injury with bile casts (*arrows*) (*A*; original magnification x400); bile duct necrosis and bile leakage into the portal tract with inflammatory response (*B*; original magnification x400); and periduct fibrosis with epithelial atrophy mimicking PSC (*C*; original magnification x400).

Pitfalls
OF DIAGNOSING ISCHEMIC
CHOLANGIOPATHY

!The most common mechanisms for ischemic biliary injury are complications of liver transplantation and HA infusion of chemotherapeutic agents; thus, sclerosing lesions with or without bile duct obliteration should always be interpreted with caution in these patients.

!MR cholangiography is highly recommended for diagnostic assistance.

REFERENCES

1. Jepsen P, Grønbæk L, Vilstrup H. Worldwide incidence of autoimmune liver disease. Dig Dis 2015; 33(Suppl 2):2–12.

2. Molodecky NA, Kareemi H, Parab R, et al. Incidence of primary sclerosing cholangitis: a systematic review and meta-analysis. Hepatology 2011;53(5): 1590–9.

3. Bambha K, Kim WR, Talwalkar J, et al. Incidence, clinical spectrum, and outcomes of primary sclerosing cholangitis in a United States community. Gastroenterology 2003;125(5):1364–9.

4. Boonstra K, Weersma RK, van Erpecum KJ, et al. Population-based epidemiology, malignancy risk, and outcome of primary sclerosing cholangitis. Hepatology 2013;58(6):2045–55.

5. Hirschfield GM, Karlsen TH, Lindor KD, et al. Primary sclerosing cholangitis. Lancet 2013;382(9904): 1587–99.

6. Chapman R, Fevery J, Kalloo A, et al. Diagnosis and management of primary sclerosing cholangitis. Hepatology 2010;51(2):660–78.

7. Tischendorf JJ, Hecker H, Krüger M, et al. Characterization, outcome, and prognosis in 273 patients with primary sclerosing cholangitis: a single center study. Am J Gastroenterol 2007;102(1):107–14.

8. Chapman MH, Thorburn D, Hirschfield GM, et al. British Society of Gastroenterology and UK-PSC guidelines for the diagnosis and management of primary sclerosing cholangitis. Gut 2019;68(8): 1356–78.

9. Palmela C, Peerani F, Castaneda D, et al. Inflammatory bowel disease and primary sclerosing cholangitis: a review of the phenotype and associated specific features. Gut Liver 2018;12(1):17–29.

10. Ji SG, Juran BD, Mucha S, et al. Genome-wide association study of primary sclerosing cholangitis identifies new risk loci and quantifies the genetic relationship with inflammatory bowel disease. Nat Genet 2017;49(2):269–73.

11. Saarinen S, Olerup O, Broomé U. Increased frequency of autoimmuno diseases in patients with primary sclerosing cholangitis. Am J Gastroenterol 2000;95(11):3195–9.

12. Weismüller TJ, Trivedi PJ, Bergquist A, et al. Patient age, sex, and inflammatory bowel disease phenotype associate with course of primary sclerosing cholangitis. Gastroenterology 2017;152(8):1975–84.e8.

13. Fung BM, Lindor KD, Tabibian JH. Cancer risk in primary sclerosing cholangitis: epidemiology, prevention, and surveillance strategies. World J Gastroenterol 2019;25(6):659–71.

14. Song J, Li Y, Bowlus CL, et al. Cholangiocarcinoma in patients with primary sclerosing cholangitis (PSC): a comprehensive review. Clin Rev Allergy Immunol 2020;58(1):134–49.

15. Soetikno RM, Lin OS, Heidenreich PA, et al. Increased risk of colorectal neoplasia in patients with primary sclerosing cholangitis and ulcerative colitis: a meta-analysis. Gastrointest Endosc 2002; 56(1):48–54.

16. Said K, Glaumann H, Bergquist A. Gallbladder disease in patients with primary sclerosing cholangitis. J Hepatol 2008;48(4):598–605.

17. Endoscopy ESoG, easloffice@easloffice.eu EAftSotLEa, Liver EAftSot. Role of endoscopy in primary sclerosing cholangitis: European Society of Gastrointestinal Endoscopy (ESGE) and European Association for the Study of the Liver (EASL) clinical guideline. J Hepatol 2017;66(6):1265–81.

18. Dave M, Elmunzer BJ, Dwamena BA, et al. Primary sclerosing cholangitis: meta-analysis of diagnostic performance of MR cholangiopancreatography. Radiology 2010;256(2):387–96.

19. Mendes FD, Jorgensen R, Keach J, et al. Elevated serum IgG4 concentration in patients with primary sclerosing cholangitis. Am J Gastroenterol 2006; 101(9):2070–5.

20. Lindor KD, Kowdley KV, Harrison ME. ACG clinical guideline: primary sclerosing cholangitis. Am J Gastroenterol 2015;110(5):646–59, [quiz: 660].

21. Hildebrand T, Pannicke N, Dechene A, et al. Biliary strictures and recurrence after liver transplantation for primary sclerosing cholangitis: a retrospective multicenter analysis. Liver Transpl 2016;22(1):42–52.

22. Boberg KM, Chapman RW, Hirschfield GM, et al. Overlap syndromes: the International Autoimmune Hepatitis Group (IAIHG) position statement on a controversial issue. J Hepatol 2011;54(2):374–85.

23. Karlsen TH, Folseraas T, Thorburn D, et al. Primary sclerosing cholangitis: a comprehensive review. J Hepatol 2017;67(6):1298–323.

24. Little R, Wine E, Kamath BM, et al. Gut microbiome in primary sclerosing cholangitis: a review. World J Gastroenterol 2020;26(21):2768–80.

25. Trottier J, Białek A, Caron P, et al. Metabolomic profiling of 17 bile acids in serum from patients

with primary biliary cirrhosis and primary sclerosing cholangitis: a pilot study. Dig Liver Dis 2012;44(4): 303–10.

26. Portmann B, Zen Y. Inflammatory disease of the bile ducts-cholangiopathies: liver biopsy challenge and clinicopathological correlation. Histopathology 2012; 60(2):236–48.

27. Sjöblom N, Boyd S, Kautiainen H, et al. Novel histological scoring for predicting disease outcome in primary sclerosing cholangitis. Histopathology 2022;81(2): 192–204.

28. Burak KW, Angulo P, Lindor KD. Is there a role for liver biopsy in primary sclerosing cholangitis? Am J Gastroenterol 2003;98(5):1155–8.

29. Kaplan GG, Laupland KB, Butzner D, et al. The burden of large and small duct primary sclerosing cholangitis in adults and children: a population-based analysis. Am J Gastroenterol 2007;102(5):1042–9.

30. Fevery J, Van Steenbergen W, Van Pelt J, et al. Patients with large-duct primary sclerosing cholangitis and Crohn's disease have a better outcome than those with ulcerative colitis, or without IBD. Aliment Pharmacol Ther 2016;43(5):612–20.

31. Björnsson E, Olsson R, Bergquist A, et al. The natural history of small-duct primary sclerosing cholangitis. Gastroenterology 2008;134(4):975–80.

32. Angulo P, Maor-Kendler Y, Lindor KD. Small-duct primary sclerosing cholangitis: a long-term follow-up study. Hepatology 2002;35(6):1494–500.

33. Broomé U, Glaumann H, Lindström E, et al. Natural history and outcome in 32 Swedish patients with small duct primary sclerosing cholangitis (PSC). J Hepatol 2002;36(5):586–9.

34. Nikolaidis NL, Giouleme OI, Tziomalos KA, et al. Small-duct primary sclerosing cholangitis: a single-center seven-year experience. Dig Dis Sci 2005; 50(2):324–6.

35. Miller GC, Clouston AD. Adult onset of genetic disorders in bile acid transport in the liver. Hum Pathol 2020;96:2–7.

36. Khosroshahi A, Stone JH. A clinical overview of IgG4-related systemic disease. Curr Opin Rheumatol 2011;23(1):57–66.

37. Deshpande V, Sainani NI, Chung RT, et al. IgG4-associated cholangitis: a comparative histological and immunophenotypic study with primary sclerosing cholangitis on liver biopsy material. Mod Pathol 2009;22(10):1287–95.

38. Ghazale A, Chari ST, Zhang L, et al. Immunoglobulin G4-associated cholangitis: clinical profile and response to therapy. Gastroenterology 2008; 134(3):706–15.

39. Culver EL, Barnes E. IgG4-related sclerosing cholangitis. Clin Liver Dis 2017;10(1):9–16.

40. Culver EL, Sadler R, Simpson D, et al. Elevated serum IgG4 levels in diagnosis, treatment response, organ involvement, and relapse in a prospective IgG4-related disease UK cohort. Am J Gastroenterol 2016;111(5):733–43.

41. Culver EL, Sadler R, Bateman AC, et al. Increases in IgE, eosinophils, and mast cells can be used in diagnosis and to predict relapse of IgG4-related disease. Clin Gastroenterol Hepatol 2017;15(9): 1444–52.e6.

42. Huggett MT, Culver EL, Kumar M, et al. Type 1 autoimmune pancreatitis and IgG4-related sclerosing cholangitis is associated with extrapancreatic organ failure, malignancy, and mortality in a prospective UK cohort. Am J Gastroenterol 2014;109(10): 1675–83.

43. Hart PA, Topazian MD, Witzig TE, et al. Treatment of relapsing autoimmune pancreatitis with immunomodulators and rituximab: the Mayo Clinic experience. Gut 2013;62(11):1607–15.

44. de Buy Wenniger LJ, Culver EL, Beuers U. Exposure to occupational antigens might predispose to IgG4-related disease. Hepatology 2014;60(4):1453–4.

45. Deshpande V, Chicano S, Chiocca S, et al. Autoimmune pancreatitis: a systemic immune complex mediated disease. Am J Surg Pathol 2006;30(12): 1537–45.

46. Lee HE, Zhang L. Immunoglobulin G4-related hepatobiliary disease. Semin Diagn Pathol 2019;36(6): 423–33.

47. Maillette de Buy Wenniger L, Rauws EA, Beuers U. What an endoscopist should know about immunoglobulin-G4-associated disease of the pancreas and biliary tree. Endoscopy 2012;44(1): 66–73.

48. Deshpande V, Zen Y, Chan JK, et al. Consensus statement on the pathology of IgG4-related disease. Mod Pathol 2012;25(9):1181–92.

49. Bateman AC, Culver EL. IgG4-related disease-experience of 100 consecutive cases from a specialist centre. Histopathology 2017;70(5): 798–813.

50. Deltenre P, Valla DC. Ischemic cholangiopathy. J Hepatol 2006;44(4):806–17.

51. Deltenre P, Valla DC. Ischemic cholangiopathy. Semin Liver Dis 2008;28(3):235–46.

Evolving Understanding of Noncirrhotic Portal Hypertension

Raymond A. Isidro, MD, PhD[a], Lei Zhao, MD, PhD[b],*

KEYWORDS

- Portal hypertension • Idiopathic noncirrhotic portal hypertension
- Porto-sinusoidal vascular disease

Key points

- Portal hypertension can result from hemodynamic perturbations occurring at multiple levels within and outside the liver but the cause of these perturbations is not always well understood.

- Porto-sinusoidal vascular disease (PSVD) is a newly developed clinical entity to include disease processes that demonstrate histologic lesions that were first identified in idiopathic noncirrhotic portal hypertension (INCPH). PSVD is likely a collection of different diseases that can cause inflammation/obstruction of porto-sinusoidal vasculature and affect portal venous pressure, with some but not all patients having full-blown clinical portal hypertension.

- Histologic lesions associated with PSVD and INCPH include vascular abnormalities (ie, portal vein stenosis, portal vein herniation, portal tract hypervascularization, abnormal periportal vessels) and parenchymal abnormalities, such as nodular regenerative hyperplasia and incomplete septal fibrosis.

- Using standardized terminology and documenting findings in detail will facilitate further studies.

ABSTRACT

Although cirrhosis is one of the most common causes of portal hypertension, noncirrhotic portal hypertension can result from hemodynamic perturbations occurring in the prehepatic, intrahepatic, and posthepatic circulation. Intrahepatic portal hypertension can be further subclassified relative to the hepatic sinusoids as presinusoidal, sinusoidal, and postsinusoidal. For many of these differential diagnoses, the etiology is known but the cause of idiopathic noncirrhotic portal hypertension, recently included in porto-sinusoidal vascular disease (PSVD), remains poorly understood. Herein, we discuss the diagnostic pathological features of noncirrhotic portal hypertension, with an emphasis on PSVD.

OVERVIEW

The clinical diagnosis of portal hypertension encompasses 2 broad categories—portal hypertension resulting from cirrhosis and noncirrhotic portal hypertension (NCPH).

NCPH can be further subdivided into cases with a known cause and those for which the cause remains elusive, or idiopathic NCPH (INCPH). Portal hypertension can also be classified based on the segment of the vasculature that is predominantly involved, thus leading to clinical signs of portal hypertension, in different disease processes (Fig. 1). An understanding of the hemodynamics of the hepatic vasculature is, therefore, essential for conceptualizing the causes of portal hypertension.

[a] Department of Pathology, Memorial Sloan Kettering Cancer Center, 1275 York Avenue, New York, NY 10065, USA; [b] Department of Pathology, Brigham and Women's Hospital, Harvard Medical School, 75 Francis Street, Boston, MA 02115, USA
* Corresponding author.
E-mail address: lzhao19@bwh.harvard.edu

Surgical Pathology 16 (2023) 549–563
https://doi.org/10.1016/j.path.2023.04.009
1875-9181/23/© 2023 Elsevier Inc. All rights reserved.

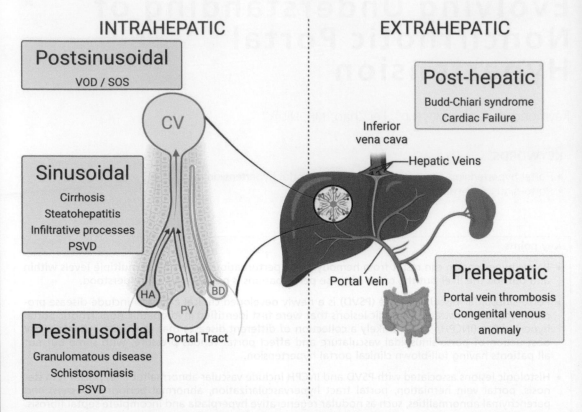

Fig. 1. Anatomic/hemodynamic classification of portal hypertension and most common causes. BD, bile duct; CV, central vein, HA, hepatic artery; PSVD, porto-sinusoidal vascular disease; PV, portal vein; SOS, sinusoidal obstruction syndrome; VOD, veno-occlusive disease. Created with Biorender.com.

The liver features a dual blood supply because it is perfused by both the systemic/arterial circulation, by way of the hepatic artery, and by the portal venous system, which collects blood from the spleen and intestines. The portal vein supplies approximately 70% of the oxygenated blood, whereas the hepatic artery provides approximately 30% of the oxygenated blood. Blood from both the portal vein and hepatic artery is distributed though the liver via the portal tracts, coalescing in the hepatic sinusoids to perfuse hepatocytes before draining into the central veins. The organization of the hepatic acinus is based on this blood flow, with zone 1 consisting of the periportal hepatocytes with the highest perfusion, and zone 3 consisting of the centrilobular hepatocytes surrounding the central veins, which have the lowest perfusion (zone 2 consists of the hepatocytes between zones 1 and 3). From the central veins, blood is drained into the inferior vena cava by way of the left, right, and middle hepatic veins. The exception to the dual blood supply is the bile ducts, which are exclusively perfused by the hepatic arteries. In contrast to the direction of blood flow from the portal tracts toward the central veins, bile flows toward the portal tracts.

As shown in **Fig. 1**, causes of portal hypertension can be anatomically and hemodynamically classified as prehepatic, intrahepatic, and posthepatic, with intrahepatic causes further classified in relation to the hepatic sinusoid as presinusoidal, sinusoidal, and postsinusoidal (**Table 1**).[1] Correlation of the histologic findings with portal pressure measurements and other clinical data can be of utmost utility when evaluating liver biopsies from patients with portal hypertension. This review will focus on the anatomic/hemodynamic classification of NCPH, with an emphasis on the pathology of INCPH and the recently proposed clinical entity porto-sinusoidal vascular disease (PSVD).

PREHEPATIC PORTAL HYPERTENSION

Two main causes of prehepatic portal hypertension include extrahepatic portal vein thrombosis and congenital venous abnormalities. It should be noted that portal vein thrombosis can be a primary cause of portal hypertension but it is more often secondary to other diseases that produce stasis and slow flow in the portal venous system. In adults, portal vein thrombosis is most common in patients with cirrhosis.[2] The risk of portal vein

Table 1
Anatomic/hemodynamic classification of portal hypertension and main differential diagnosis

	Prehepatic	Intrahepatic			Posthepatic
		Presinusoidal	Sinusoidal	Postsinusoidal	
Etiology	Portal vein thrombosis (chronic) Congenital venous anomaly	Granulomatous disease (PBC, sarcoidosis, TB) Schistosomiasis PSVD	Cirrhosis Steatohepatitis Infiltrative processes (EMH, amyloid, neoplasms, other) PSVD	VOD/SOS	Budd-Chiari syndrome Cardiac failure
FHVP	Normal	Normal	Normal	Normal	High
WHVP	Normal	Normal	High	High	High
HVPG	Normal	Normal	High	High	Normal or high
PVP	High	High	High	High	High
Histologic findings	Unremarkable Mild portal fibrosis Hepatocyte atrophy Portal vein thrombosis ± webs NRH Dilatation of hepatic arterioles, central veins, sinusoids Portal vein and hepatic artery structural changes	Granulomata ± other features *Schistosoma* eggs *Histologic lesions of PSVD*—vascular alterations (see Fig. 2), NRH, incomplete septal cirrhosis	*Cirrhosis*—regenerative nodules bound by fibrous septa *Steatohepatitis*—steatosis, ballooning degeneration, inflammation, fibrosis *Infiltrative processes*—sinusoidal infiltration by hematopoietic precursors, amyloid, neoplastic cells, other *Histologic lesions of PSVD*	Dilated and congested sinusoids Fibrous occlusion of central veins and small venules Intimal fibrosis Sclerosis of the venular wall Centrilobular necrosis Zone 3 sinusoidal fibrosis	Sinusoidal dilatation Hepatocyte atrophy Centrilobular necrosis

Abbreviations: EMH, extramedullary hematopoiesis; FHVP, free hepatic vein pressure; HVPG, hepatic vein pressure gradient; NRH, nodular regenerative hyperplasia; PBC, primary biliary cholangitis; PSVD, porto-sinusoidal vascular disease; PVP, portal vein pressure; SOS, sinusoidal obstruction syndrome; TB, tuberculosis; VOD, veno-occlusive disease.

thrombosis is increased with prothrombotic/hypercoagulable states, local, or systemic inflammation and/or infection, vascular injury, congenital anomaly, and malignancy.[3] Extrahepatic portal vein thrombosis can be clinically and histologically silent because of the liver's dual blood supply. Nonetheless, portal hypertension, splenomegaly, variceal bleeding, and cavernous transformation may ensue in the chronic setting.[3] Microscopic features may range from unremarkable hepatic parenchyma to mild portal fibrosis, hepatocyte atrophy, portal vein thrombosis with or without recanalization, and portal vein webs. The histologic findings may also include nodular regenerative hyperplasia (NRH),[4] which will be discussed further in the presinusoidal intrahepatic portal hypertension section. Rush and colleagues[5] have proposed that diffuse, obvious dilatation of the sinusoids, central veins, and hepatic arterioles as well as centrilobular hepatic cord thinning and structural changes to the portal veins and hepatic arteries are histologic features of extrahepatic portal vein thrombosis. Congenital venous anomalies can increase portal pressure by increasing resistance to blood flow and by increasing the risk of portal vein thrombosis. Congenital venous anomalies include agenesis, atresia, and/or hypoplasia of the portal veins, portosystemic shunt, and Abernathy malformation. Abernathy malformation is characterized by congenital extrahepatic portosystemic shunts resulting from absent or hypoplastic portal veins, with histology showing absent veins, malformed veins, or vein remnants within portal tracts.[6] This condition is associated with hepatic neoplasia.[6,7]

INTRAHEPATIC PORTAL HYPERTENSION

PRESINUSOIDAL

Presinusoidal causes of portal hypertension mainly include granulomatous diseases, such as primary biliary cholangitis (PBC), sarcoidosis, and tuberculosis; schistosomiasis; and idiopathic conditions. The presence of necrotizing granulomata with demonstration of acid-fast bacilli or Mycobacterial organisms through special stains or immunohistochemistry distinguishes tuberculosis from other granulomatous diseases. PBC and sarcoidosis can be distinguished by the presence of ductopenia in the former and its absence in the latter, as well as by the presence of extrahepatic sarcoidal disease. Identification of Schistosoma species eggs is essential for establishing the diagnosis of schistosomiasis. The free and wedged hepatic vein pressures (FHVP and WHVP, respectively) as well as the hepatic vein pressure gradient (HVPG, calculated as the difference between the WHVP

and FHVP) are normal in presinusoidal portal hypertension, despite elevated portal vein pressure (PVP). This hemodynamic profile is shared with prehepatic portal hypertension.

Idiopathic Noncirrhotic Portal Hypertension and Porto-Sinusoidal Vascular Disease

It is thought that the first reported cases of INCPH were described by Guido Banti in the late 1880s, likely as a part of a cohort that included other liver and vascular diseases.[8,9] Subsequent studies in India used the term idiopathic portal fibrosis to describe portal hypertension without intrahepatic or extrahepatic obstruction.[10] Thereafter, the term idiopathic portal hypertension was introduced to describe similar presentations.[11] INCPH was proposed by Schouten and colleagues[9] as a term to collectively and uniformly refer to conditions with portal hypertension and without cirrhosis or an identifiable cause (Fig. 2). INCPH manifests with the signs or complications of portal hypertension, such as esophageal varices, portal hypertensive bleeding, splenomegaly, or hypersplenism, and normal to mildly altered liver tests (including alkaline phosphatase levels). Imaging may reveal portosystemic collaterals, a nodular liver surface, and thickening of the portal vein wall. Portal pressure measurement shows a normal to minimally increased WHVP and HVPG. Liver stiffness on transient elastography is usually lower than what is typically observed in cirrhotic patients (mean 8.45 kPa in INCPH versus >14 kPa in cirrhosis).[12]

Many conditions have been associated with INCPH.[13] Immunological disorders, such as systemic sclerosis, systemic lupus erythematosus, celiac disease, inflammatory bowel disease, human immunodeficiency virus infection, primary hypogammaglobulinemia, and rheumatoid arthritis, represent one broad disease category that has been associated with INCPH. Repeated gastrointestinal infections have also been linked to INCPH. Indeed, repeated injections of Escherichia coli into the gastrosplenic vein or repeated intramuscular injections of splenic extract in rabbits led to increased portal pressures and splenomegaly without significant histopathologic or biochemical evidence of disease.[14,15] INCPH has also been associated with the HLA-DR3 gene, the p.V450L gain of function missense mutation in KCNN3, the p.N46S loss of function missense mutation in DGUOK, missense mutations in FOPV, Adams-Oliver syndrome, and Turner syndrome.[16–24] Prothrombotic conditions and hematologic disorders have also been associated with INCPH. Finally, treatment with didanosine, azathioprine, tioguanine, and oxaliplatin, as well as

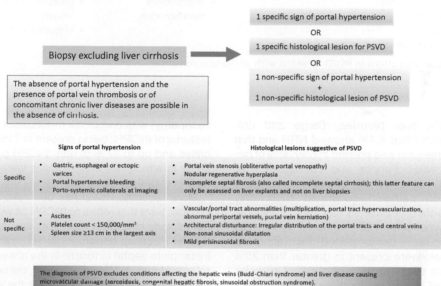

Diagnostic Criteria of Idiopathic Noncirrhotic Portal Hypertension[a] (Schouten et al. 2011)

1. Clinical signs of portal hypertension (any one of the following[b])
   - Splenomegaly/hypersplenism
   - Esophageal varices
   - Ascites (nonmalignant)
   - Increased hepatic venous pressure gradient
   - Porto-systemic collaterals
2. Exclusion of cirrhosis on liver biopsy
3. Exclusion of chronic liver disease causing cirrhosis or noncirrhotic portal hypertension[c])
   - Chronic viral hepatitis B and / or C
   - Nonalcoholic steatohepatitis/alcoholic steatohepatitis
   - Autoimmune hepatitis
   - Wilson's disease
   - Primary biliary cirrhosis
4. Exclusion of conditions causing noncirrhotic portal hypertension
   - Congenital liver fibrosis
   - Sarcoidosis
   - Schistosomiasis
5. Patent portal and hepatic veins (Doppler ultrasound or computed tomography scanning)

[a]All five criteria must be fulfilled to diagnose idiopathic noncirrhotic portal hypertension
[b]Splenomegaly must be accompanied by additional signs of portal hypertension to fulfill this criterion
[c]Chronic liver disease must be excluded, because severe fibrosis might be understaged on liver biopsy

Diagnostic Criteria of Porto-sinusoidal Vascular Disease (De Gottardi et al. 2022)

Biopsy excluding liver cirrhosis →

1 specific sign of portal hypertension
OR
1 specific histological lesion for PSVD
OR
1 non-specific sign of portal hypertension
+
1 non-specific histological lesion of PSVD

The absence of portal hypertension and the presence of portal vein thrombosis or of concomitant chronic liver diseases are possible in the absence of cirrhosis.

	Signs of portal hypertension	Histological lesions suggestive of PSVD
Specific	• Gastric, esophageal or ectopic varices • Portal hypertensive bleeding • Porto-systemic collaterals at imaging	• Portal vein stenosis (obliterative portal venopathy) • Nodular regenerative hyperplasia • Incomplete septal fibrosis (also called incomplete septal cirrhosis); this latter feature can only be assessed on liver explants and not on liver biopsies
Not specific	• Ascites • Platelet count < 150,000/mm³ • Spleen size ≥13 cm in the largest axis	• Vascular/portal tract abnormalities (multiplication, portal tract hypervascularization, abnormal periportal vessels, portal vein herniation) • Architectural disturbance: Irregular distribution of the portal tracts and central veins • Non-zonal sinusoidal dilatation • Mild perisinusoidal fibrosis

The diagnosis of PSVD excludes conditions affecting the hepatic veins (Budd-Chiari syndrome) and liver disease causing microvascular damage (sarcoidosis, congenital hepatic fibrosis, sinusoidal obstruction syndrome).

Fig. 2. Diagnostic criteria for INCPH[9] and PSVD.[37]

exposure to arsenic, has been reported in association with INCPH.

A liver biopsy is essential to exclude cirrhosis. Hepatoportal sclerosis,[25] NRH,[26] and incomplete septal cirrhosis[27] are among the most common histologic terms that have been described in liver specimens from patients with INCPH. Of note, many other terms had been used to describe findings that are related to hepatoportal sclerosis, including obliterative portal venopathy, phlebosclerosis, portal vein obliteration, and portal vein herniation (**Fig. 3**). However, it has been recognized that none of these changes (hepatoportal sclerosis, NRH, or incomplete septal cirrhosis) are pathognomonic for INCPH because these alterations can be encountered in other entities and disease processes. Wanless found NRH in 2.5% of livers from 2500 autopsies, only one of which had clinically documented portal hypertension.[28] Zuo and colleagues[29] reported NRH in 36% of 81 biopsies, 50 of which were performed incidentally and intraoperatively and 31 that were performed for fatty liver disease without portal hypertension or cirrhosis; 90% of all biopsies contained at least one feature of INCPH and 10% of cases demonstrated 5 to 6 features of INCPH.

Vascular alterations in PSVD

Normal
Portal Tract

Portal Vein Stenosis

Portal Vein Herniation

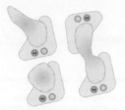

Portal Tract
Hypervascularization

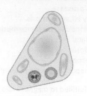

Abnormal periportal vessels

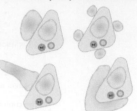

Other unfavored terms
- Phlebosclerosis
- Obliterative portal venopathy
- Portal vein obliteration
- Small portal vein obliteration
- Hepatoportal sclerosis

Other unfavored terms
- Shunt vessel
- Hepatoportal sclerosis

Other unfavored terms
- Portal tract angiomatosis
- Angiomatoid lesion
- Angiomatous transformation

Other unfavored terms
- Aberrant vessels
- Cavernous transformation
- Paraportal shunting vessels
- Megasinusoids

Fig. 3. Vascular alterations in PSVD. Created with BioRender.com.[32,38]

Among 3600 liver biopsies, Barge and colleagues[30] found that 4.4% showed NRH and that portal hypertension was present in only 38% of patients with NRH. Penrice and colleagues[31] reported that in a cohort of 167 consecutive patients with pathology-confirmed NRH, only around one-third of patients had clinical features of portal hypertension at diagnosis. Krasinskas and colleagues[32] demonstrated that abnormal portal vessels were present in greater than 25% of the portal tracts in 88% of a set of biopsies composed of 46 native liver biopsies and 48 allograft biopsies, with a significant number of biopsies from patients without portal hypertension. Notably, over half of the biopsies included in this study were from patients infected with the hepatitis C virus (HCV). Kmeid and colleagues[33] reported that among 34 liver cases (15 INCPH, 19 control) interobserver agreement among 7 liver pathologists was very low and that up to 37% of cases without a clinical history of INCPH were classified as INCPH based on histologic findings. In a study by Guido and colleagues,[34] portal vein stenosis (obliterative portal venopathy) was identified in 19.5% of 482 biopsies from patients without portal hypertension and 100% of 20 patients with INCPH. Similarly, Liang and colleagues[35] found that portal vein stenosis (obliterative portal

venopathy) was one of the most useful pathologic features of INCPH, being present in 71% of INCPH cases and up to 27% of non- INCPH controls in a study in which 104 liver biopsies were evaluated by 6 liver pathologists.

More recently, PSVD has been proposed as a broader term that refers to INCPH as well as histopathologic changes that are associated with INCPH (such as hepatoportal sclerosis, NRH, or incomplete septal cirrhosis) in the absence of portal hypertension.[36] In other words, the unifying factor between INCPH and PSVD is the absence of cirrhosis and the presence of the abovementioned histologic change(s). The biggest difference between INCPH and PSVD is that portal hypertension is not required for a diagnosis of PSVD (see **Fig. 2**). In addition, unlike INCPH, the concomitant presence of other chronic liver disease such as metabolic syndrome, alcohol-related liver disease, viral hepatitis, and portal vein thrombosis do not exclude the diagnosis of PSVD. To be used as a clinical entity, disease conditions that should be included and excluded under the diagnosis of PSVD will continue to be further refined. The landmark articles by De Gottardi and colleagues[36,37] systematically summarized the histologic lesions related to porto-sinusoidal vascular and microvascular injury and recognized that these lesions are likely the result of various causes and may also be a subcomponent of other chronic liver diseases. Hereafter, we focus on the histologic aspect of PSVD because accurate characterization of these histologic lesions is key for further studies to improve our understanding of PSVD.

PSVD manifests as a combination of vascular and parenchymal alterations that may be unevenly distributed throughout the liver. These vascular alterations were collectively classified under the term hepatoportal sclerosis. They are centered within and around the portal tracts and include portal vein stenosis and herniation, portal tract hypervascularization, and the presence of abnormal periportal vessels (see **Fig. 3**; **Fig. 4**).[38] Portal vein stenosis is defined as luminal narrowing or obliteration of portal venules, with or without wall thickening, and usually occurring within fibrotic portal tracts. Portal vein herniation refers to an eccentric portal vein that extends beyond the limits of the portal tract and abuts hepatocytes. Portal tract hypervascularization is present as increased thin-walled vessels or vascular spaces within portal tracts, whereas abnormal periportal veins are thin-walled vessels or vascular spaces that abut, but are external to, the portal tracts. As noted in **Fig. 3**, multiple other terms have been used to refer to these changes but we prefer and recommend the terminology described herein as proposed by Guido and colleagues[38] from the International Liver Pathology Study Group.

The parenchymal alterations include NRH and incomplete septal fibrosis/cirrhosis (**Figs. 5** and **6**). NRH is characterized by hyperplastic nodules with thickened hepatocyte plates alternating with compressed and/or atrophic hepatocytes plates. Notably, significant fibrosis should be absent. These changes can be appreciated on hematoxylin-eosin (H&E) but are nicely highlighted by reticulin stains. Sinusoidal dilation may also be present, and it may be nonzonal. Incomplete septal fibrosis consists of thin fibrous septa, which may delineate nodular parenchyma. Importantly, well-formed regenerative nodules as seen in cirrhosis, are not present. Incomplete septal fibrosis/cirrhosis has been postulated to also represent regressed/regressing cirrhosis in other clinical scenarios.[39–42] Other parenchymal alterations include portal and periportal fibrosis and abnormal spacing between portal tracts and central veins.

The presence of the histologic features of PSVD in patients without portal hypertension raises the question of whether these patients truly have pre-hypertensive INCPH or whether the findings are not actually indicative of PSVD/INCPH. In all likelihood, the histologic changes of PSVD are present to a certain degree before portal hypertension becomes clinically apparent. As the histologic burden of disease increases in severity and distribution, the liver's ability to compensate for this increased vascular resistance decreases, leading to progressively increasing portal pressures that will eventually result in portal hypertension and signs thereof (**Fig. 7**A). Other conditions that can also show the histologic changes seen in PSVD, such as HCV and nonalcoholic steatohepatitis, may feature a component of PSVD but likely ultimately progress to portal hypertension by way of increased fibrotic burden and, ultimately, cirrhosis (**Fig. 7**B). The respective contribution of PSVD and other chronic liver disease to the development of portal hypertension is difficult to delineate due to underdocumentation of histologic lesions of PSVD in other chronic liver diseases. A systemic documentation of the vascular and parenchymal changes will aid in devising future studies that could potentially address these and other questions. In **Box 1**, we outline our recommended approach for documenting such findings in the pathology report.

SINUSOIDAL

Sinusoidal causes of portal hypertension include cirrhosis, steatohepatitis, and sinusoidal infiltrative processes. Portal hypertension is a well-recognized consequence of cirrhosis, in which normal flow through sinusoids is impeded by the presence of fibrotic bands separating regenerative nodules. Several studies have demonstrated that portal hypertension can occur in the absence of cirrhosis in alcoholic and nonalcoholic fatty liver disease.[43–47] In steatohepatitis, the flow through sinusoids is disrupted by a combination of hepatocyte enlargement that results from steatosis and ballooning degeneration, sinusoidal/perisinusoidal fibrosis that usually begins in zone 3, and inflammatory and microthrombotic processes that result in sinusoidal dysfunction and increased intrahepatic vascular resistance.[46] The latter process likely contributes to the presence of histologic lesions of PSVD in some of the steatohepatitis cases. **Fig. 8** shows a focus of dense hyaline sclerosis and extensive pericellular/sinusoidal fibrosis from a patient with alcoholic steatohepatitis and noncirrhotic portal hypertension. Sinusoidal infiltrative processes, such as extramedullary hematopoiesis (**Fig. 9**A-B), amyloidosis (**Fig. 9**C-E), sickle cell disease, hypervitaminosis A, Gaucher disease, histiocytic and mast cell neoplasms (Rosai-Dorfman disease, Langerhans cell histiocytosis, mastocytosis), vascular neoplasms (angiosarcoma, epithelioid hemangioendothelioma),

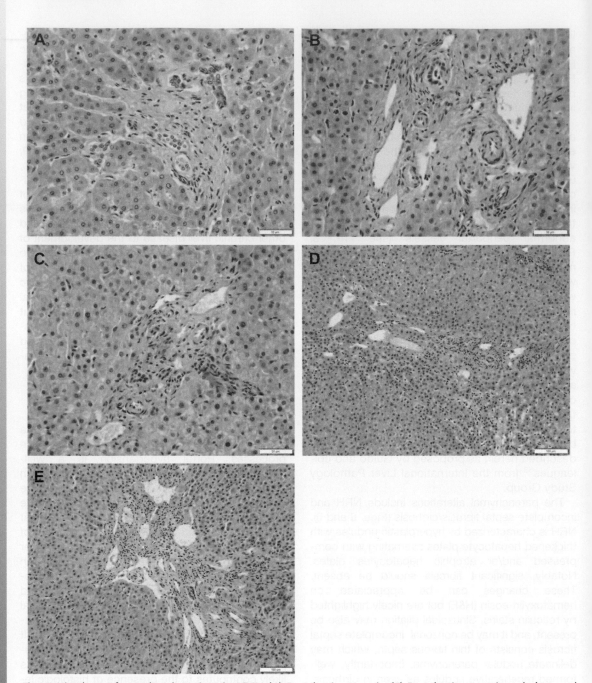

Fig. 4. Histology of vascular alterations in PSVD. (A) Portal vein stenosis. (B) Portal vein stenosis and abnormal periportal vessel. (C) Portal vein stenosis and abnormal periportal vessel. (D) Abnormal periportal vessel. (E) Portal tract hypervascularization and abnormal periportal vessel.

and metastatic neoplasms, cause sinusoidal hypertension by restricting flow through the hepatic sinusoids.

POSTSINUSOIDAL

Veno-occlusive disease (VOD) or sinusoidal obstruction syndrome (SOS) is a systemic

endothelial disease that presents after myeloablative conditioning for stem cell transplantation, chemotherapy (particularly oxaliplatin), or exposure to pyrrolizidine alkaloids.[48] As has been shown in an animal model, sinusoidal endothelial injury leads to endothelial cell sloughing and central vein obstruction, causing postsinusoidal hypertension.[49] Centrilobular necrosis and zone 3 sinusoidal

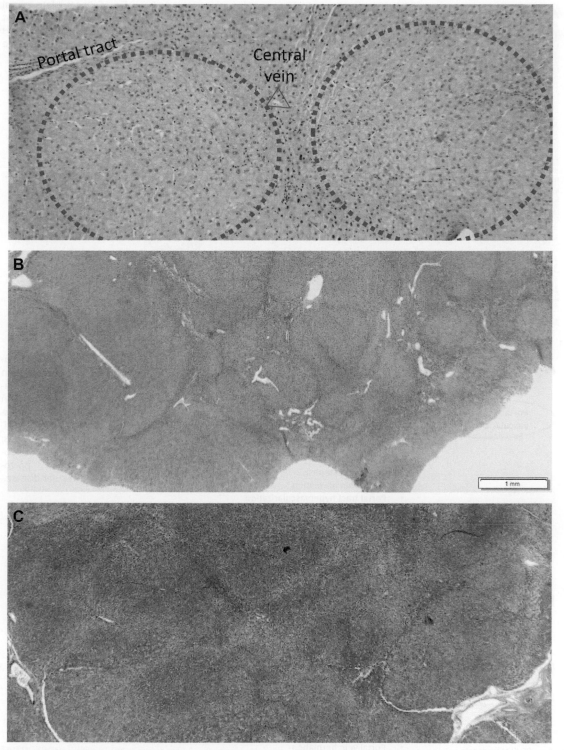

Fig. 5. NRH in PSVD. (*A*) Dotted circles demarcated hypertrophic areas with intervening atrophic hepatocytes. Low-power view of diffuse nodularity on H&E (*B*) and trichrome (*C*) stains.

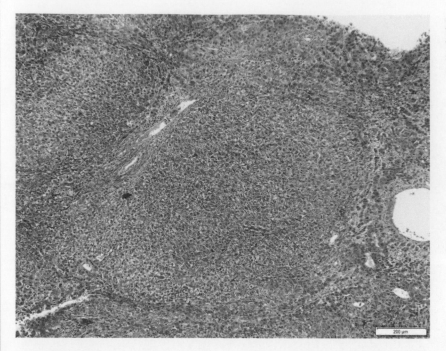

Fig. 6. Incomplete septal fibrosis in a liver explant from a patient with INCPH secondary to azathioprine use.

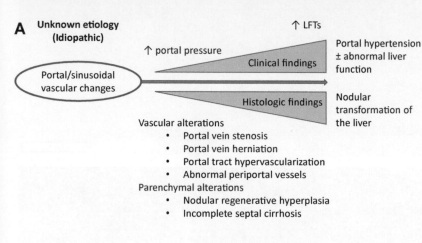

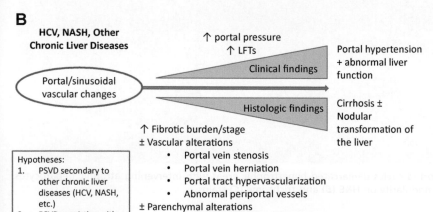

Fig. 7. Proposed mechanism for disease evolution in PSVD occurring in isolation (*A*) or in association with other chronic liver diseases (*B*). HCV, hepatitis C virus; LFT, liver function tests; NASH, nonalcoholic steatohepatitis; PSVD, portosinusoidal vascular disease.

> **Box 1**
> **Recommended approach for documenting the histologic features of porto-sinusoidal vascular disease**
>
> If vascular changes and hepatocyte regenerative changes are the predominant findings.
>
> - Features suggestive of PSVD
>   - If portal hypertension is present clinically
>   - Findings supportive of clinical diagnosis of INCPH
>   - If no clinical portal hypertension
>   - Findings may represent early/preclinical INCPH
>
> If other findings also present, such as chronic hepatitis or steatohepatitis
>
> - Document vascular changes in detail, but no need to comment on or conclude relationship to PSVD/INCPH; grade and stage chronic liver disease according to its respective criteria/guideline

fibrosis may also ensue. Other histologic findings include dilated and congested sinusoids, fibrous occlusion of central veins and small venules, intimal fibrosis, and sclerosis of the venular wall. Differential diagnoses to consider are causes of venous outflow obstruction, such as Budd-Chiari syndrome, and vascular occlusion due to neoplastic invasion, as may occur with epithelioid hemangioendothelioma. In contrast to presinusoidal and prehepatic hypertension, postsinusoidal

hypertension features an elevated WHVP and high HVPG, as is also seen in sinusoidal portal hypertension.

POSTHEPATIC

The 2 main causes of posthepatic portal hypertension are congestive hepatopathy and Budd-Chiari syndrome. Congestive hepatopathy, resulting from congestive heart failure or constrictive

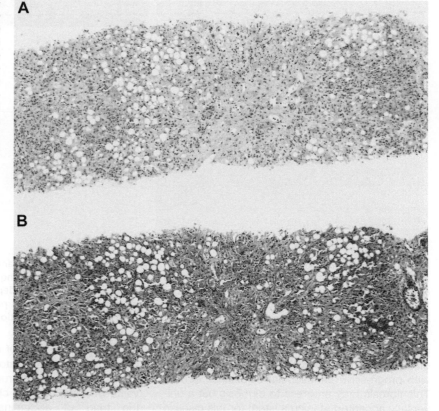

Fig. 8. Alcoholic steatohepatitis with sclerosing hyaline necrosis and extensive pericellular fibrosis as a cause of noncirrhotic portal hypertension. The patient presented with jaundice, fever, leukocytosis, ascites, and elevated wedged hepatic venous pressure (13.6 mm Hg). H&E (*A*) and trichrome (*B*) stains.

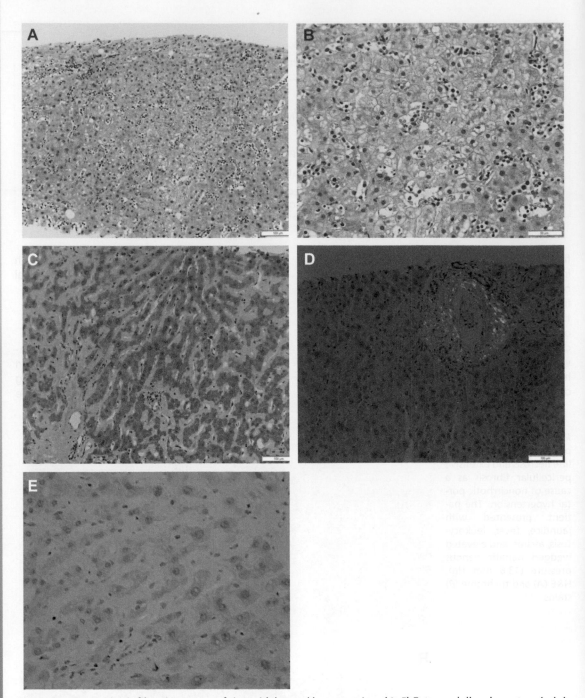

Fig. 9. Representative infiltrative causes of sinusoidal portal hypertension. (*A, B*) Extramedullary hematopoiesis in a patient with polycythemia vera harboring a JAK2 p.V617F mutation and presenting with portal hypertension and significant hepatosplenomegaly. (*C–E*) Sinusoidal and perivascular amyloid deposition in a liver biopsy from a patient with AL lambda light chain amyloidosis presenting with abdominal pain, unintentional weight loss, scleral icterus, varices, and ascites (*C*, H&E; *D-E*, congo red stains with polarization).

pericarditis, characteristically shows an irregular distribution of sinusoidal dilatation and congestion with progressive centrilobular sinusoidal fibrosis. This fibrosis may progress to cirrhosis but a universally accepted staging system for this disease is lacking at present. Of note, NRH may also be seen in congestive hepatopathy. Budd-Chiari syndrome results from obstruction of the large hepatic veins or the IVC and classically presents with the triad of abdominal pain, ascites, and

Fig. 10. Marked sinusoidal dilatation and congestion in a case of Budd-Chiari syndrome presenting with acute liver failure (*A, B*).

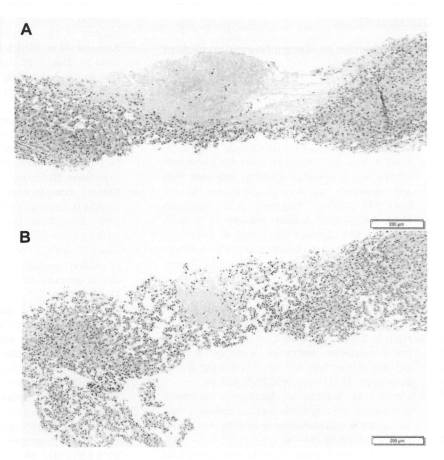

hepatomegaly. Cases of chronic obstruction may present with signs of portal hypertension. However, some cases may be asymptomatic because of collateral circulation. The diagnosis is usually established by imaging modalities. Obstruction can be primary, in which vascular injury or hypercoagulable states lead to thrombosis, or secondary, in which compression or neoplastic invasion restricts blood flow. Primary Budd-Chiari syndrome is associated with polycythemia vera/myeloproliferative neoplasms, JAK2 mutation, pregnancy, use of oral contraceptives, and lupus anticoagulants. Budd-Chiari syndrome shows many of the same histologic features observed in congestive hepatopathy (**Fig. 10**). Posthepatic portal hypertension features an elevated FHVP, WHVP, and PVP. HVPG may be normal or high.

In conclusion, when interpreting liver histology in patients with portal hypertension, utilizing clinical information to deduce the anatomic level of disease can effectively narrow down the differential diagnosis. Using standardized terminology to document vascular and parenchymal changes will further improve our understanding of portosinusoidal vascular disorders.

CLINICS CARE POINTS

- Integrating histologic findings with clinical information, such as hemodynamic parameters, can help narrow the differential diagnosis in cases of portal hypertension.

- PSVD has been proposed as a broad term to refer to the histopathologic changes associated with INCPH, regardless of whether portal hypertension is present.

- PSVD can manifest with vascular alterations centered in the portal tract and sinusoids (portal vein stenosis and/or herniation, portal tract hypervascularization, abnormal periportal vessels) and parenchymal alterations (NRH and incomplete septal fibrosis).

- The histologic changes of PSVD can be seen in other chronic liver conditions, but the role of PSVD in disease progression and the development of portal hypertension in other chronic liver conditions remains unclear.

DISCLOSURE

The authors have no relevant financial conflicts of interest to disclose.

REFERENCES

1. Bosch J, Iwakiri Y. The portal hypertension syndrome: etiology, classification, relevance, and animal models. Hepatol Int 2018;12(Suppl 1):1–10.
2. Malik A, Sharma S, Young M, Giwa AO. Portal Vein Obstruction. StatPearls Publishing. StatPearls Web site. Available at: https://www.ncbi.nlm.nih.gov/books/NBK541134/. Published 2022. Updated November 28, 2022. Accessed November 14, 2022.
3. Intagliata NM, Caldwell SH, Tripodi A. Diagnosis, development, and treatment of portal vein thrombosis in patients with and without cirrhosis. Gastroenterology 2019;156(6):1582–1599 e1581.
4. Tublin ME, Towbin AJ, Federle MP, et al. Altered liver morphology after portal vein thrombosis: not always cirrhosis. Dig Dis Sci 2008;53(10):2784–8.
5. Rush N, Sun H, Nakanishi Y, et al. Hepatic arterial buffer response: pathologic evidence in noncirrhotic human liver with extrahepatic portal vein thrombosis. Mod Pathol 2016;29(5):489–99.
6. Lisovsky M, Konstas AA, Misdraji J. Congenital extrahepatic portosystemic shunts (Abernethy malformation): a histopathologic evaluation. Am J Surg Pathol 2011;35(9):1381–90.
7. Baiges A, Turon F, Simon-Talero M, et al. Congenital extrahepatic portosystemic shunts (abernethy malformation): an international observational study. Hepatology 2020;71(2):658–69.
8. Riggio O, Gioia S, Pentassuglio I, et al. Idiopathic noncirrhotic portal hypertension: current perspectives. Hepat Med 2016;8:81–8.
9. Schouten JN, Garcia-Pagan JC, Valla DC, et al. Idiopathic noncirrhotic portal hypertension. Hepatology 2011;54(3):1071–81.
10. Sama SK, Bhargava S, Nath NG, et al. Noncirrhotic portal fibrosis. Am J Med 1971;51(2):160–9.
11. Boyer JL, Sen Gupta KP, Biswas SK, et al. Idiopathic portal hypertension. Comparison with the portal hypertension of cirrhosis and extrahepatic portal vein obstruction. Ann Intern Med 1967;66(1):41–68.
12. Siramolpiwat S, Seijo S, Miquel R, et al. Idiopathic portal hypertension: natural history and long-term outcome. Hepatology 2014;59(6):2276–85.
13. Hernandez-Gea V, Baiges A, Turon F, et al. Idiopathic portal hypertension. Hepatology 2018;68(6):2413–23.
14. Kathayat R, Pandey GK, Malhotra V, et al. Rabbit model of non-cirrhotic portal fibrosis with repeated immunosensitization by rabbit splenic extract. J Gastroenterol Hepatol 2002;17(12):1312–6.
15. Omanwar S, Rizvi MR, Kathayat R, et al. A rabbit model of non-cirrhotic portal hypertension by repeated injections of E.coli through indwelling cannulation of the gastrosplenic vein. Hepatobiliary Pancreat Dis Int 2004;3(3):417–22.
16. Sarin SK, Mehra NK, Agarwal A, et al. Familial aggregation in noncirrhotic portal fibrosis: a report of four families. Am J Gastroenterol 1987;82(11):1130–3.
17. Bauer CK, Schneeberger PE, Kortum F, et al. Gain-of-function mutations in KCNN3 encoding the small-conductance Ca(2+)-activated K(+) Channel SK3 cause zimmermann-laband syndrome. Am J Hum Genet 2019;104(6):1139–57.
18. Koot BG, Alders M, Verheij J, et al. A de novo mutation in KCNN3 associated with autosomal dominant idiopathic non-cirrhotic portal hypertension. J Hepatol 2016;64(4):974–7.
19. Girard M, Amiel J, Fabre M, et al. Adams-Oliver syndrome and hepatoportal sclerosis: occasional association or common mechanism? Am J Med Genet 2005;135(2):186–9.
20. Pouessel G, Dieux-Coeslier A, Wacrenier A, et al. Association of Adams-Oliver syndrome and hepatoportal sclerosis: an additional case. Am J Med Genet 2006;140(9):1028–9.
21. Swartz EN, Sanatani S, Sandor GG, et al. Vascular abnormalities in Adams-Oliver syndrome: cause or effect? Am J Med Genet 1999;82(1):49–52.
22. Vilarinho S, Sari S, Yilmaz G, et al. Recurrent recessive mutation in deoxyguanosine kinase causes idiopathic noncirrhotic portal hypertension. Hepatology 2016;63(6):1977–86.
23. Roulot D, Degott C, Chazouilleres O, et al. Vascular involvement of the liver in Turner's syndrome. Hepatology 2004;39(1):239–47.
24. Besmond C, Valla D, Hubert L, et al. Mutations in the novel gene FOPV are associated with familial autosomal dominant and non-familial obliterative portal venopathy. Liver Int 2018;38(2):358–64.
25. Mikkelsen WP, Edmondson HA, Peters RL, et al. Extra- and intrahepatic portal hypertension without cirrhosis (hepatoportal sclerosis). Ann Surg 1965;162(4):602–20.
26. Steiner PE. Nodular regenerative hyperplasia of the liver. Am J Pathol 1959;35:943–53.
27. Sciot R, Staessen D, Van Damme B, et al. Incomplete septal cirrhosis: histopathological aspects. Histopathology 1988;13(6):593–603.
28. Wanless IR. Micronodular transformation (nodular regenerative hyperplasia) of the liver: a report of 64 cases among 2,500 autopsies and a new classification of benign hepatocellular nodules. Hepatology 1990;11(5):787–97.
29. Zuo C, Chumbalkar V, Ells PF, et al. Prevalence of histological features of idiopathic noncirrhotic portal hypertension in general population: a retrospective study of incidental liver biopsies. Hepatol Int 2017;11(5):452–60.

30. Barge S, Grando V, Nault JC, et al. Prevalence and clinical significance of nodular regenerative hyperplasia in liver biopsies. Liver Int 2016;36(7): 1059–66.

31. Penrice DD, Thakral N, Kezer CA, et al. Outcomes of idiopathic versus secondary nodular regenerative hyperplasia of the liver: a longitudinal study of 167 cases. Liver Int 2022;42(6):1379–85.

32. Krasinskas AM, Goldsmith JD, Burke A, et al. Abnormal intrahepatic portal vasculature in native and allograft liver biopsies: a comparative analysis. Am J Surg Pathol 2005;29(10):1382–8.

33. Kmeid M, Zuo C, Lagana SM, et al. Interobserver study on histologic features of idiopathic noncirrhotic portal hypertension. Diagn Pathol 2020; 15(1):129.

34. Guido M, Sarcognato S, Sonzogni A, et al. Obliterative portal venopathy without portal hypertension: an underestimated condition. Liver Int 2016;36(3): 454–60.

35. Liang J, Shi C, Dupont WD, et al. Key histopathologic features in idiopathic noncirrhotic portal hypertension: an interobserver agreement study and proposal for diagnostic criteria. Mod Pathol 2021;34(3):592–602.

36. De Gottardi A, Rautou PE, Schouten J, et al. Portosinusoidal vascular disease: proposal and description of a novel entity. Lancet Gastroenterol Hepatol 2019;4(5):399–411.

37. De Gottardi A, Sempoux C, Berzigotti A. Porto-sinusoidal vascular disorder. J Hepatol 2022;77(4): 1124–35.

38. Guido M, Alves VAF, Balabaud C, et al. Histology of portal vascular changes associated with idiopathic non-cirrhotic portal hypertension: nomenclature and definition. Histopathology 2019;74(2):219–26.

39. Khan S, Saxena R. Regression of hepatic fibrosis and evolution of cirrhosis: a concise review. Adv Anat Pathol 2021;28(6):408–14.

40. Schinoni MI, Andrade Z, de Freitas LA, et al. Incomplete septal cirrhosis: an enigmatic disease. Liver Int 2004;24(5):452–6.

41. Theise ND, Jia J, Sun Y, et al. Progression and regression of fibrosis in viral hepatitis in the treatment era: the Beijing classification. Mod Pathol 2018;31(8):1191–200.

42. Wanless IR, Nakashima E, Sherman M. Regression of human cirrhosis. Morphologic features and the genesis of incomplete septal cirrhosis. Arch Pathol Lab Med 2000;124(11):1599–607.

43. Mendes FD, Suzuki A, Sanderson SO, et al. Prevalence and indicators of portal hypertension in patients with nonalcoholic fatty liver disease. Clin Gastroenterol Hepatol 2012;10(9):1028–1033 e1022.

44. Rodrigues SG, Montani M, Guixe-Muntet S, et al. Patients With Signs of Advanced Liver Disease and Clinically Significant Portal Hypertension Do Not Necessarily Have Cirrhosis. Clin Gastroenterol Hepatol 2019;17(10):2101–2109 e2101.

45. Vonghia L, Magrone T, Verrijken A, et al. Peripheral and hepatic vein cytokine levels in correlation with non-alcoholic fatty liver disease (NAFLD)-related metabolic, histological, and haemodynamic features. PLoS One 2015;10(11):e0143380.

46. Ryou M, Stylopoulos N, Baffy G. Nonalcoholic fatty liver disease and portal hypertension. Explor Med 2020;1:149–69.

47. Karasawa T, Chedid A. Sclerosing hyaline necrosis in noncirrhotic chronic alcoholic hepatitis. Am J Clin Pathol 1976;66(5):802–9.

48. Bonifazi F, Barbato F, Ravaioli F, et al. Diagnosis and Treatment of VOD/SOS After Allogeneic Hematopoietic Stem Cell Transplantation. Front Immunol 2020;11:489.

49. DeLeve LD, Ito Y, Bethea NW, et al. Embolization by sinusoidal lining cells obstructs the microcirculation in rat sinusoidal obstruction syndrome. Am J Physiol Gastrointest Liver Physiol 2003;284(6):G1045–52.

Inflammatory Pseudotumor of the Liver

Donghai Wang, MD, PhD[a], Joseph Misdraji, MD[b],*

KEYWORDS

- Liver • Inflammatory pseudotumor • Abscess • IgG4-related disease
- Inflammatory myofibroblastic tumor • Follicular dendritic cell tumor • Syphilis • Hodgkin lymphoma

Key points

- Inflammatory pseudotumor (IPT) describes a heterogeneous group of lesions that comprise a mixture of fibroblasts and inflammatory cells.
- Hepatic IPTs are most often idiopathic but presumed to be an exuberant response to infection, healing abscesses, or cholangitis.
- In specific clinical circumstances, pathologists must consider ancillary techniques to exclude specific infectious organisms such as mycobacteria, Candida, and Syphilis.
- A subset of hepatic IPTs with numerous plasma cells may be a manifestation of IgG4-related disease.
- Neoplasms that mimic hepatic IPTs must be excluded using appropriate ancillary studies, including inflammatory myofibroblastic tumor, follicular dendritic cell tumor, inflammatory angiomyolipoma, Hodgkin lymphoma, and inflammatory hepatocellular carcinoma.

ABSTRACT

Hepatic inflammatory pseudotumor (IPT) describes a mass lesion composed of fibroblasts or myofibroblasts with a dense inflammatory infiltrate comprising lymphocyte, plasma cells, and histiocytes. These lesions are presumed to be an exuberant response to an infectious organism, although in most cases the causative agent is unknown. In specific circumstances, pathologists should consider ancillary techniques to exclude specific infections, such as mycobacteria, Candida, or syphilis. IgG4-related disease may cause a plasma-cell rich IPT. Finally, true neoplasms can mimic IPTs and must be excluded with appropriate ancillary studies, including inflammatory myofibroblastic tumor, follicular dendritic cell tumor, inflammatory angiomyolipoma, Hodgkin lymphoma, and inflammatory hepatocellular carcinoma.

OVERVIEW

Inflammatory pseudotumors (IPTs) are mass-forming lesions composed of fibroblasts or myofibroblasts and inflammatory cells that occur in various organs and have been described using a variety of terms including plasma cell granuloma, fibroxanthoma, and histiocytoma.[1] In the liver, these lesions are more often encountered when a biopsy or resection of a mass lesion is performed due to clinical concern of a primary hepatic tumor or a metastatic tumor. One of the challenges to understanding the nature of IPTs is that this term encompasses a heterogeneous group of lesions that include infectious and inflammatory disorders. Furthermore, many studies on hepatic IPT predate recognition of neoplastic entities that mimic IPTs.

Most IPTs are presumed to be an exuberant response to cholangitis or infection, although in most cases, the infectious agent is unknown. In

[a] Department of Pathology, New York University Grossman School of Medicine, NYU Langone Health, 560 First Avenue TH-483, New York, NY 10016, USA; [b] Department of Pathology, Yale School of Medicine, Yale New Haven Hospital, 20 York Street EP2-611, New Haven, CT 06510, USA
* Corresponding author.
E-mail address: joseph.misdraji@yale.edu

Surgical Pathology 16 (2023) 565–580
https://doi.org/10.1016/j.path.2023.04.010

occasional cases, the infectious agent is identified, such as in treponemal or candidal infection. Before rendering a diagnosis of IPT, pathologists must exclude neoplastic entities that resemble IPTs, including neoplasms that were called IPT until their neoplastic nature was recognized, namely inflammatory myofibroblastic tumor (IMT) and follicular dendritic cell tumor. Other neoplasms infrequently have a morphologic resemblance to IPT, such as angiomyolipoma (AML) or Hodgkin lymphoma.

In this review, the first section will discuss general hepatic IPTs, including their morphologic features, histologic classification, and association with cholangitis and abscesses. We will also review those infections and inflammatory conditions that can cause hepatic IPT but that can be specifically recognized by pathologists. This section is followed by a review of the most common neoplasms that enter the differential diagnosis. Our goal is to provide pathologists with a useful guide to evaluating a biopsy of a hepatic lesion when it resembles an IPT.

INFLAMMATORY PSEUDOTUMOR

General Features

Hepatic IPT is rare, accounting for less than 1% of liver tumors.[2] Patient age range is broad, with an average age of approximately 50 years.[3,4] Some studies report that both sexes are affected equally,[3] whereas some report slight male predilection.[5,6] Most patients have a single lesion but occasional patients have multiple lesions.[5,7] The right lobe is affected more often than the left.[3,5,6] Common symptoms include fever, abdominal pain, and weight loss; however, occasional lesions are found on imaging in asymptomatic patients being investigated for neoplasia.[4–7] Large centrally located lesions may result in obstructive jaundice and occlusive portal phlebitis.[8] Some patients have elevated C-reactive protein, erythrocyte sedimentation rate, and neutrophil count.[4,6] A minority has elevated liver tests. Most patients do not have cirrhosis.[5] A history of biliary disease or cholangitis is fairly common,[5] including reports of hepatic IPT in the setting of primary sclerosing cholangitis, primary biliary cholangitis, and recurrent pyogenic cholangitis.[9–12] They have also been reported in patients with Crohn disease and Sjogren syndrome,[13–16] disorders that can be associated with cholangiopathy.

Macroscopically, the tumors are grayish white to tan-white and firm. Foci of hemorrhage or necrosis can be present.[17] The size range is broad, from less than 1 cm to more than 20 cm, with most falling within the range of 2 to 5 cm.[3,5,17]

Histologically, IPTs consist of a proliferation of fibroblasts or myofibroblasts arranged in a whorled, storiform, or short fascicular pattern with admixed inflammation (Fig. 1). The fibroblasts can demonstrate a reactive appearance with mildly enlarged vesicular nuclei and small nucleoli but significant atypia is not a feature of hepatic IPT and should raise concern for a true neoplasm. Rare mitoses can be found in the spindle cells. The inflammatory component includes histiocytes, plasma cells, lymphocytes, and neutrophils with some cases demonstrating microabscesses.[3,17] Occasional cases have multinucleated giant cells or granulomatous inflammation.[3] Individual cases can have more fibrosis or more inflammation, and some pseudotumors demonstrate significant heterogeneity within the same lesion. Various stages of obliterative phlebitis can be seen within the lesion and in the adjacent liver parenchyma.[18] Cholangitis is also a feature of some cases, and can involve the extrahepatic or intrahepatic bile ducts adjacent to the tumor (Fig. 2), as well as peribiliary glands. Affected ducts show fibrous thickening of the bile duct wall with chronic inflammation.[19]

The inflammatory composition in hepatic IPTs has been the basis of their histologic classifications. In 1978, Someren[18] called attention to 3 histologic patterns of IPT based on descriptions in the literature: those with a prominent histiocytic component (xanthogranuloma type); those with a prominent plasma cell component (plasma cell granuloma type); and those with markedly sclerotic features (sclerosing pseudotumors). However, this report generated little interest, partly due to the perception that tumoral heterogeneity accounted for some of the perceived differences and made it difficult to classify individual lesions, and also because no attempt was made to attach clinical relevance to the various subtypes. In 2007, Zen and colleagues[20] classified 16 cases of hepatic IPTs into fibrohistiocytic and lymphoplasmacytic variants (Table 1). Fibrohistiocytic hepatic IPTs had a prominent histiocytic inflammatory infiltrate, including foamy macrophages and multinucleated giant cells. The lymphoplasmacytic type showed prominent lymphocytes and plasma cells, and most showed increased eosinophils as well. In their series, both types showed venous occlusive changes, but the fibrohistiocytic type showed occluded large veins with little or no inflammation whereas the lymphoplasmacytic type showed occlusion of smaller veins with an inflammatory cell infiltrate (obliterative phlebitis). Cholangitis was seen in both types but inflammatory cholangitis, characterized by periductal lymphoplasmacytic infiltration without periductal concentric fibrosis, was observed only in the

Fig. 1. A biopsy of a fibrohistiocytic IPT shows a mass lesion composed of spindle cells, lymphocytes, and numerous macrophages including foamy macrophages.

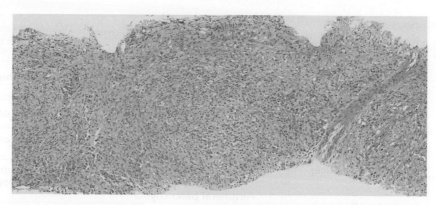

fibrohistiocytic type. Sclerosing cholangitis with periductal inflammation and concentric periductal fibrosis was only seen in the lymphoplasmacytic type. Both types had numerous IgG-positive plasma cells by immunohistochemistry but the lymphoplasmacytic type also had numerous IgG4-positive plasma cells throughout the lesion, and high IgG4:IgG ratio. In contrast, most fibrohistiocytic IPTs had very few IgG4-positive plasma cells and low IgG4:IgG ratio.

Significantly, the clinical characteristics between the 2 types differed.[20] Fibrohistiocytic hepatic IPTs occurred in men and women equally. The right and left lobes of the liver were equally affected, and the lesions were more often peripheral in the liver, with a mass-forming growth pattern that mimicked a mass-forming intrahepatic cholangiocarcinoma. In contrast, in their cohort, lymphoplasmacytic hepatic IPTs occurred only in men. The lesions were more often in the left lobe, near the hilum, where they followed the course of large ducts, similar to periductal infiltrating type of cholangiocarcinoma. The authors concluded that lymphoplasmacytic type of hepatic IPT is a distinct lesion that belongs within the IgG4-related disease spectrum.

In a subsequent study of 22 hepatic IPTs, Ahn and colleagues[21] found that 3 of 5 patients with lymphoplasmacytic IPT had clinical findings of IgG4-related cholangitis but all of them resolved without steroid therapy. In contrast, 17 fibrohistiocytic IPTs had negative IgG4 immunohistochemical stains. Obstructive phlebitis and lymphoid follicle formation occurred more often in the lymphoplasmacytic type but not to a statistically significant degree. They were unable to show an association between the subtype of IPT and its location, clinical presentation, or laboratory findings. The authors agreed that hepatic IPTs can be classified by the number of IgG4-positive plasma cells but were uncertain about whether lymphoplasmacytic IPTs represent an autoimmune process.

Hepatic IPT can be managed conservatively because many tumors respond to antibiotics or resolve spontaneously.[3,4,7,21] IPTs may also respond to steroids.[4,7] Still, a significant number of IPTs are resected, either because malignancy cannot be excluded based on a biopsy or because no presurgical biopsy is performed. Although resection is curative, it can result in complications, particularly when the lesion approximates hilar

Fig. 2. Cholangitis involving a large duct adjacent to an IPT, with periductal mononuclear inflammation (left). Note the narrowing of the vein lumen nearby as well (lower right).

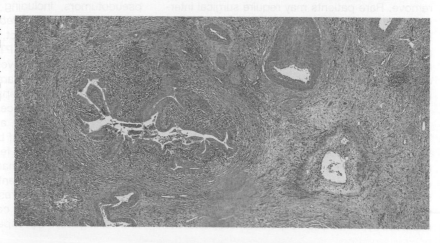

Table 1
General pathologic and clinical characteristics of fibrohistiocytic and lymphoplasmacytic types of hepatic inflammatory pseudotumors[20]

	Fibrohistiocytic Type	Lymphoplasmacytic Type
Gender	Equal sex distribution	Predominantly men
Clinical presentation	More often associated with subjective symptoms such as fever, abdominal pain, and malaise	More often incidental or identified due to liver test abnormalities
Location within liver	Equal involvement of right and left lobes Peripheral parenchyma	Predominantly left lobe Hilar location
Growth pattern	Mass-forming pattern	Periductal infiltrating pattern
Cell composition	Abundant histiocytes, including xanthogranulomatous inflammation and multinucleated giant cells Numerous plump stromal cells expressing smooth muscle actin	Abundant lymphoplasmacytic inflammation Eosinophil infiltration
IgG4 expression	Few IgG4-positive plasma cells Low IgG4:IgG ratio	Many IgG4-positive plasma cells throughout the lesion High IgG4:IgG ratio
Venous changes	Obliteration of large veins with little inflammation	Venous occlusion with inflammatory cell infiltrate
Duct changes	Bile ducts within the lesion are destroyed Adjacent ducts with periductal lymphoplasmacytic infiltration without periductal concentric fibrosis	Bile ducts within the lesion show preserved bile duct epithelium despite intense inflammation Adjacent ducts with sclerosing cholangitis with periductal inflammation and concentric edematous fibrosis Sclerosing inflammation of peribiliary glands

Adapted from Zen Y, Fujii T, Sato Y, Masuda S, Nakanuma Y. Pathological classification of hepatic inflammatory pseudotumor with respect to IgG4-related disease. Mod Pathol 2007;20:884-94.

structures and requires hemihepatectomy to remove. Rare patients may require surgical intervention if the lesion fails to respond to conservative management, enlarges, or compresses adjacent structures.[4] Reports of IPTs acting in a malignant fashion likely represent misdiagnosis of a more aggressive lesion such as IMT or follicular dendritic cell tumor.[22,23]

Hepatic Inflammatory Pseudotumor and Infections

Many cases of IPT are idiopathic in nature. However, there are several features of hepatic IPTs that suggest an infectious cause, including clinical signs such as fever, elevated neutrophil counts, multifocality, antibiotic responsiveness, and the fact that organisms have been isolated from rare pseudotumors, including various Gram-positive cocci, Bacteroides, *Klebsiella pneumoniae*, or *Escherichia coli*.[3,6] In fact, one proposed explanation for some hepatic IPTs is resolving liver abscess.[24,25] Although several authors have noted the different imaging characteristics of a liquefactive liver abscess and hepatic IPTs,[3,4] abscess remains the clinical concern in several reported cases.[6,24,25] In practice, a biopsy of a lesion that is clinically suspected of being an abscess occasionally demonstrates features of hepatic IPT with numerous foamy macrophages and fibrosis, and presumably represents the healing phase; in some cases, there is residual purulent material (**Fig. 3**). In one of the cases reported by Tsou and colleagues,[24] a preoperative biopsy of a lesion

Fig. 3. Hepatic abscess. At right, the biopsy shows purulent inflammation consistent with abscess cavity. The remainder of the biopsy shows the fibroblastic response that is reminiscent of IPT.

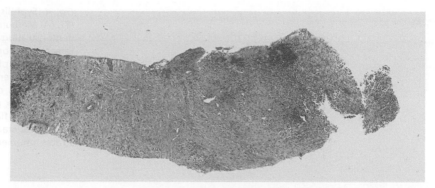

that demonstrated abundant neutrophils consistent with an abscess evolved into IPT by the time of resection. Even when a biopsy demonstrates abscess, the adjacent liver tissue commonly shows foamy macrophages and fibrosis, features indistinguishable from hepatic IPT. The association of hepatic IPT with biliary disease[5,19] suggests that IPTs may be an exuberant response to cholangitis. Cholangitis is one cause of hepatic abscess, and therefore, all of these conditions may reflect different stages of the same process.

Despite the theory that hepatic IPTs are related to infection, the infectious agent is often elusive, notwithstanding the rare example in which an infectious agent is identified. However, there are important infectious agents that have to be considered when a biopsy demonstrates what appears to be an IPT because several organisms can, on occasion, cause inflammatory masses that are identified on imaging and either biopsied or resected. These include various mycobacteria, *Brucella*, *Bartonella*, syphilis, *Candida*, and *Actinomyces*. Patient characteristics and clinical history are important considerations when one of these agents is being considered, and whether ancillary testing is warranted. Histologic features of the tumor may also provide important clues as to the nature of the lesion, and which ancillary tests to pursue.

Mycobacterium tuberculosis can cause a localized lesion that may be either a tuberculoma or tuberculous abscess. A tuberculoma is composed of confluent granulomas and contains few organisms, whereas a tuberculous abscess is centrally suppurative and contains numerous organisms. The former is more likely in immune competent hosts, whereas the latter is generally seen in immunocompromised individuals.[26] A brucelloma is typically seen in patients who had brucellosis years previously, suggesting reactivation. Histologically, a brucelloma shows necrotic areas surrounded by a palisaded histiocytic reaction but rarely it may show only fibrosis and chronic inflammation.[26]

Bartonella henselae is the agent of cat scratch disease; hepatic cat scratch disease generally affects children aged from 5 to 10 years. Patients usually have abdominal lymphadenopathy but the classic axial lymphadenopathy and skin papule of cat scratch disease is often absent. The lesions are often multiple, hard, and mimic malignancy. Resection of these lesions shows irregular stellate abscesses surrounded by palisading histiocytes, lymphocytes, and a rim of fibrotic tissue. Depending on the age of the lesion, there may be more necrosis with less organization or, in older lesions, confluent granulomas with scarring and scant necrosis. Biopsies may show any of these features, and thus may be mistaken for an hepatic IPT if the areas of necrosis are not sampled.[26]

Syphilis has a range of histologic findings when it involves the liver.[27] In 2014, Hagen and colleagues[28] reported 2 cases of hepatic IPTs in human immunodeficiency virus (HIV)-positive homosexual men. Others have reported hepatic IPT in syphilis in HIV-negative patients.[29] Patients may not have the classic rash of secondary syphilis, and therefore, a high index of suspicion is necessary to consider this infection. A history of high-risk sexual activity, homosexual sex, earlier history of syphilis, or anal HPV disease may be relevant when evaluating an IPT. Patients may have disproportionately high alkaline phosphatase relative to the transaminase elevations. Biopsies show areas of plump fibroblasts admixed with lymphocytes, plasma cells, and neutrophils, as well as hypocellular areas composed of edematous hyalinized fibrous tissue (**Fig. 4**). Residual neutrophilic collections can be present, either as small microabscesses or as expanding necrotic lesions within the tumor. An important clue to the diagnosis of syphilis is the presence of periductal edema and neutrophilic pericholangitis in portal tracts outside the IPT. Immunohistochemical stain for *Treponema* shows innumerable organisms in these pseudotumors. Silver stains such as Steiner stain are too insensitive to exclude syphilis in these cases.

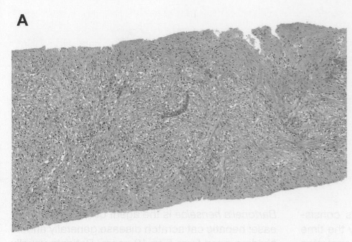

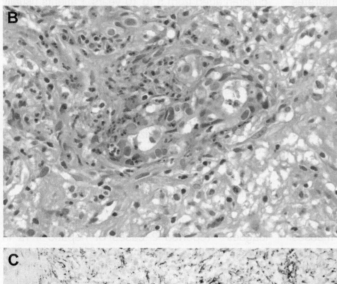

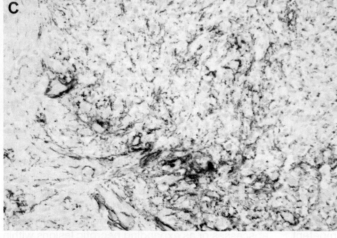

Fig. 4. Syphilis manifesting as a hepatic IPT. (*A*) Medium power view of the lesion demonstrating fibroblasts arranged as intersecting short fascicles admixed with lymphocytes, plasma cells, and histiocytes. (*B*) High-power view of a bile duct nearby to the lesion demonstrates neutrophilic inflammation, duct injury, and periductal edema and inflammation. (*C*) Immunohistochemical stain for *Treponema* demonstrates innumerable organisms.

Hepatic candidiasis is an infection that is particularly likely to affect patients with leukemia. In fact, in patients who carry a diagnosis of acute leukemia who develop hepatic or splenic lesions, candidiasis has to be aggressively excluded. Histologic features include necrotizing granulomas, abscesses or necrotic foci with histiocytes at the edge, often surrounded by a fibrotic wall, or, in the late stages, fibrotic lesions with few organisms (**Fig. 5**).[26] In this setting, Grocott's Methenamine

Silver (GMS) stain should be performed to exclude *Candida*.

Actinomycosis is a chronic suppurative disease that results in a markedly fibrotic mass lesion with draining sinuses. Within the pus, colonies of Actinomyces can appear grossly as yellow flecks, known as sulfur granules. Abdominal actinomycosis can involve the liver as large hepatic fibrotic masses that can be mistaken for an IPT.[30] Some of the reported cases affected women with intrauterine device use.[31,32] Microscopic evaluation demonstrates dense fibrotic masses with abscesses

and marked inflammation consisting of lymphocytes, plasma cells, and foamy macrophages.[31] Characteristic colonies of filamentous organisms may be found in the abscesses, and can be highlighted with GMS stain or Gram stain.

IgG4-related disease associated hepatic inflammatory pseudotumor

IgG-related disease (IgG4-RD) is a disorder associated with autoimmune pancreatitis and multiple organ involvement, including the liver, in which

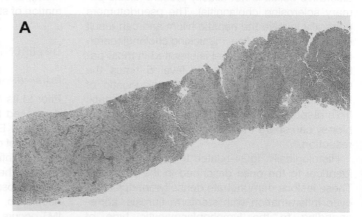

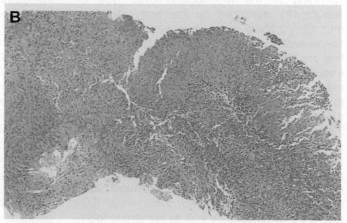

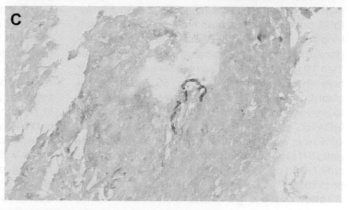

Fig. 5. Hepatic candidiasis in a patient with leukemia. (*A*) Low-power view demonstrates an area of intense inflammation (right) with adjacent areas resembling IPT. (*B*) High-power view of the area of abscess demonstrates a granulomatous component. (*C*) GMS stain demonstrates rare fragmented pseudohyphae consistent with *Candida*.

the most common manifestation is a form of sclerosing cholangitis. Patients can develop one or more hepatic IPTs, possibly due to an exuberant nodular inflammatory response to affected ducts.[33,34] Hepatic IPTs may occur together with sclerosing cholangitis or the hepatic tumor may dominate the clinical presentation with the cholangitis becoming evident at the time of microscopic evaluation of the resected specimen.[33]

IgG4-related hepatic IPTs affect older patients with a strong male predominance.[3,34] Diabetes mellitus is a common comorbidity.[34] A history of ulcerative colitis is not usually present (unlike primary sclerosing cholangitis). The pseudotumors generally involve the hepatic hilum and can result in obstructive jaundice, mimicking cholangiocarcinoma.[34] Serum IgG4 level is elevated in most patients with IgG4-RD, and a level 5 times the upper limit of normal is virtually diagnostic of IgG4-RD.[35] IgG4-RD and its associated hepatic IPTs respond to steroids; therefore, diagnosis on biopsy can spare the patient complicated hepatic resection.

Histologically, IgG4-related IPTs in the liver are identical to the ones described in the pancreas. These lesions demonstrate dense lymphoplasmacytic inflammation with storiform fibrosis, corresponding to the lymphoplasmacytic type of hepatic IPT described by Zen and colleagues (Fig. 6).[20,34] Many cases show eosinophil infiltration as well. Lymphoid follicles with germinal centers are often observed.[36] Obliterative phlebitis is frequently seen, particularly in resection specimens, although an elastic stain may be necessary to recognize these obliterated veins within the tumor.[20] In resection specimens, the inflammatory infiltrate involves adjacent tissue. Adjacent ducts show luminal narrowing and periductal lymphoplasmacytic inflammation but in contrast with primary sclerosing cholangitis, the duct epithelial lining is preserved.[33] Immunohistochemical evaluation for IgG and IgG4 shows numerous IgG-positive plasma cells as well as numerous IgG4-positive plasma cells. Diagnostic thresholds for IgG4-positive plasma cells have been set for both biopsies and resection specimens of various organs. In biopsies and resection specimens, greater than 10 IgG4-positive plasma cells per high power field (HPF) and greater than 50 IgG4-positive plasma cells per HPF, respectively, is suggested to arrive at a diagnosis of IgG4-RD. Moreover, the IgG4:IgG plasma cell ratio should be higher than 40%. It is worth noting that most IgG4-related hepatic IPTs harbor many more IgG4-positive plasma cells (>100 per HPF) and show higher IgG4:IgG ratio (>50%).[20,36] Conversely, about a third of hepatic IPTs not related to IgG4-RD, or mimics such as IMT,

will reach thresholds described above.[34,36] Therefore, it may be difficult in borderline cases to determine if the hepatic IPT is related to IgG4-RD based only on histology and immunohistochemistry, and the mere presence of numerous plasma cells and even IgG4-positive plasma cells does not exclude certain infections or IPT mimics such as IMT. A diagnosis of IgG4-RD hepatic IPT should be made after considering infections such as syphilis and excluding IPT mimics, and in conjunction with clinical data such as IgG4 serum level, extrahepatic organ involvement (particularly pancreatic involvement), and, if steroids have been initiated, confirmation of steroid responsiveness.

DIFFERENTIAL DIAGNOSIS

Inflammatory Myofibroblastic Tumor

Prior to its recognition in the 1990s, IMT was often diagnosed as IPT. A report in the early 1990s by Meis and Enzinger described aggressive behavior in a subset of IPTs, and the authors labeled these tumors as "inflammatory fibrosarcoma."[37] The recognition that they often harbored clonal rearrangements of chromosome 2p confirmed that these tumors are neoplastic, and today they are classified as IMT. IMT occurs most often in young to middle-aged patients. They occur in the abdominopelvic region, lung, and retroperitoneum; hepatic IMT is uncommon, accounting for less than 10% of IMTs.[38,39] Similar to IPT, patients can present with constitutional symptoms such as fever, weight loss and malaise, and these symptoms resolve following resection.[39]

The gross features of IMT are similar to IPT, with a firm, fleshy, or gelatinous white or tan cut surface.[38] Microscopically, IMTs show a proliferation of myofibroblastic spindle cells in a fibrotic stroma, with prominent inflammatory cell infiltration comprising numerous plasma cells and lymphocytes, with occasional eosinophils and neutrophils (Fig. 7). Lymphoid follicles with germinal centers are seen in a minority of cases.[36] Significantly, IgG4-positive plasma cells can be present, even reaching the threshold that has been set for IgG4-related IPT, although generally the number is lower than the threshold, and the IgG4:IgG ratio is low.[36] Another reported difference between IMT and IgG4-related IPT is that the inflammatory infiltrate in IMT is not prominent in peritumoral tissue.[36] Otherwise, there can be considerable variation in the morphology, ranging from areas that resemble nodular fasciitis, to areas with compact spindle cells and numerous plasma cells, and fibromatosis-like areas with elongate spindle cells in a densely collagenous background with only scattered lymphocytes.[39]

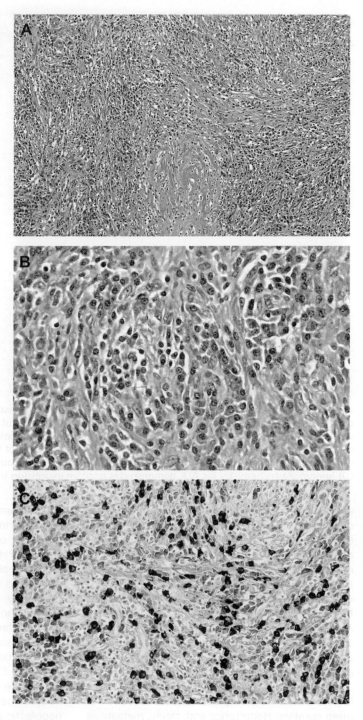

Fig. 6. IgG4-related IPT. (*A*) Medium-power view of a lymphoplasmacytic IPT demonstrates storiform fibrosis and lymphoplasmacytic infiltrate. (*B*) High-power view demonstrates numerous plasma cells in the IPT. (*C*) Immunohistochemical stain for IgG4 shows numerous IgG4-positive plasma cells.

Ganglion-like cells similar to those seen in proliferative fasciitis can be seen. Mitotic figures can be seen but atypical mitoses are not found.[38] The tumor may evolve into a high-grade sarcoma, and these tumors can show spindle, epithelioid, or round cell morphology.

Immunohistochemistry demonstrates that the spindle cells are usually positive for smooth muscle actin (SMA), and the majority express desmin and calponin, at least focally.[38] About one-third of cases show focal reactivity for keratin. About half of the tumors harbor a clonal translocation

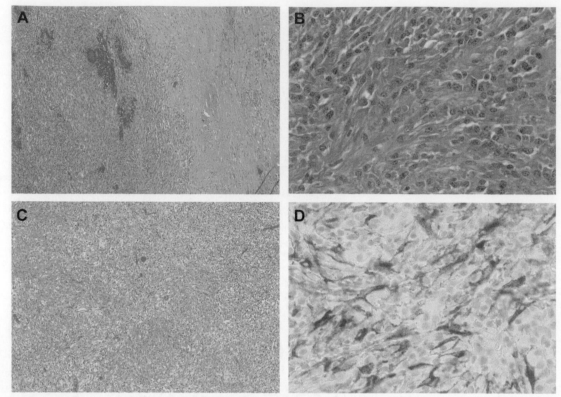

Fig. 7. IMT, variable features. (*A*) Low-power view of an IMT shows variable cellularity, with hypercellular areas composed of plump spindle cells with lymphocytic infiltrate (left), and areas of hypocellular collagenous stroma with delicate spindle cells (right). (*B*) High-power view of this example of IMT demonstrates numerous plasma cells, which can raise confusion with IgG4-related IPT. (*C*) Example of IMT that demonstrates numerous plump, mildly atypical myofibroblasts with relatively mild inflammatory component and patchy tumor cell necrosis. (*D*) Immunohistochemistry for ALK demonstrates positive expression in the tumor cells.

involving the anaplastic lymphoma kinase (ALK)-receptor tyrosine kinase gene located at 2p23 locus; multiple fusion partners to *ALK* have been described.[40] *ALK* rearrangement-negative tumors may have other genetic rearrangements, such as *ROS1*.[40] The presence of *ALK* or *ROS1* rearrangement can be helpful in the diagnosis of IMT, and these tumors will frequently show expression of ALK or ROS1 by immunohistochemistry, facilitating diagnosis.[36] However, it is worth noting that the absence of a known genetic fusion does not exclude the diagnosis of IMT.

IMT is considered a tumor of intermediate biological potential. Complete surgical resection is often curative. Recurrence and, rarely, metastasis are largely described in those tumors that, by fault of their location, cannot be completely excised.

Inflammatory Pseudotumor-Like Follicular Dendritic Cell Tumor

In the 1990s, several investigators reported Epstein-Barr virus (EBV) expression in IPTs.[41–43]

Shortly thereafter, it was recognized that the spindle cells in these EBV-positive IPTs expressed markers of follicular dendritic cells (FDCs). Demonstration that the episomal EBV genome is monoclonal supports that the FDC proliferation is neoplastic.[23,41] EBV-positive FDC tumors are rare; they occur almost exclusively in the liver and spleen and have a marked female predilection. Systemic inflammatory symptoms such as weight loss and fever are common.[44] Radiologic and macroscopic features are similar to IPT. Histologically, EBV-driven FDC tumors resemble an IPT, unlike their counterparts in peripheral lymph nodes. The tumor is composed of spindle or oval neoplastic cells with a brisk inflammatory cell infiltrate comprising lymphocytes, plasma cells, and histiocytes. The FDCs usually show only minimal atypia but some tumors demonstrate neoplastic FDCs that have enlarged vesicular nuclei, nuclear irregularity, and prominent nucleoli. Binucleated tumor cells with prominent nucleoli can be mistaken for Reed-Sternberg cells (**Fig. 8**). Rare tumors have areas that resemble conventional

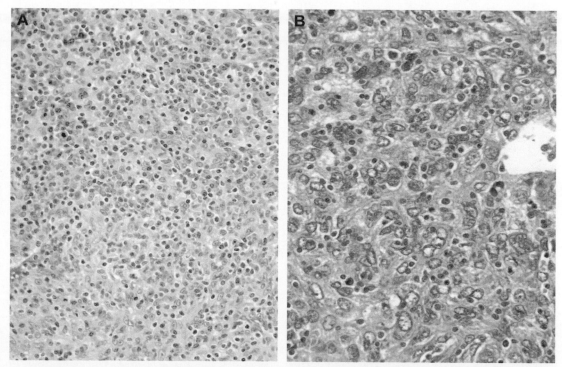

Fig. 8. IPT-like follicular dendritic cell tumor. (*A*) Medium-power view shows numerous oval pale cells with small central nucleoli in a background of numerous lymphocytes and plasma cells (Courtesy of Dr Sanjay Kakar). (*B*) High-power view demonstrates atypical FDCs with enlarged, vesicular and occasionally binucleate tumor cells that can resemble Reed-Sternberg cells, with scattered lymphocytes (Courtesy of Dr Vikram Deshpande).

FDC tumors, with syncytial spindle cells in a storiform pattern, lightly sprinkled with lymphocytes.[44] Many cases exhibit vascular ectasia with deposition of fibrinous material in the vessel wall.[44]

Immunohistochemistry shows that the tumor cells are positive for FDC markers, although staining can be patchy or focal, and therefore a panel of antibodies is advisable.[44] CD21 and CD35 are the

Fig. 9. Inflammatory variant of AML. A minority of AMLs show a striking lymphocytic inflammatory infiltrate that, together with the spindled tumor cells, mimics IPT.

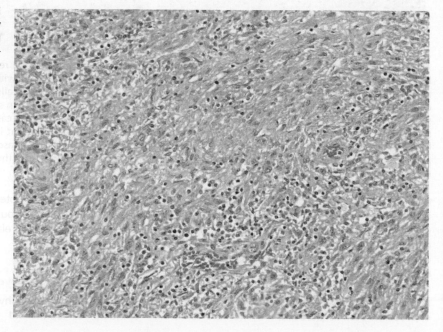

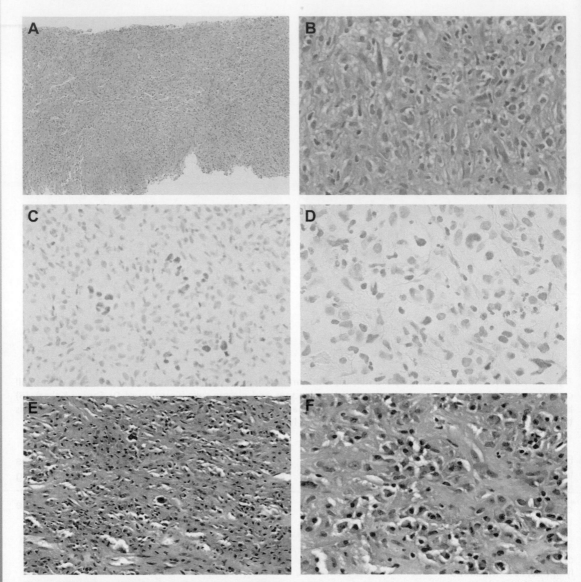

Fig. 10. Hodgkin lymphoma mimicking IPT. (*A*) Medium-power view of a tumor that resembles a fibrohistiocytic IPT. (*B*) High-power view of the same tumor demonstrates many histiocyte-like cells, with nuclear irregularity and abnormal forms, although the atypical cells are not diagnostic of Reed-Sternberg cells. (*C*) PAX5 immunohistochemical stain demonstrates nuclear staining of the large neoplastic cells. (*D*) EBER in situ hybridization demonstrates staining in the large neoplastic cells. (*E*) Medium-power view of a different case of Hodgkin lymphoma resembling a lymphoplasmacytic IPT. Large hyperchromatic atypical cells are present in a background of fibroblasts, lymphocytes, and numerous plasma cells. (*F*) High-power view of the same case demonstrates numerous plasma cells that can cause confusion with IgG4-related IPT. Note the large cell with the atypical hyperchromatic nucleus (far left).

most reliable of the commonly available antibodies, and CD23 may be less sensitive.[44] EBV expression has been reported in the vast majority of IPT-like FDC tumors and is confined to the spindle cells.[23,41,44] In fact, EBV expression is considered a very sensitive method of screening an IPT, and if the tumor proves to be EBV positive, immunohistochemical staining with markers of FDC expression can be pursued. IPT-like FDC tumors

have a low malignant potential. Resection is curative in most patients but some patients suffer recurrence and tumor-related deaths have been recorded.[23,44]

Inflammatory Angiomyolipoma

AML is a benign mesenchymal tumor composed of spindled or epithelioid smooth muscle cells,

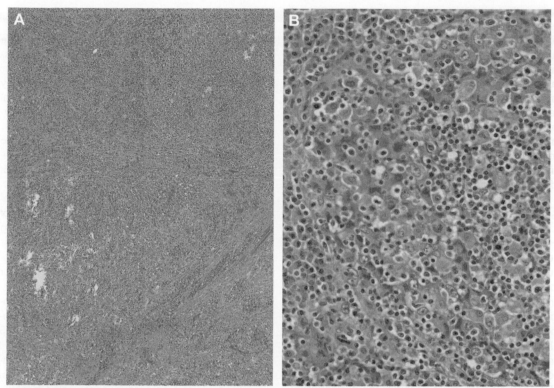

Fig. 11. Hepatocellular carcinoma, inflammatory type. (*A*) Low-power view of a tumor that demonstrates marked lymphoplasmacytic infiltrate and resembles an IPT. (*B*). High-power examination betrays the large epithelial cells with vesicular nuclei and eosinophilic nucleoli that are obscured by the intense inflammation.

adipocytes, and thick-walled vessels that occurs more often in the kidney, and rarely in the liver. Hepatic AMLs rarely show an exuberant inflammatory component, and this variant is known as inflammatory AML.[25,45] In those tumors with spindled myocytes, the heavy but variable infiltrate of lymphocytes, plasma cells, and histiocytes can mimic IPT, particularly on biopsy material (Fig. 9). Immunohistochemical staining for Human Melanoma Black-45 (HMB-45) confirms the diagnosis of AML.

Lymphoma

Involvement of the liver by Hodgkin lymphoma can create an appearance that resembles an IPT (Fig. 10). Similarly, large B-cell lymphomas that induce an inflammatory infiltrate (eg, T-cell/histiocyte rich large B-cell lymphoma) can mimic IPT. Usually, patients carry a history of lymphoma but rarely they present with hepatic involvement. In most cases, careful assessment of the lesion will demonstrate scattered large atypical lymphoid cells but, in some cases, the neoplastic cells can be easily overlooked, particularly when they resemble histiocytes. In suspicious cases, markers for B-cells (cluster of differentiation

[CD]-20 and Pax-5) may be useful. Large B-cell lymphoma will generally express CD20. Reed-Sternberg cells do not express CD20 but retain Pax-5.[46] Multiple Myeloma-1 (MUM-1) is also often positive in the neoplastic cells in Hodgkin lymphoma. In situ hybridization for EBV-encoded RNA (EBER) is also helpful to highlight neoplastic cells because a significant number of Hodgkin lymphomas and large B-cell lymphomas are associated with EBV. Although Reed-Sternberg cells are well known to express CD15 and CD30, screening IPTs with those 2 markers can be misleading because inflammatory cells can express CD15, and CD30 can mark activated lymphocytes.

Lymphoepithelioma-like Hepatocellular Carcinoma (Inflammatory Hepatocellular Carcinoma)

A variety of terms have been used to describe rare hepatocellular carcinomas (HCC) that are associated with a dense infiltrate of lymphoid cells, including lymphoepithelioma-like HCC, inflammatory HCC, and HCC with lymphoid stroma. These tumors show varying proportions of neoplastic cells and inflammatory cells; a biopsy from a region that has a paucity of neoplastic cells and massive infiltration of immune cells may resemble an IPT (**Fig. 11**). The inflammatory infiltrate varies among cases, with most examples showing numerous lymphocytes and rare cases showing a predominance of plasma cells.[47,48] In these tumors, the neoplastic cells often have large vesicular nuclei, prominent nucleoli, and relatively abundant eosinophilic cytoplasm; the tumor cells frequently express Hep Par 1. The neoplastic cells in lymphoepithelioma-like HCC are EBV negative,[47,48] although one EBV-positive case was described in a liver explant.[49]

SUMMARY

Hepatic IPT is a term for a heterogeneous group of tumor-like lesions that share similar histologic features, namely a proliferation of fibroblasts or myofibroblasts and an inflammatory infiltrate. The inflammatory infiltrate is typically mononuclear but can include granulomas or giant cells, neutrophils or abscesses, and eosinophils. Although many of these lesions are presumed to be a response to infection, the organism responsible is only rarely identified. However, when confronted with a hepatic IPT, pathologists must consider the clinicopathologic scenario to determine the appropriateness of various techniques to exclude specific infections such as mycobacterial infection, fungal infection, or syphilis. When the lesion contains numerous plasma cells, assessing for IgG and IgG4 may be of use to investigate for IgG4-related IPT, although this diagnosis should be made in conjunction with clinical findings. Finally, the possibility of a neoplastic mimic of IPT should be considered. IMT may show expression of ALK or ROS1 by immunohistochemistry. Follicular dendritic cell tumor may demonstrate expression of follicular dendritic cell antigens or EBV by in situ hybridization for EBV-encoded RNA. EBER can also be useful to identify some types of lymphoma that can resemble a hepatic IPT. Inflammatory AML can be excluded with HMB-45 stain and the possibility of an underlying inflammatory hepatocellular carcinoma can be evaluated with Hep Par 1 or appropriate keratin stains. Ultimately, hepatic IPT is a diagnosis of exclusion that requires consideration of specific infections and neoplastic mimics, and the application of selected ancillary studies to investigate for these possibilities in the context of the clinical circumstances and particular histologic appearance of the tumor.

DISCLOSURES

The authors have no relevant financial disclosures.

REFERENCES

1. Anthony PP. Inflammatory pseudotumour (plasma cell granuloma) of lung, liver and other organs. Histopathology 1993;23:501–3.
2. Torzilli G, Inoue K, Midorikawa Y, et al. Inflammatory pseudotumors of the liver: prevalence and clinical impact in surgical patients. Hepato-Gastroenterology 2001;48:1118–23.
3. Arora KS, Anderson MA, Neyaz A, et al. Fibrohistiocytic variant of hepatic pseudotumor: an antibiotic responsive tumefactive lesion. Am J Surg Pathol 2021;45:1314–23.
4. Goldsmith PJ, Loganathan A, Jacob M, et al. Inflammatory pseudotumours of the liver: a spectrum of presentation and management options. Eur J Surg Oncol 2009;35:1295–8.
5. Yang X, Zhu J, Biskup E, et al. Inflammatory pseudotumors of the liver: experience of 114 cases. Tumour Biol 2015;36:5143–8.
6. Park JY, Choi MS, Lim YS, et al. Clinical features, image findings, and prognosis of inflammatory pseudotumor of the liver: a multicenter experience of 45 cases. Gut Liver 2014;8:58–63.
7. Koea JB, Broadhurst GW, Rodgers MS, et al. Inflammatory pseudotumor of the liver: demographics, diagnosis, and the case for nonoperative management. J Am Coll Surg 2003;196:226–35.
8. Lee SL, DuBois JJ. Hepatic inflammatory pseudotumor: case report, review of the literature, and a proposal for morphologic classification. Pediatr Surg Int 2001;17:555–9.
9. Tsui WM, Chan YK, Wong CT, et al. Hepatolithiasis and the syndrome of recurrent pyogenic cholangitis: clinical, radiologic, and pathologic features. Semin Liver Dis 2011;31:33–48.
10. Toda K, Yasuda I, Nishigaki Y, et al. Inflammatory pseudotumor of the liver with primary sclerosing cholangitis. J Gastroenterol 2000;35:304–9.
11. Endo S, Watanabe Y, Abe Y, et al. Hepatic inflammatory pseudotumor associated with primary biliary cholangitis and elevated alpha-fetoprotein lectin 3 fraction mimicking hepatocellular carcinoma. Surg Case Rep 2018;4:114.
12. Rai T, Ohira H, Tojo J, et al. A case of hepatic inflammatory pseudotumor with primary biliary cirrhosis. Hepatol Res 2003;26:249–53.
13. Mouelhi L, Abbes L, Houissa F, et al. Inflammatory pseudotumor of the liver associated with Crohn's disease. J Crohns Colitis 2009;3:305–8.
14. Amankonah TD, Strom CB, Vierling JM, et al. Inflammatory pseudotumor of the liver as the first manifestation of Crohn's disease. Am J Gastroenterol 2001;96:2520–2.
15. Papachristou GI, Wu T, Marsh W, et al. Inflammatory pseudotumor of the liver associated with Crohn's disease. J Clin Gastroenterol 2004;38:818–22.

16. Hosokawa A, Takahashi H, Akaike J, et al. A case of Sjogren's syndrome associated with inflammatory pseudotumor of the liver. Nihon Rinsho Meneki Gakkai Kaishi 1998;21:226–33.

17. Shek TW, Ng IO, Chan KW. Inflammatory pseudotumor of the liver. Report of four cases and review of the literature. Am J Surg Pathol 1993;17:231–8.

18. Someren A. "Inflammatory pseudotumor" of liver with occlusive phlebitis: report of a case in a child and review of the literature. Am J Clin Pathol 1978;69:176–81.

19. Nakanuma Y, Tsuneyama K, Masuda S, et al. Hepatic inflammatory pseudotumor associated with chronic cholangitis: report of three cases. Hum Pathol 1994;25:86–91.

20. Zen Y, Fujii T, Sato Y, et al. Pathological classification of hepatic inflammatory pseudotumor with respect to IgG4-related disease. Mod Pathol 2007;20:884–94.

21. Ahn KS, Kang KJ, Kim YH, et al. Inflammatory pseudotumors mimicking intrahepatic cholangiocarcinoma of the liver; IgG4-positivity and its clinical significance. J Hepatobiliary Pancreat Sci 2012;19:405–12.

22. Zavaglia C, Barberis M, Gelosa F, et al. Inflammatory pseudotumour of the liver with malignant transformation. Report of two cases. Ital J Gastroenterol 1996;28:152–9.

23. Shek TW, Ho FC, Ng IO, et al. Follicular dendritic cell tumor of the liver. Evidence for an Epstein-Barr virus-related clonal proliferation of follicular dendritic cells. Am J Surg Pathol 1996;20:313–24.

24. Tsou YK, Lin CJ, Liu NJ, et al. Inflammatory pseudotumor of the liver: report of eight cases, including three unusual cases, and a literature review. J Gastroenterol Hepatol 2007;22:2143–7.

25. Horiuchi R, Uchida T, Kojima T, et al. Inflammatory pseudotumor of the liver. Clinicopathologic study and review of the literature. Cancer 1990;65:1583–90.

26. Masia R, Misdraji J. Liver and bile duct infections. In: Kradin RL, editor. Diagnostic pathology of infectious disease. 2nd Edition. Philadelphia: Elsevier; 2018. p. 272–322.

27. Malvar G, Cardona D, Pezhouh MK, et al. Hepatic secondary syphilis can cause a variety of histologic patterns and may be negative for treponeme immunohistochemistry. Am J Surg Pathol 2022;46:567–75.

28. Hagen CE, Kamionek M, McKinsey DS, et al. Syphilis presenting as inflammatory tumors of the liver in HIV-positive homosexual men. Am J Surg Pathol 2014;38:1636–43.

29. DeRoche TC, Huber AR. The great imitator: syphilis presenting as an inflammatory pseudotumor of liver. Int J Surg Pathol 2018;26:528–9.

30. Tambay R, Cote J, Bourgault AM, et al. An unusual case of hepatic abscess. Can J Gastroenterol 2001;15:615–7.

31. White JE, Chase CW, Kelley JE, et al. Inflammatory pseudotumor of the liver associated with extrahepatic infection. Southampt Med J 1997;90:23–9.

32. Kim HS, Park NH, Park KA, et al. A case of pelvic actinomycosis with hepatic actinomycotic pseudotumor. Gynecol Obstet Invest 2007;64:95–9.

33. Nakanuma Y, Zen Y. Pathology and immunopathology of immunoglobulin G4-related sclerosing cholangitis: The latest addition to the sclerosing cholangitis family. Hepatol Res 2007;37(Suppl 3):S478–86.

34. Zen Y, Harada K, Sasaki M, et al. IgG4-related sclerosing cholangitis with and without hepatic inflammatory pseudotumor, and sclerosing pancreatitis-associated sclerosing cholangitis: do they belong to a spectrum of sclerosing pancreatitis? Am J Surg Pathol 2004;28:1193–203.

35. Oseini AM, Chaiteerakij R, Shire AM, et al. Utility of serum immunoglobulin G4 in distinguishing immunoglobulin G4-associated cholangitis from cholangiocarcinoma. Hepatology 2011;54:940–8.

36. Yamamoto H, Yamaguchi H, Aishima S, et al. Inflammatory myofibroblastic tumor versus IgG4-related sclerosing disease and inflammatory pseudotumor: a comparative clinicopathologic study. Am J Surg Pathol 2009;33:1330–40.

37. Meis JM, Enzinger FM. Inflammatory fibrosarcoma of the mesentery and retroperitoneum. A tumor closely simulating inflammatory pseudotumor. Am J Surg Pathol 1991;15:1146–56.

38. Gleason BC, Hornick JL. Inflammatory myofibroblastic tumours: where are we now? J Clin Pathol 2008;61:428–37.

39. Coffin CM, Watterson J, Priest JR, et al. Extrapulmonary inflammatory myofibroblastic tumor (inflammatory pseudotumor). A clinicopathologic and immunohistochemical study of 84 cases. Am J Surg Pathol 1995;19:859–72.

40. Antonescu CR, Suurmeijer AJ, Zhang L, et al. Molecular characterization of inflammatory myofibroblastic tumors with frequent ALK and ROS1 gene fusions and rare novel RET rearrangement. Am J Surg Pathol 2015;39:957–67.

41. Selves J, Meggetto F, Brousset P, et al. Inflammatory pseudotumor of the liver. Evidence for follicular dendritic reticulum cell proliferation associated with clonal Epstein-Barr virus. Am J Surg Pathol 1996;20:747–53.

42. Arber DA, Kamel OW, van de Rijn M, et al. Frequent presence of the Epstein-Barr virus in inflammatory pseudotumor. Hum Pathol 1995;26:1093–8.

43. Arber DA, Weiss LM, Chang KL. Detection of Epstein-Barr Virus in inflammatory pseudotumor. Semin Diagn Pathol 1998;15:155–60.

44. Cheuk W, Chan JK, Shek TW, et al. Inflammatory pseudotumor-like follicular dendritic cell tumor: a distinctive low-grade malignant intra-abdominal

neoplasm with consistent Epstein-Barr virus association. Am J Surg Pathol 2001;25:721–31.

45. Tsui WM, Colombari R, Portmann BC, et al. Hepatic angiomyolipoma: a clinicopathologic study of 30 cases and delineation of unusual morphologic variants. Am J Surg Pathol 1999;23:34–48.

46. Choi WT, Gill RM. Hepatic lymphoma diagnosis. Surg Pathol Clin 2018;11:389–402.

47. Patel KR, Liu TC, Vaccharajani N, et al. Characterization of inflammatory (lymphoepithelioma-like)

hepatocellular carcinoma: a study of 8 cases. Arch Pathol Lab Med 2014;138:1193–202.

48. Emile JF, Adam R, Sebagh M, et al. Hepatocellular carcinoma with lymphoid stroma: a tumour with good prognosis after liver transplantation. Histopathology 2000;37:523–9.

49. Si MW, Thorson JA, Lauwers GY, et al. Hepatocellular lymphoepithelioma-like carcinoma associated with epstein barr virus: a hitherto unrecognized entity. Diagn Mol Pathol 2004;13:183–9.

Evaluating Liver Biopsies with Well-Differentiated Hepatocellular Lesions

Sarah E. Umetsu, MD, PhD*, Sanjay Kakar, MD

KEYWORDS

• Well-differentiated • Hepatocellular • Adenoma • Carcinoma • Focal nodular hyperplasia

Key Points

- The differential diagnosis for well-differentiated hepatocellular lesions includes focal nodular hyperplasia (FNH), hepatocellular adenoma (HCA), and well-differentiated hepatocellular carcinoma (HCC) in noncirrhotic liver.
- Due to morphologic overlap of FNH and inflammatory hepatocellular adenoma, routine use of immunohistochemical stains for glutamine synthetase and Serum amyloid A/C-reactive protein (or both) is recommended, especially for biopsies.
- A small subset of cases show borderline atypical features such as cytoarchitectural abnormalities, reticulin pattern and glutamine synthetase staining pattern that are not sufficient for diagnosis of HCC; these cases should be classified as "atypical hepatocellular neoplasms."

ABSTRACT

Needle core biopsies of liver lesions can be challenging, particularly in cases with limited material. The differential diagnosis for well-differentiated hepatocellular lesions includes focal nodular hyperplasia, hepatocellular adenoma, and well-differentiated hepatocellular carcinoma (HCC) in noncirrhotic liver, while dysplastic nodules and well-differentiated HCC are the primary considerations in cirrhotic liver. The first part of this review focuses on histochemical and immunohistochemical stains as well as molecular assays that are useful in the differential diagnosis. The second portion describes the features of hepatocellular adenoma subtypes and focuses on the differential diagnoses in commonly encountered clinicopathologic scenarios.

ROLE OF ANCILLARY STAINS AND MOLECULAR STUDIES

RETICULIN

Abnormalities in reticulin framework such as focal wide trabeculae, fragmentation, and loss are hallmarks of hepatocellular carcinoma (HCC; **Fig. 1A**). Abnormal reticulin framework is present in most well-differentiated HCC as well. If the abnormalities are focal and confined to a small area, they are not diagnostic of HCC, especially in the absence of significant cytoarchitectural atypia. Multifocal reticulin loss is a more reliable feature for HCC diagnosis. A small subset of well-differentiated HCC may not have overt reticulin abnormalities.[1] Of note, reticulin abnormalities can be seen in benign settings. Loss and fragmentation of reticulin is frequently seen in areas of steatosis in both neoplastic and nonneoplastic liver (**Fig. 1B**).[2] Areas adjacent to hemorrhage or infarction frequently show reticulin loss. Reticulin stain often shows "packeting" of small groups of tumor cells in hepatocyte nuclear factor 1-alpha (*HNF1A*)-inactivated HCA (H-HCA) (**Fig. 1C**), and this finding alone should not raise concern for HCC.[3]

CD34

Arterialization of the blood supply can lead to acquisition of the characteristics of capillary endothelium by the sinusoidal lining cells, which start expressing CD34. This leads to diffuse sinusoidal

Department of Pathology, University of California San Francisco, 505 Parnassus Avenue, Box 0102, San Francisco, CA 94143, USA

* Corresponding author.

E-mail address: sarah.umetsu@ucsf.edu

Surgical Pathology 16 (2023) 581–598

https://doi.org/10.1016/J.path.2023.04.011

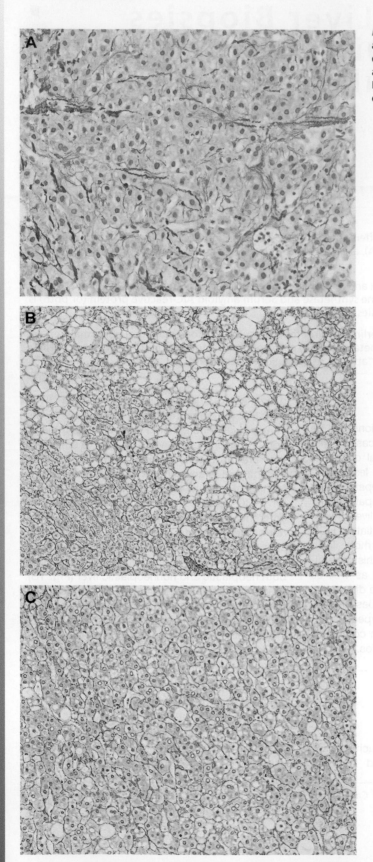

Fig. 1. Reticulin stain. (*A*) Reticulin loss and fragmentation in well-differentiated HCC. (*B*) Reticulin loss in areas of fat in nonneoplastic liver. (*C*) In H-HCA, reticulin stain often shows "packeting" of small groups of tumor cells.

CD34 staining with immunohistochemistry (IHC), a common finding in HCC. However, varying degrees of increase in sinusoidal CD34 staining can also be seen in focal nodular hyperplasia (FNH) and HCA and is not a reliable feature to distinguish benign entities from HCC. CD34 can be useful in small biopsies as a tool for identifying lesional versus nonlesional liver because staining in nonlesional liver should be confined to periportal sinusoids, whereas lesional areas will show increased sinusoidal staining. Hepatocellular tumors with CTNNB1 exon 7 mutations often show a peripheral rim of glutamine synthetase (GS) staining; sinusoidal CD34 staining is seen in the central portion of these lesions but has been described as being absent in the rim.[4]

GLYPICAN-3

Glypican-3 is an oncofetal antigen that is expressed in the majority of HCCs but not in normal adult liver or benign entities. Diffuse staining for glypican-3 can be useful in the diagnosis of HCC, especially on small biopsies.[5,6] Glypican-3 has a high sensitivity for poorly differentiated HCC (80%–83%), whereas the sensitivity for well-differentiated HCC is lower (56%–62%).[5,7] Thus, the stain is only useful if it is positive, and a negative result does not exclude the diagnosis. It should be noted that glypican-3 is not specific for HCC and can be expressed by a variety of other tumors, including melanoma, squamous cell carcinoma, germ cell tumors, and a small subset of intrahepatic cholangiocarcinoma.[5,8]

ARGINASE-1

Arginase-1 is expressed in both benign and malignant hepatocytes and is the most sensitive and specific marker of hepatocellular differentiation.[7] It should always be obtained when evaluating a tumor for hepatocellular differentiation. Arginase-1 has high sensitivity of 80%-90% in poorly differentiated HCC and can be negative in small subset of well-differentiated HCC.[9]

HEAT SHOCK PROTEIN-70

Heat shock protein (HSP)-70 is an antiapoptotic protein that is overexpressed in 50% to 70% of HCCs.[10–12] The combined use of HSP-70, GS, and glypican-3 has been advocated for the distinction of high-grade dysplastic nodules (HGDN) from HCC. In our experience, HSP70 is positive in a small subset of HCC cases and the diagnosis is evident in most of these cases based on hematoxylin and eosin (H&E) and reticulin stains. The utility of HSP70 is limited in this setting.

IMMUNOHISTOCHEMISTRY USED IN HCA SUBTYPING

a. Liver fatty acid binding protein (LFABP): HNF1A-inactivated HCAs (H-HCAs) show complete loss of LFABP expression by IHC (**Fig. 2**A), whereas normal liver and other variants of HCA show diffuse cytoplasmic LFABP expression (**Table 1**). The diagnosis of H-HCA should be based on a combination of overall morphologic features and LFABP stain result because decreased expression or complete loss of LFABP staining can be seen in HCC, even in cases without associated HCA (**Fig. 2**B).[3,13,14] Downregulation of LFABP can occur in other HCA subtypes such as sonic hedgehog-activated HCA (shHCA) leading to decrease in LFABP expression but complete loss of LFABP typically does not occur in other HCA subtypes.[15]

b. Serum amyloid A (SAA)/C-reactive protein (CRP): Diffuse strong cytoplasmic staining with SAA and CRP IHC is characteristic of inflammatory HCA (I-HCA) because of activation of the Janus kinase/signal transducers and activators of transcription (JAK-STAT) pathway.[16] SAA is more specific, although somewhat less sensitive, as approximately 10% to 20% of I-HCA are negative for SAA.[17] CRP has higher sensitivity and is positive in nearly 100% of I-HCA. Patchy CRP staining is common in FNH and tends to be more prominent in periseptal hepatocytes. Both SAA and CRP can be positive in nonneoplastic hepatocytes adjacent to a mass lesion, especially in the setting of metabolic syndrome but staining is often less intense.[17] Increased staining with SAA and CRP in the lesional hepatocytes compared with the background liver is more reliable for a diagnosis of I-HCA (**Fig. 2**C and D).

c. β-catenin: Activation of the Wnt signaling pathway is observed in many hepatocellular neoplasms, and most commonly occurs as a result of mutations/deletions involving CTNNB1 exon 3. However, mutations in exons 7/8 as well as mutations in other components of Wnt signaling pathway (APC, AXIN) can occur in a small number of cases. Wnt activation leads to nuclear translocation of β-catenin, which can be identified by IHC as nuclear staining.[18] However, this finding is not sensitive for β-catenin activation, as staining for β-catenin is often absent or limited to rare hepatocytes, particularly on biopsies (**Fig. 2**E).[19]

d. Glutamine synthetase (GS): GS is an enzyme that is expressed in pericentral hepatocytes in normal liver. Nuclear translocation of β-catenin

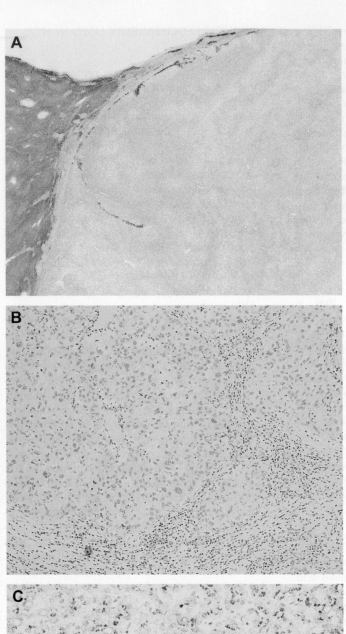

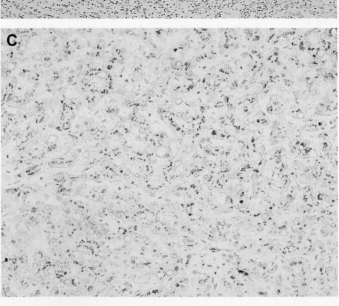

Fig. 2. Immunohistochemical stains used for HCA subtyping. (*A*) H-HCA with complete loss of LFABP in the tumor (right side) as compared to the background liver (left). (*B*) Moderately differentiated HCC with loss of LFABP staining. (*C*) I-HCA with diffuse staining for SAA and

Fig. 2. (continued). (D) CRP. (E) Rare hepatocytes showing positive nuclear staining with β-catenin, consistent with β-catenin activation.

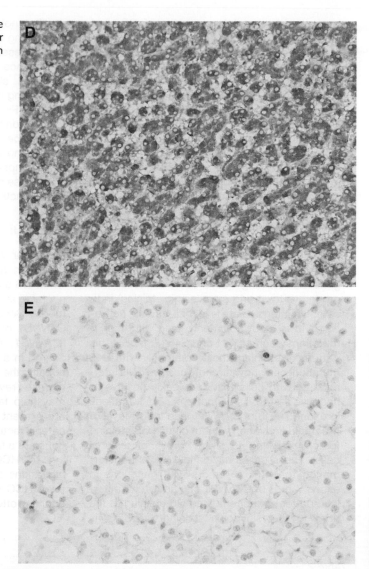

Table 1
Immunohistochemical features of focal nodular hyperplasia and hepatocellular adenoma

IHC	FNH	Inflammatory HCA	HNF1-α Inactivated HCA	β-Catenin Activated HCA/AHN	shHCA
GS	Strong, map-like	Perivascular/patchy	Perivascular/patchy	Diffuse (homogeneous or heterogeneous)	Perivascular/patchy
β-catenin	Membranous	Membranous	Membranous	Nuclear (subset)	Membranous
SAA	Focal or negative	Diffuse	Negative	Negative	Negative
CRP	Periseptal	Diffuse	Negative	Negative	Negative
LFABP	Intact	Intact	Lost	Intact	Intact
Reticulin	Intact	Intact	Intact, may show packeting	Intact/focal loss	Intact

Abbreviations: AHN, atypical hepatocellular neoplasm; HCA, hepatocellular adenoma.

leads to increased transcription of GS, and diffuse GS staining is an excellent surrogate marker of β-catenin activation.[18–20] Diffuse GS staining is defined as moderate-to-strong cytoplasmic staining in greater than 50% of lesional hepatocytes.[18] It is divided into diffuse homogeneous and diffuse heterogeneous patterns, which is a reflection of different levels of activation of the Wnt pathway and often correlates with the type of *CTNNB1* mutation (**Table 2**).[4,17,21] Diffuse homogeneous staining (more than 90% of tumor cells with moderate-to-strong cytoplasmic staining, **Fig. 3**A) indicates a high level of β-catenin activation and is most commonly seen with deletions in exon 3 of *CTNNB1*, as well as mutations in D32-S37 region, and is associated with a high risk for the development of HCC.[21] Diffuse heterogeneous staining (50%–90% of cells with moderate-to-strong cytoplasmic staining) indicates an intermediate level of β-catenin activation and is most commonly seen with exon 3 mutations such as T41 and S45 (**Fig. 3**B). This pattern of staining (most commonly with S45 mutation) can show strongly positive cells intermingled with cells that are weakly positive or negative ("starry sky" pattern).[21,22] Mutations in exons 7 or 8 of *CTNNB1* lead to low level of β-catenin activation without diffuse GS staining (patchy staining involving <50% of lesional cells). These cases have a low risk of transformation to HCC.[21] Tumors with mutations in exons 7 or 8 of *CTNNB1* can show characteristic pattern of accentuated GS staining at the rim (**Fig. 3**C); sinusoidal staining with CD34 is often not seen in these areas of enhanced GS staining at the rim while diffuse CD34 staining is present in the central portions.[4] In the absence of β-catenin activation, most HCA cases show patchy weak-to-moderate GS staining involving less than 50% of the lesional cells (**Fig. 3**D). In a small subset of cases (especially on biopsies), the GS staining is indeterminate because it is difficult to determine if GS staining involves more than or less than 50% of tumor cells. Molecular studies are necessary in these cases to determine the status of β-catenin activation.

MOLECULAR STUDIES

Molecular assays and/or cytogenetics may be helpful in a small subset of cases, particularly when GS staining is indeterminate, and if β-catenin activation status would influence management. Sequencing can identify mutations in *CTNNB1* or other Wnt signaling pathway genes (*CTNNB1*, *APC*, *AXIN1*, and *AXIN2*), which are altered in a small subset of these tumors.[3] Additionally, the identification of mutations in the telomerase reverse-transcriptase (*TERT*) promoter may help favor HCC. *TERT* promoter mutations are present in 40% to 50% of HCC,[23] and in β-catenin activated tumors, *TERT* promoter mutations are a frequent second molecular event leading to HCC.[24,25] Characteristic copy number alterations such as gains of 1q, 8q, and 7q also favor HCC because they are infrequent in HCAs and are often present even in well-differentiated HCC.[26]

Table 2
Patterns of glutamine synthetase staining

Terminology	Pattern	β-Catenin Activation	*CTNNB1* Mutation
Diffuse homogeneous	Moderate to strong cytoplasmic staining in 90%–100% of lesional cells	Strongly correlates with β-catenin activation	Exon 3 deletions and some exon 3 non-S45 mutations
Diffuse heterogeneous	Moderate cytoplasmic staining in 50%–90% of lesional cells	β-catenin activation in most cases	Some exon 3 mutations (T41, S45), rare cases with mutations in exon 7 and 8
Patchy, perivascular, or peripheral enhancement	Patchy, focal, or faint	Weak	Exon 7 and 8 mutations, minority of Exon 3 S45
Patchy, perivascular	Perivascular and patchy staining	Absent	Exon 7 and 8 mutations, or no mutations
Indeterminate	Difficult to determine diffuse versus patchy pattern	Not clear	Not clear; consider molecular analysis if necessary

Fig. 3. Staining patterns of GS. (*A*) Diffuse homogenous GS staining correlates strongly with β-catenin activation. (*B*) Diffuse heterogeneous GS staining correlates with an intermediate level of β-catenin activation.

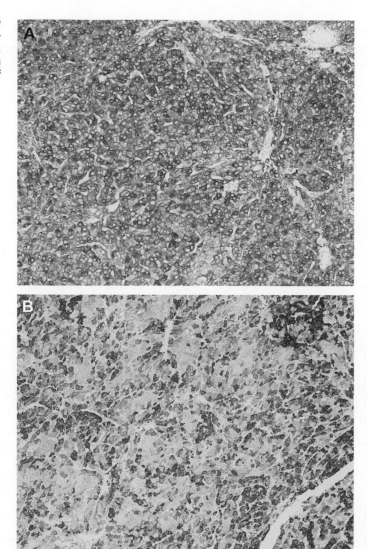

SUBTYPES OF HEPATOCELLULAR ADENOMA

There are 4 well-defined subtypes of HCA based on established molecular pathways: (1) inactivation of *HNF1A*,[27,28] (2) activation of JAK/STAT pathway,[24,29,30] (3) activation of Wnt pathway,[28,31,32] and (4) activation of sonic hedgehog pathway.[15,33,34] Many of these subtypes demonstrate distinctive immunophenotypes that allow for classification of most cases by IHC without molecular testing (Table 3).[18,20] A small subset (5%–10%) of HCA lack any of the known genetic changes and are categorized as "unclassified" subtype.

The vast majority of HCAs are seen in young to middle-aged women with either exogenous estrogen use through oral contraceptives or fatty liver disease.[20,35] Given the risk of hemorrhage in lesions large than 5 cm, resection is generally recommended for all lesions greater than 5 cm in size.[36] It is also recommended that all HCAs in male patients be resected irrespective of size, due to the higher risk of malignant transformation.[35,37] If no therapeutic intervention is pursued, HCAs require follow-up imaging at 6 to 12-month intervals.[37,38]

Histologically, all subtypes consist of well-differentiated hepatocytes with thin cell plates (1–2 cells thick) and unpaired arterioles in the absence of portal tracts. There is little to no cytologic or architectural atypia. There may be hemorrhage, inflammation, and/or ductular reaction. The reticulin framework is largely intact. IHC is necessary to confirm the subtype. Although size and clinical findings are the basis for clinical management, pathologic HCA subtyping can help to guide clinical

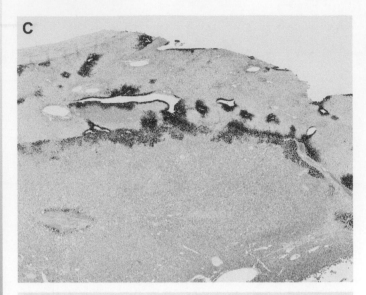

Fig. 3. (*continued*). (*C*) A strong rim of GS staining at the peripheral junction of tumor (bottom) with normal liver (top) is often seen with *CTNNB1* exon 7/8 mutations. (*D*) Patchy staining of GS does not support β-catenin activation.

management strategies, particular in situations with ambiguous imaging characteristics, inadequate follow-up, comorbidities that make surgical resection risky, or patient reluctance for resection.

Some patients present with numerous HCAs, which can represent different HCA subtypes.[33] The presence of 10 or more adenomas is designated *adenomatosis* and is associated with glycogen storage disease, as well as germline mutations in *HNF1A* and maturity onset diabetes of the young (MODY3).[39–41]

INFLAMMATORY HEPATOCELLULAR ADENOMA

Inflammatory hepatocellular adenoma (I-HCA) is the most common HCA subtype, and accounts

for 30% to 50% of all HCAs.[20,42] Metabolic syndrome and fatty liver disease are known risk factors.[18]

Sinusoidal dilatation and congestion or hemorrhage are more commonly seen in this subtype (**Fig. 4**A)[18] but are not always present. Small fibrous septa are often seen with mild ductular reaction and this often mimics FNH (**Fig. 4**B).[17,28] Steatosis is not common but can be present; the background liver can show features of fatty liver disease. Diffuse strong staining with SAA and CRP is typically seen (see **Fig. 2**C and D).

Almost all inflammatory adenomas have activation of the JAK/STAT pathway resulting from mutation in *IL6ST*, *STAT3*, *JAK1*, *GNAS*, or *FRK* gene.[24,29,30,43,44] In addition, mutations in *CTNNB1* exon 3 can be seen in 10% of cases

Table 3
Clinical, histologic, and molecular features of hepatocellular adenoma subtypes

	Inflammatory HCA	*HNF1A*-Inactivated HCA	AHN/β-Catenin Activated HCA	Sonic Hedgehog HCA
Clinical setting	Female, obesity, metabolic syndrome	Female, MODY3	Male	Female, metabolic syndrome, high risk of bleeding
Histologic features	Inflammation, sinusoidal dilatation, ductular reaction	Steatosis, occasional pseudoglands	Increased cytoarchitectural atypia	Hemorrhage
IHC	CRP, Serum amyloid associated protein (SAA)	Loss of LFABP	Nuclear β-catenin, diffuse GS	Not established (ASS1, PTGDS have been proposed)
HCC risk	Uncommon (10% have/β-catenin mutation)	Rare	High risk (~40%)	Rare
Genetic alteration	JAK/STAT pathway, *IL6RT*, *FRK*, *STAT3*, *GNAS*	*HNF1A*	*CTNNB1*, *APC*, *AXIN*	*INHBE:GLI1* fusion

Abbreviations: ASS1, argininosuccinate synthase 1; HCA, hepatocellular adenoma; HCC, hepatocellular carcinoma; IHC, immunohistochemistry; LFABP, liver fatty acid binding protein; MODY3, maturity onset diabetes of the young; PTGDS, prostaglandin D synthetase.

and is accompanied by diffuse GS staining. The risk of HCC in these cases is similar to other HCAs with β-catenin activation.[24,29] GS should be performed on all cases of I-HCA in order to identify cases with β-catenin activation.

HEPATOCYTE NUCLEAR FACTOR 1-ALPHA-INACTIVATED HEPATOCELLULAR ADENOMA

HNF1A-inactivated hepatocellular adenomas (H-HCA) account for 30% to 40% of all HCAs.[20,28,42,45] The majority of cases show sporadic biallelic inactivation of *HNF1A* but rare cases occur in individuals with germline mutations in *HNF1A*. The latter occur in younger individuals, often with numerous adenomas, and can be associated with MODY3.[40,41] Histologically, the majority of H-HCA show moderate-to-severe steatosis (Fig. 5A). Fat may be sparse or absent in 10% to 15% of cases. Most cases show a mixture of lightly eosinophilic cytoplasm and cells with cytoplasmic clearing. Scattered pseudoglands can be seen in a minority of cases (Fig. 5B). If there is extensive or multifocal pseudoglandular architecture, a diagnosis of HCC should be considered.

Marked deposition of lipofuscin can be seen in rare cases of H-HCA (Fig. 5C).[3,46] Rarely, H-HCA show a loose eosinophilic matrix or myxoid change, which stains positively with Alcian blue (myxoid HCA).[47–49] Reticulin stain often highlights a "packeted" appearance in which the reticulin framework encircles small clusters of hepatocytes (see Fig. 1C) but overt loss of reticulin staining is not seen. Inactivation of *HNF1A* leads to downregulation of LFABP, a lipid trafficking protein expressed in the cytoplasm of normal hepatocytes.[16,20] This downregulation can be reliably detected as complete loss of expression by IHC (see Fig. 2A) and is the defining feature for the diagnosis of H-HCA.

Other than *HNF1A* mutations and loss of heterozygosity at chromosome 12q in a subset of cases, most cases of H-HCA show no other recurrent genetic abnormalities.[24] However, malignant transformation can occur in rare cases (2% or less), especially in patients aged older than 60 years.[3,47,50] Lack of fat, pseudoglandular architecture, heavy pigmentation, and myxoid change are considered high-risk factors for HCC.[3,46] Alterations of Wnt signaling have not been identified in H-HCA, even

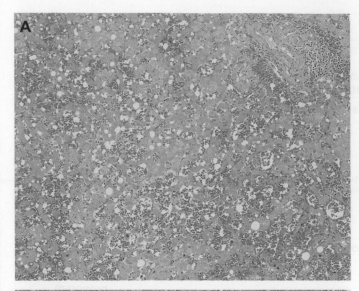

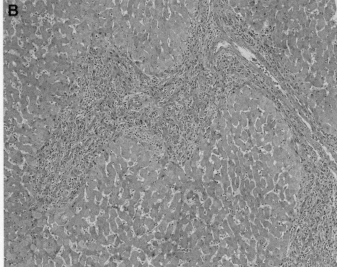

Fig. 4. I-HCA. (*A*) Sinusoidal dilatation and congestion is commonly seen. (*B*) Small fibrous septa with mild ductular reaction can be seen in some cases that can mimic FNH.

in cases demonstrating diffuse expression of GS; the significance of this staining is unclear.[3,47]

β-CATENIN-ACTIVATED HEPATOCELLULAR ADENOMAS

β-catenin-activated hepatocellular adenomas (B-HCAs) represent 5% to 10% of all HCAs. This subtype occurs more commonly in men, particularly in the setting of anabolic steroid use or hereditary glycogen storage disease. The vast majority of these tumors result from *CTNNB1* exon 3 mutations/deletions and less commonly from mutations in other Wnt signaling genes such as *APC* and *AXIN1/2*. These B-HCAs have a high rate of malignant transformation, and association with

concurrent or subsequent HCC is seen in up to 40% of cases.[18,28,51] Hence resection is recommended when this subtype is identified on biopsy.[37] In view of the high risk of association with HCC, it has been proposed that β-catenin activated lesions should not be categorized as HCAs but should be referred to as atypical hepatocellular neoplasms (AHNs).[19,26] The term "hepatocellular neoplasm with uncertain malignant potential" has also been proposed for these tumors.[52] B-HCA frequently show cytoarchitectural abnormalities, such as small cell change, prominent pseudoacinar formation, and cytologic atypia, although these features are not always seen.[18,28] Due to the lack of sensitivity of nuclear staining for β-catenin by IHC, diffuse staining by

Fig. 5. *HNF1A*-inactivated hepatocellular adenoma. (*A*) Typical cases show moderate-to-severe steatosis. (*B*) Occasional pseudoglands can be seen. (*C*) Prominent pigment can be seen in H-HCA and is associated with an increased risk of malignant transformation.

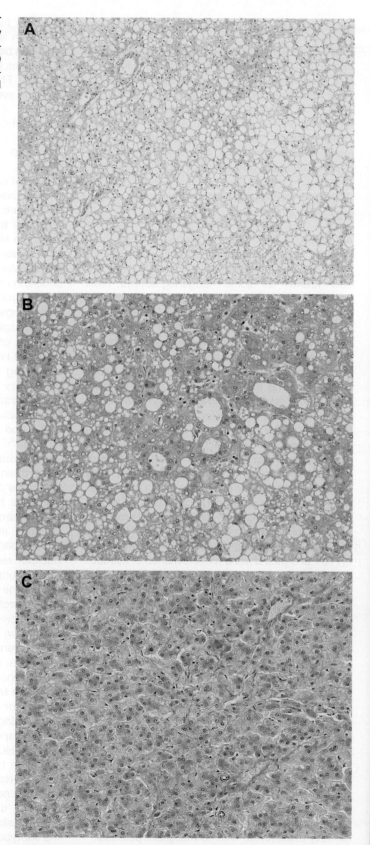

GS is used as a surrogate marker to indicate β-catenin activation.[18,20]

A small subset of these tumors have *CTNNB1* exons 7 or 8 mutations. These tumors typically lack cytoarchitectural atypia and do not show nuclear β-catenin or diffuse GS staining on IHC. Thus, if IHC is used for subtyping HCA, these tumors will end up in the "unclassified" category. These tumors are thought to have a low-malignant potential but these mutations have been identified in rare cases of HCC.[3,21]

SONIC HEDGEHOG HEPATOCELLULAR ADENOMA

Activation of the sonic hedgehog pathway has recently been identified in approximately 4% of HCAs, which were previously unclassified, and are now known as sonic hedgehog-actived HCA (shHCA).[15,33,34] These cases have a fusion of the promoter of inhibin beta E chain (*INHBE*) with *GLI1*, resulting in upregulation of GLI expression, which in turn activates the sonic hedgehog pathway. This adenoma subtype is associated with long-term oral contraceptives, particularly those with metabolic syndrome and nonalcoholic steatohepatitis, and a higher risk of bleeding as compared with other HCA subtypes.[33] Histologically, these HCAs frequently show hemorrhage, and often have no inflammation, ductular reaction, or steatosis. It has been reported that this subtype shows overexpression of argininosuccinate synthase 1 (ASS1),[15,53] a protein involved in the urea cycle that is physiologically expressed in periportal hepatocytes. ASS1 can be detected by IHC[15,53,54] and has been proposed as a useful marker to identify shHCA.[34] However, ASS1 can be positive in other HCA subtypes and in FNH, and thus is not a specific marker of this subtype.[15,53] IHC for prostaglandin D synthetase (PTGDS) has also been proposed for the identification of this subtype but may have low sensitivity and needs to be validated in additional studies.[15,34]

UNCLASSIFIED HEPATOCELLULAR ADENOMA

Approximately 5% of all HCAs lack distinctive morphologic, immunohistochemical or molecular features, and are categorized as unclassified.

COMMON DIFFERENTIAL DIAGNOSTIC CONSIDERATIONS

FOCAL NODULAR HYPERPLASIA VERSUS HEPATOCELLULAR ADENOMA

FNH is a reactive and hyperplastic lesion, often incidentally discovered, with no malignant potential.[55]

Although the diagnosis of FNH on an excisional specimen is often straightforward, a biopsy specimen can be more difficult, especially with a limited sample, as the histologic features can overlap with HCA.[3,56] FNH does not require resection unless large or symptomatic. In contrast, HCA is often resected if there are high-risk features (male gender, β-catenin activation), risk of bleeding (size >5 cm), rupture, or malignant transformation. Follow-up is recommended if the tumor is not resected.

In most cases, FNH presents as a solitary lesion smaller than 5 cm but multiple lesions in a single patient are not uncommon. FNH likely forms in response to an underlying vascular injury, which results in shunting between arteries and veins. In rare cases, FNH can develop adjacent to other mass-lesions. FNH can be found in patients with underlying vascular liver diseases, such as Budd-Chiari syndrome, obliterative portal venopathy, and congenital disorders, including hereditary hemorrhagic telangiectasia, and congenital absence of the portal vein.[57] It is important to note that HCAs can also develop in the setting of underlying vascular liver disease, and some patients may have both types of lesions. FNH can be accurately diagnosed by imaging in many cases, including both computed tomography and MRI, and liver biopsy is not always performed.[36,37,58] Biopsy may be necessary if the imaging features are not typical of FNH, which is most often seen in fatty FNH and small FNHs where the central scar is often missing.[58]

FNH is typically well circumscribed, shows a nodular architecture and has a central scar that contains abnormal thick-walled blood vessels. Fibrous bands containing mixed inflammation and ductular reaction are typically present (Fig. 6A). Normal portal tracts are not present within the lesion. The lesional hepatocytes show minimal or no cytoarchitectural atypia. The central scar and large thick-walled vessels are often not sampled on biopsy, and the nodular architecture may not be apparent, resulting in a picture indistinguishable from HCA. The finding of small aberrant arterioles in the absence of fibrous stroma is less common in FNH and favors HCA. GS is the most useful IHC marker for FNH and shows a characteristic map-like staining pattern (Fig. 6B), which is both sensitive and specific for FNH.[16,17,59] Additional IHC to exclude HCA (especially I-HCA) such as SAA and CRP can be performed (see Table 1). CRP can show periseptal staining in FNH (Fig. 6C) but is typically not diffuse. SAA is typically negative, although can show focal staining. In HCA, GS shows patchy or diffuse staining, depending on the subtype but map-like staining is not observed.

Fig. 6. FNH. (*A*) Wide fibrous bands containing mixed inflammation and ductular reaction. (*B*) Characteristic map-like staining pattern of GS. (*C*) CRP can show staining of periseptal hepatocytes.

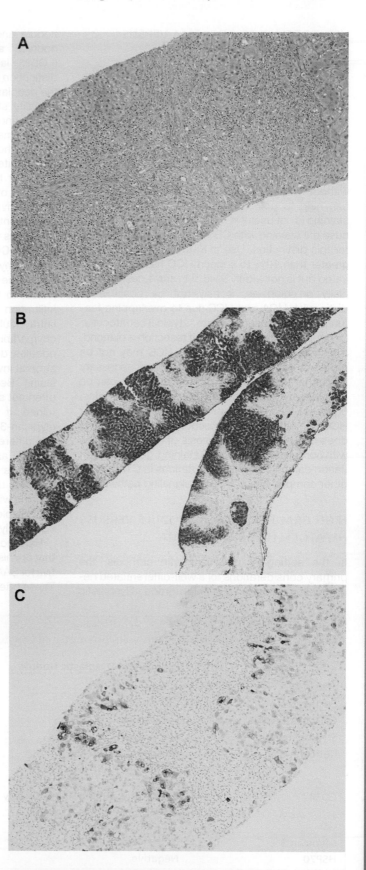

HEPATOCELLULAR ADENOMA VERSUS HEPATOCELLULAR CARCINOMA

The distinction of HCC from HCA is largely based on cytoarchitectural atypia and reticulin loss. Thick cell plates, small cell change, crowding and high cell density, prominent pseudoacinar architecture, cytologic atypia, and multifocal reticulin loss favor HCC. Some cases can show borderline features such as focal cytoarchitectural atypia and/or focal reticulin loss. In such cases, diffuse GS staining (with or without nuclear β-catenin) and glypican-3 staining can help to point toward HCC, whereas HSP70 staining is not useful in most cases.[60] Increase in sinusoidal staining with CD34 is not a reliable feature for this distinction. Use of Ki-67 proliferation index greater than 10% to support HCC has been advocated but is not widely used.[61] In some cases especially on biopsies, it may not be possible to distinguish HCA and HCC due to overlapping features. We have used the term "atypical hepatocellular neoplasm" for such cases. If resection is planned, a distinction between HCA and HCC may not be required. If a more definite diagnosis is necessary for further management, molecular studies can be helpful as cytogenetic changes such as 1q/8q gains, 6q loss, and TERT promoter mutations favor HCC,[3,24] although the absence of these changes does not exclude the diagnosis of HCC. For cases with borderline pattern of GS staining, genomic evaluation can help to identify mutations in CTNNB1 or other components of the Wnt signaling pathway.[3]

HIGH-GRADE DYSPLASTIC NODULE VERSUS HEPATOCELLULAR CARCINOMA

In the setting of a patient with cirrhosis, the primary considerations for a well-differentiated hepatocellular lesion are high-grade dysplastic nodule and HCC (Table 4). Large regenerative nodules and low-graded dysplastic nodules (LGDN) lack cytoarchitectural atypia and the distinction between these entities is difficult unless the neoplastic nature of LGDN is demonstrated by clonality studies. From the practical standpoint, this distinction is not clinically significant and we do not make a diagnosis of LGDN in practice. HGDN show occasional unpaired arterioles and cytoarchitectural atypia but the changes are not sufficient for an unequivocal diagnosis of HCC. Features of HGDN may be focal within the nodule, or may involve the entire nodule. Portal tracts can be present, but reduced in number in HGDN.

Lesions with size larger than 2 cm are more likely to be HCC. Significant cytoarchitectural atypia and/or any more than focal loss of reticulin favors HCC. The earliest feature in the progression of HGDN to HCC is stromal invasion evidenced by infiltration of neoplastic cells into portal tracts (intranodular or extranodular) or adjacent parenchyma/fibrous septa (Fig. 7).[62] Unlike regenerative nodules, ductular reaction is absent in the areas of stromal invasion and can be highlighted with CK7 stain.[63] Because stromal invasion can be focal, it is often not sampled and additional IHC may be obtained if necessary. Combined use of GS, glypican-3, and HSP70 has been advocated for this differential diagnosis.[11,12] Diffuse expression of GS and glypican-3 favor HCC, whereas HSP70 is not helpful in most cases and is not routinely used in our practice. Diffuse sinusoidal staining with CD34 also favors HCC. Focal staining with glypican-3 can be seen in HGDN and less commonly in cirrhotic nodules.[6]

Rare nodules have been described in cirrhosis that are histologically similar to I-HCA and are positive for SAA and CRP without loss of reticulin.[54,64–66] These often show mutations in IL6ST, STAT3, and

Table 4		
High-grade dysplastic nodule versus well-differentiated hepatocellular carcinoma		
	High-Grade Dysplastic Nodule	**Well-Differentiated HCC**
Size	<2 cm	≥2 cm
Portal tracts	Can be present	Typically absent
Cytoarchitectural atypia	Focal/mild	Multifocal/diffuse
Stromal invasion	Not present	Can be present
Reticulin	Mostly intact, focal fragmentation/loss may be seen	Multifocal loss, fragmentation, or extensive irregularity
CD34	Patchy sinusoidal staining, usually in the periphery	Diffuse staining can be present
GS	Typically patchy	Diffuse staining may be present
Glypican-3	Negative/focal	Diffuse
HSP70	Negative	Can be positive

Fig. 7. HCC showing stromal invasion into and around a portal tract. Nonneoplastic cirrhotic liver is seen on the left of the image.

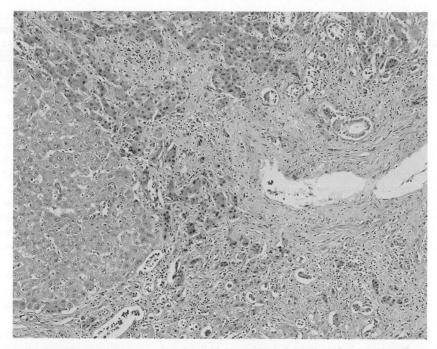

GNAS, similar to I-HCA in the noncirrhotic setting.[64,66] These tumors were initially described in the setting of alcoholic cirrhosis but can also occur in cirrhosis due to other causes. The natural history of these I-HCA-like lesions in cirrhosis is not clear and it is prudent to regard them as HGDN for management.

SUMMARY

The diagnosis of well-differentiated hepatocellular lesions plays an important role in guiding the clinical management. Due to morphologic overlap of FNH and I-HCA, routine use of IHC for GS and SAA/CRP (or both) is recommended, especially for biopsies. Reticulin and GS stains are important for risk stratification of HCA and its distinction from HCC. Additional stains such as glypican-3 and β-catenin can be obtained depending on the overall features. If a confident diagnosis of HCA can be made and β-catenin activation is excluded by GS stain, further subtyping is not clinically necessary. However, the use of IHC to subtype HCAs (LFABP, SAA, CRP, GS) is helpful to confirm the diagnosis and is routinely performed in our practice. In a small subset of cases, there are borderline atypical features such as cytoarchitectural abnormalities, reticulin pattern, and GS staining pattern that are not sufficient for diagnosis of HCC. These cases are classified as "AHNs" and resection/close follow-up is recommended for these cases depending on the clinical setting. Molecular

abnormalities such as copy number alterations, *TERT* promoter mutation and *CTNNB1* mutation can help to classify these borderline lesions.

CLINICS CARE POINTS

- Reticulin and GS stains are the most critical stains for risk stratification of HCA and its distinction from HCC.

- If a confident diagnosis of HCA can be made and β-catenin activation is excluded by GS stain, further subtyping is not clinically necessary.

- If there are borderline atypical features present on biopsy such as cytoarchitectural abnormalities, reticulin pattern, and GS staining pattern that are not sufficient for diagnosis of HCC, resection or close follow-up is recommended for these cases depending on the clinical setting.

REFERENCES

1. Yasir S, Chen ZE, Said S, et al. Biopsies of hepatocellular carcinoma with no reticulin loss: an important diagnostic pitfall. Hum Pathol 2021;107:20–8.
2. Singhi AD, Jain D, Kakar S, et al. Reticulin loss in benign fatty liver: an important diagnostic pitfall

when considering a diagnosis of hepatocellular carcinoma. Am J Surg Pathol 2012;36(5):710–5.

3. Joseph NM, Blank A, Shain AH, et al. Hepatocellular neoplasms with loss of liver fatty acid binding protein: clinicopathologic features and molecular profiling. Hum Pathol 2022;122:60–71.

4. Sempoux C, Gouw ASH, Dunet V, et al. Predictive patterns of glutamine synthetase immunohistochemical staining in CTNNB1-mutated hepatocellular adenomas. Am J Surg Pathol 2021;45(4):477–87.

5. Krings G, Ramachandran R, Jain D, et al. Immunohistochemical pitfalls and the importance of glypican 3 and arginase in the diagnosis of scirrhous hepatocellular carcinoma. Mod Pathol 2013;26(6):782–91.

6. Shafizadeh N, Ferrell LD, Kakar S. Utility and limitations of glypican-3 expression for the diagnosis of hepatocellular carcinoma at both ends of the differentiation spectrum. Mod Pathol 2008;21(8):1011–8.

7. Nguyen T, Phillips D, Jain D, et al. Comparison of 5 immunohistochemical markers of hepatocellular differentiation for the diagnosis of hepatocellular carcinoma. Arch Pathol Lab Med 2015;139(8):1028–34.

8. Nakatsura T, Nishimura Y. Usefulness of the novel oncofetal antigen glypican-3 for diagnosis of hepatocellular carcinoma and melanoma. BioDrugs 2005;19(2):71–7.

9. Clark I, Shah SS, Moreira R, et al. A subset of well-differentiated hepatocellular carcinomas are Arginase-1 negative. Hum Pathol 2017;69:90–5.

10. Nguyen TB, Roncalli M, Di Tommaso L, et al. Combined use of heat-shock protein 70 and glutamine synthetase is useful in the distinction of typical hepatocellular adenoma from atypical hepatocellular neoplasms and well-differentiated hepatocellular carcinoma. Mod Pathol 2016;29(3):283–92.

11. Di Tommaso L, Destro A, Seok JY, et al. The application of markers (HSP70 GPC3 and GS) in liver biopsies is useful for detection of hepatocellular carcinoma. J Hepatol 2009;50(4):746–54.

12. Di Tommaso L, Franchi G, Park YN, et al. Diagnostic value of HSP70, glypican 3, and glutamine synthetase in hepatocellular nodules in cirrhosis. Hepatology 2007;45(3):725–34.

13. Cho SJ, Ferrell LD, Gill RM. Expression of liver fatty acid binding protein in hepatocellular carcinoma. Hum Pathol 2016;50:135–9.

14. Liu L, Shah SS, Naini BV, et al. Immunostains used to subtype hepatic adenomas do not distinguish hepatic adenomas from hepatocellular carcinomas. Am J Surg Pathol 2016;40(8):1062–9.

15. Nault JC, Couchy G, Caruso S, et al. Argininosuccinate synthase 1 and periportal gene expression in sonic hedgehog hepatocellular adenomas. Hepatology 2018;68(3):964–76.

16. Bioulac-Sage P, Cubel G, Taouji S, et al. Immunohistochemical markers on needle biopsies are helpful for the diagnosis of focal nodular hyperplasia and hepatocellular adenoma subtypes. Am J Surg Pathol 2012;36(11):1691–9.

17. Joseph NM, Ferrell LD, Jain D, et al. Diagnostic utility and limitations of glutamine synthetase and serum amyloid-associated protein immunohistochemistry in the distinction of focal nodular hyperplasia and inflammatory hepatocellular adenoma. Mod Pathol 2014;27(1):62–72.

18. Bioulac-Sage P, Rebouissou S, Thomas C, et al. Hepatocellular adenoma subtype classification using molecular markers and immunohistochemistry. Hepatology 2007;46(3):740–8.

19. Hale G, Liu X, Hu J, et al. Correlation of exon 3 beta-catenin mutations with glutamine synthetase staining patterns in hepatocellular adenoma and hepatocellular carcinoma. Mod Pathol 2016;29(11):1370–80.

20. Bioulac-Sage P, Laumonier H, Couchy G, et al. Hepatocellular adenoma management and phenotypic classification: the Bordeaux experience. Hepatology 2009;50(2):481–9.

21. Rebouissou S, Franconi A, Calderaro J, et al. Genotype-phenotype correlation of CTNNB1 mutations reveals different ss-catenin activity associated with liver tumor progression. Hepatology 2016;64(6):2047–61.

22. Board WCoTE. WHO classification of tumours, 5th edition, vol. 1: Digestive system tumours. 5th ed. 2019. p. 224-5. chap Hepatocellular adenoma.

23. Cancer Genome Atlas Research Network. Electronic address wbe, Cancer Genome Atlas Research N. Comprehensive and Integrative Genomic Characterization of Hepatocellular Carcinoma. Cell 2017;169(7):1327–1341 e23.

24. Pilati C, Letouze E, Nault JC, et al. Genomic profiling of hepatocellular adenomas reveals recurrent FRK-activating mutations and the mechanisms of malignant transformation. Cancer Cell 2014;25(4):428–41.

25. Nault JC, Mallet M, Pilati C, et al. High frequency of telomerase reverse-transcriptase promoter somatic mutations in hepatocellular carcinoma and preneoplastic lesions. Nat Commun 2013;4:2218.

26. Evason KJ, Grenert JP, Ferrell LD, et al. Atypical hepatocellular adenoma-like neoplasms with beta-catenin activation show cytogenetic alterations similar to well-differentiated hepatocellular carcinomas. Hum Pathol 2013;44(5):750–8.

27. Bluteau O, Jeannot E, Bioulac-Sage P, et al. Bi-allelic inactivation of TCF1 in hepatic adenomas. Nat Genet 2002;32(2):312–5.

28. Zucman-Rossi J, Jeannot E, Nhieu JT, et al. Genotype-phenotype correlation in hepatocellular adenoma: new classification and relationship with HCC. Hepatology 2006;43(3):515–24.

29. Rebouissou S, Amessou M, Couchy G, et al. Frequent in-frame somatic deletions activate gp130

in inflammatory hepatocellular tumours. Nature 2009; 457(7226):200–4.

30. Nault JC, Fabre M, Couchy G, et al. GNAS-activating mutations define a rare subgroup of inflammatory liver tumors characterized by STAT3 activation. J Hepatol 2012;56(1):184–91.

31. Chen YW, Jeng YM, Yeh SH, et al. P53 gene and Wnt signaling in benign neoplasms: beta-catenin mutations in hepatic adenoma but not in focal nodular hyperplasia. Hepatology 2002;36(4 Pt 1): 927–35.

32. Rebouissou S, Couchy G, Libbrecht L, et al. The beta-catenin pathway is activated in focal nodular hyperplasia but not in cirrhotic FNH-like nodules. J Hepatol 2008;49(1):61–71.

33. Nault JC, Couchy G, Balabaud C, et al. Molecular classification of hepatocellular adenoma associates with risk factors, bleeding, and malignant transformation. Gastroenterology 2017;152(4):880–894 e6.

34. Sala M, Gonzales D, Leste-Lasserre T, et al. ASS1 overexpression: a hallmark of sonic hedgehog hepatocellular adenomas; recommendations for clinical practice. Hepatol Commun 2020;4(6):809–24.

35. Dokmak S, Paradis V, Vilgrain V, et al. A single-center surgical experience of 122 patients with single and multiple hepatocellular adenomas. Gastroenterology 2009;137(5):1698–705.

36. Marrero JA, Ahn J, Rajender Reddy K, et al. ACG clinical guideline: the diagnosis and management of focal liver lesions. Am J Gastroenterol 2014; 109(9):1328–47, [quiz :1348].

37. (EASL) EAftSotL. EASL Clinical Practice Guidelines on the management of benign liver tumours. J Hepatol 2016;65(2):386–98.

38. Belghiti J, Cauchy F, Paradis V, et al. Diagnosis and management of solid benign liver lesions. Nat Rev Gastroenterol Hepatol 2014;11(12):737–49.

39. Flejou JF, Barge J, Menu Y, et al. Liver adenomatosis. An entity distinct from liver adenoma? Gastroenterology 1985;89(5):1132–8.

40. Reznik Y, Dao T, Coutant R, et al. Hepatocyte nuclear factor-1 alpha gene inactivation: cosegregation between liver adenomatosis and diabetes phenotypes in two maturity-onset diabetes of the young (MODY)3 families. J Clin Endocrinol Metab 2004;89(3):1476–80.

41. Bacq Y, Jacquemin E, Balabaud C, et al. Familial liver adenomatosis associated with hepatocyte nuclear factor 1alpha inactivation. Gastroenterology 2003;125(5):1470–5.

42. Shafizadeh N, Genrich G, Ferrell L, et al. Hepatocellular adenomas in a large community population, 2000 to 2010: reclassification per current World Health Organization classification and results of long-term follow-up. Hum Pathol 2014;45(5):976–83.

43. Pilati C, Amessou M, Bihl MP, et al. Somatic mutations activating STAT3 in human inflammatory hepatocellular adenomas. J Exp Med 2011;208(7): 1359–66.

44. Poussin K, Pilati C, Couchy G, et al. Biochemical and functional analyses of gp130 mutants unveil JAK1 as a novel therapeutic target in human inflammatory hepatocellular adenoma. OncoImmunology 2013;2(12):e27090.

45. Deniz K, Umetsu SE, Ferrell L, et al. Hepatocellular adenomas in the Turkish population: reclassification according to updated World Health Organization criteria. Histopathology 2021;79(1):23–33.

46. Mounajjed T, Yasir S, Aleff PA, et al. Pigmented hepatocellular adenomas have a high risk of atypia and malignancy. Mod Pathol 2015;28(9):1265–74.

47. Putra J, Ferrell LD, Gouw ASH, et al. Malignant transformation of liver fatty acid binding protein-deficient hepatocellular adenomas: histopathologic spectrum of a rare phenomenon. Mod Pathol 2020; 33(4):665–75.

48. Rowan DJ, Yasir S, Chen ZE, et al. Morphologic and molecular findings in myxoid hepatic adenomas. Am J Surg Pathol 2021;45(8):1098–107.

49. Salaria SN, Graham RP, Aishima S, et al. Primary hepatic tumors with myxoid change: morphologically unique hepatic adenomas and hepatocellular carcinomas. Am J Surg Pathol 2015;39(3): 318–24.

50. Yasir S, Chen ZE, Jain D, et al. Hepatic adenomas in patients 60 and older are enriched for HNF1A inactivation and malignant transformation. Am J Surg Pathol 2022;46(6):786–92.

51. Kakar S, Grenert JP, Paradis V, et al. Hepatocellular carcinoma arising in adenoma: similar immunohistochemical and cytogenetic features in adenoma and hepatocellular carcinoma portions of the tumor. Mod Pathol 2014;27(11):1499–509.

52. Bedossa P, Burt AD, Brunt E, et al. Well-differentiated hepatocellular neoplasm of uncertain malignant potential–reply. Hum Pathol 2015;46(4):635–6.

53. Henriet E, Abou Hammoud A, Dupuy JW, et al. Argininosuccinate synthase 1 (ASS1): a marker of unclassified hepatocellular adenoma and high bleeding risk. Hepatology 2017;66(6):2016–28.

54. Sasaki M, Yoneda N, Kitamura S, et al. Characterization of hepatocellular adenoma based on the phenotypic classification: The Kanazawa experience. Hepatol Res 2011;41(10):982–8.

55. Rebouissou S, Bioulac-Sage P, Zucman-Rossi J. Molecular pathogenesis of focal nodular hyperplasia and hepatocellular adenoma. J Hepatol 2008;48(1): 163–70.

56. Makhlouf HR, Abdul-Al HM, Goodman ZD. Diagnosis of focal nodular hyperplasia of the liver by needle biopsy. Hum Pathol 2005;36(11):1210–6.

57. Sempoux C, Paradis V, Komuta M, et al. Hepatocellular nodules expressing markers of hepatocellular adenomas in Budd-Chiari syndrome and other rare

hepatic vascular disorders. J Hepatol 2015;63(5): 1173–80.

58. LeGout JD, Bolan CW, Bowman AW, et al. focal nodular hyperplasia and focal nodular hyperplasia-like lesions. Radiographics 2022;42(4):1043–61.

59. Bioulac-Sage P, Laumonier H, Rullier A, et al. Over-expression of glutamine synthetase in focal nodular hyperplasia: a novel easy diagnostic tool in surgical pathology. Liver Int 2009;29(3):459–65.

60. Choi WT, Kakar S. Atypical Hepatocellular Neoplasms: Review of Clinical, Morphologic, Immunohistochemical, Molecular, and Cytogenetic Features. Adv Anat Pathol 2018;25(4):254–62.

61. Jones A, Kroneman TN, Blahnik AJ, et al. Ki-67 "hot spot" digital analysis is useful in the distinction of hepatic adenomas and well-differentiated hepatocellular carcinomas. Virchows Arch 2021;478(2):201–7.

62. International Consensus Group for Hepatocellular NeoplasiaThe International Consensus Group for Hepatocellular N. Pathologic diagnosis of early hepatocellular carcinoma: a report of the international consensus group for hepatocellular neoplasia. Hepatology 2009;49(2):658–64.

63. Park YN, Kojiro M, Di Tommaso L, et al. Ductular reaction is helpful in defining early stromal invasion, small hepatocellular carcinomas, and dysplastic nodules. Cancer 2007;109(5):915–23.

64. Sasaki M, Yoneda N, Sawai Y, et al. Clinicopathological characteristics of serum amyloid A-positive hepatocellular neoplasms/nodules arising in alcoholic cirrhosis. Histopathology 2015;66(6):836–45.

65. Sasaki M, Yoneda N, Kitamura S, et al. A serum amyloid A-positive hepatocellular neoplasm arising in alcoholic cirrhosis: a previously unrecognized type of inflammatory hepatocellular tumor. Mod Pathol 2012;25(12):1584–93.

66. Calderaro J, Nault JC, Balabaud C, et al. Inflammatory hepatocellular adenomas developed in the setting of chronic liver disease and cirrhosis. Mod Pathol 2016;29(1):43–50.

Challenges in Diagnosing and Reporting Cholangiocarcinoma

Tony El Jabbour, MD[a], Attila Molnar, MD[b], Stephen M. Lagana, MD[c],*

KEYWORDS

- Cholangiocarcinoma • Intrahepatic • iCCA • Small duct type iCCA • Large duct type iCCA
- Bile duct hamartoma • Biliary duct adenoma • cHCC-CCA

Key points

- Benign/pre-neoplastic lesions and bland looking subtypes/forms of cholangiocarcinomas share multiple morphologic features. Usage of well-established microscopic criteria and ancillary tests along with clinical and radiological data is crucial to avoid diagnostic pitfalls.
- Every option should be used when classifying poorly differentiated malignancies of the liver, as some entities may have a specific therapeutic strategy or/and targeted therapy.
- Historically, combined hepatocellular-cholangiocarcinoma were difficult to define and to diagnose. The last WHO classification of digestive tumors has simplified this concept rendering the diagnosis and subsequent staging of combined hepatocellular-cholangiocarcinoma more feasible.

ABSTRACT

Intrahepatic cholangiocarcinoma is a challenge to the practicing surgical pathologist for several reasons. It is rare in many parts of the world, and thus practical exposure may be limited. Related to the fact of its rarity is the fact that more common tumors which frequently metastasize to the liver can be morphologically indistinguishable (eg, pancreatic ductal adenocarcinoma). Immunohistochemical testing is generally noncontributory in this context. Other difficulties arise from the protean morphologic manifestations of cholangiocarcinoma (ie, small duct vs. large duct) and the existence of combined cholangiocarcinoma and hepatocellular carcinoma. These, and other issues of concern to the practicing diagnostic pathologist are discussed herein.

OVERVIEW

Cholangiocarcinoma (CCA) is a heterogeneous group of tumors composed of malignant epithelial neoplasms arising from the bile ducts and showing biliary differentiation.[1] Based on their anatomical origin they can be classified as intrahepatic cholangiocarcinoma (iCCA), perihilar cholangiocarcinoma (pCCA) or extrahepatic cholangiocarcinoma (eCCA).[1] This article is devoted to iCCA and its mimics with a special emphasis on the challenges they can possibly bring to surgical pathologists.

HISTOLOGIC FEATURES OF INTRAHEPATIC CHOLANGIOCARCINOMAS

iCCA is a type of invasive adenocarcinoma which generally displays variable sized tubular, acinar, and or micropapillary structures.[2–4] The malignant cells are usually small to medium sized, cuboidal more than columnar, and demonstrate clear or eosinophilic cytoplasm, closely resembling biliary epithelial cells.[2–4] The nuclei are frequently small, and the nucleoli are not especially prominent. The tumors may produce mucin, and do not produce bile. These characteristics are usually the opposite in

[a] West Virginia University; [b] Mount Sinai Morningside and Mount Sinai West, Department of Pathology, 1000 Tenth Avenue, First floor, Room G183, New York, NY 10019, USA; [c] New York-Presbyterian /Columbia University, Irving Medical Center, 622 W168th St, Vc14-209, New York, NY 10032, USA
* Corresponding author.
E-mail address: sml2179@cumc.columbia.edu

Surgical Pathology 16 (2023) 599–608
https://doi.org/10.1016/j.path.2023.04.012
1875-9181/23/© 2023 Elsevier Inc. All rights reserved.

hepatocellular carcinoma (HCC).[5] Moreover, distinctive features of invasion such as desmoplasia, perineural invasion and proximity of glands to larger arteries are common findings supporting the diagnosis of malignancy.[5,6] On a scant biopsy material however, a few glands may only be available for evaluation. In such cases, the main differential is the normal biliary glands, and the main goal is to establish a diagnosis of malignancy. Multiple studies attempted to provide guidance for such scenarios, specifically when the above listed invasive features, are absent.[7–9] Immunohistochemistry is not typically useful in this distinction, although studies on the topic are available. For example, the Ki 67 proliferation index may be considered, given benign glands often have a Ki67 index less than 10% while in some cases of iCCA this index is higher.[10] Aberrant (mutational) p53 immunoreactivity (strong diffuse staining or complete absence of staining) certainly increases the likelihood that a proliferation is malignant.[11,12] However many iCCAs exhibit a normal (wild type) p53 staining pattern (scattered nuclear reactivity), and so p53 is meaningful only when it is clearly abnormal.[13] Cytokeratins (CK), such as pan-CK cocktails, CK7, and CK19 strongly mark benign and malignant biliary proliferations (typically), but they may be useful to highlight single cells within fibrotic stroma, or to better illustrate an invasive pattern. Identification of a rare single cell does not entirely establish the diagnosis of malignancy either, as the possibility of benign entrapped cells and a glancing cut of the "start" of a duct profile need to be excluded.[14–17] Loss of nuclear BAP1 occurs in 16-32% of iCCA and virtually never in benign biliary glands.[18,19] Thus, sensitivity is poor, but specificity is high (nearly 100%). Other malignancies may lose BAP1, in particular mesothelioma, so the tumor must be determined to be of biliary phenotype before interpreting BAP1 loss by immunohistochemistry.

Assuming a malignant primary tumor of liver with biliary phenotype has been established, the 5th edition of WHO, has further categorized iCCAs into small or large duct types.[20] While the etiology in many cases of iCCAs is unknown, some risk factors seem to contribute more to the formation of one type over to the other. Furthermore, some of these risk factors contribute to both subtypes or are shared with HCCs or eCCAs, see **Table 1**.[21–25] The characteristics and mimickers of each iCCA subtype will be detailed in the following sections.

INTRAHEPATIC CHOLANGIOCARCINOMA, LARGE DUCT TYPE

Large duct type iCCA recapitulates the large intrahepatic ducts and the peribiliary glands.[2] Histologically, the tumor is formed by ductal or tubular mucin secreting glands appearing as large cancerous bile ducts with columnar to cuboidal epithelial lining and surrounding desmoplastic stroma.[26,27] Intracellular or luminal mucin secretion is significantly more frequent in large duct type iCCA.[28] One particular location is critical for these tumors: the intrahepatic portions of the right and left hepatic ducts. Due to their proximity to the hilar region, tumors arising in the intrahepatic portions of the right and left hepatic ducts may present as hilar masses, confounding a practicing pathologist to incorrectly classify them as pCCA. However, the correct classification of such tumors is iCCA large duct type. The term perihilar cholangiocarcinoma is reserved for the tumors arising from the extrahepatic portion of the right or left hepatic ducts or the common hepatic duct.[4] The difference between these two anatomic locations is illustrated in **Fig. 1**. This differentiation is crucial since iCCAs

---

Table 1
Examples of subtype-specific risk factors for iCCA

Small Duct Type iCCA[a]	Large Duct Type iCCA[b]	Both Small and Large Duct Type iCCA
HBV	Caroli disease	Asbestos
HCV	Bile duct cyst	Nitrosamine
Alcoholic liver disease	Congenital hepatic fibrosis	Dioxins
Obesity/Metabolic syndrome/ Diabetes	Opisthorchis viverrini/Clonorchis sinensis	Vinyl chlorides
Hemochromatosis	PSC	Thorotrast
Wilson's disease	Choledocholithiasis/Cholangitis	
	Hepatolithiasis	

Abbreviations: HBV, hepatitis B virus; HCV, hepatitis B virus; PSC, primary sclerosing cholangitis.
[a] Shared risk factors with HCC.
[b] Shared risk factors with eCCA.

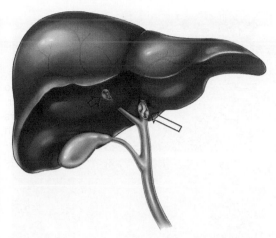

Fig. 1. Short arrow: Tumor of the right hepatic duct localized intrahepatically: this tumor can present as a perihilar mass and should be classified as intrahepatic cholangiocarcinoma. Long arrow: Tumor of the left hepatic duct localized extrahepatically: this tumor will present as a perihilar mass and should be classified as perihilar cholangiocarcinoma.

and pCCAs are established as two separate entities.[29] They are also different at the molecular level and are staged differently according to the AJCC cancer manual (8th edition).[29,30] *KRAS* mutation seems to be an important driver of oncogenesis in iCCA especially in large duct types.[31] When *KRAS* is mutated, it means constant activation of MAPK and AKT pathways, leading to signal independent cell proliferation and mitosis as well as increased metastatic activity.[32,33] Moreover, mutations in *KRAS, TP53* and *CDKN2A* were shown to predict worse overall survival in patients with iCCA, regardless of stage and treatment status.[34]

INTRAHEPATIC CHOLANGIOCARCINOMA, SMALL DUCT TYPE

Small duct iCCAs arise in the peripheral parts of the liver recapitulating septal and interlobular bile ducts.[2] Histologically they display small tubules lined by cuboidal to low columnar cells.[26] While not exactly stated in the last edition of the WHO, it seems that the vast majority of small iCCA do not need to be further subtyped and are referred to as iCCA, small duct type (conventional).[20] That said, iCCA small duct type can be further classified as cholangiolocarcinoma or small duct type iCCA with ductal plate malformation (DPM) pattern.[2,20,35]

Small duct type iCCA, cholangiolocarcinoma subtype (or simply cholangiolocarcinoma) has features resembling reactive bile ductules.[26] The possible origin of these tumors is postulated to

be the hepatic progenitor cells and stem cells of the canals of Herring or the stem cells of bile ductules.[2] As the name implies, small duct type iCCA with DPM pattern are markedly different and resemble ductal plate malformation.[26,35] Fig. 2 summarizes the three patterns of small duct iCCA in comparison to large duct iCCA. Isocytrate dehydrogenase 1 (*IDH1*) mutation is displayed by many carcinomas including iCCA.[36] Multiple studies show that small duct type iCCA more frequently harbors *IDH1* mutation than large duct type iCCA, raising the possibility of using it as a potential biomarker in the diagnostic process.[2,4,36–38] The gain of function mutation of *IDH1* results in the accumulation of D-2-hydroxy glutarate (D-2HG).[36,39] The accumulation of this metabolite appears to inhibit hepatocellular differentiation and leads to the uncontrolled proliferation of liver progenitor cells.[40] Based on the above findings it is suggested that *IDH1* mutation can be an initial step in the carcinogenesis of iCCA, whether by itself or in combination with other genetic changes remains unclear.[41]

MIMICKERS OF CHOLANGIOLOCARCINOMAS: BILE DUCT HAMARTOMA, BILIARY DUCT ADENOMA AND BILIARY ADENOFIBROMA

As previously described, cholangiolocarcinoma is a small duct type iCCA where the tumor displays homogenous growth with a small tubular or acinar pattern and well to moderately differentiated cells, resembling proliferating bile ductules.[26] Consequently, the main mimickers of this lesion are benign and pre-neoplastic lesions that are formed by bland looking ducts or ductules such as: bile duct hamartoma (BDH) also known as Von Meyenburg complex (VMC), bile duct adenoma (BDA) and biliary adenofibroma (BAF).

The characteristics of these entities in comparison to cholangiolocarcinoma are summarized in **Table 2** and demonstrated in **Fig. 3**. This diagnosis is very difficult to establish on biopsy, as tissue invasion is the feature most likely to allow for diagnosis.

INTRAHEPATIC CHOLANGIOCARCINOMA VERSUS METASTATIC PANCREATOBILIARY ADENOCARCINOMA TO THE LIVER: AN ONGOING DIAGNOSTIC DILEMMA

Adenocarcinomas of the biliary tree and the pancreatic duct (including perihilar cholangiocarcinoma, extrahepatic/distal cholangiocarcinoma, pancreatic ductal adenocarcinoma (PDAC) and ampullary/periampullary adenocarcinoma with

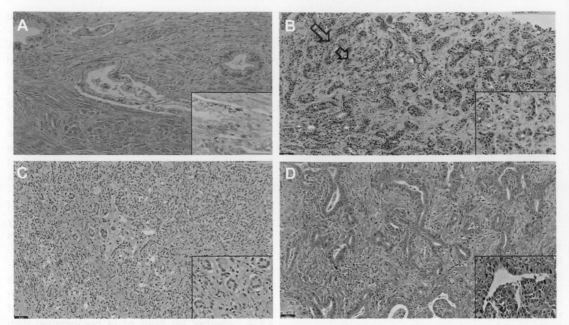

Fig. 2. (*A*). Large duct type iCCA (20x) showing cancerous large caliber bile ducts with irregular shapes. The lumen is lined by multilayered tumor cells displaying relatively small and pale nuclei with occasional, small nucleoli as shown in the insert (60x). (*B*). Small duct type iCCA (20x) displays small tubular and focally anastomosing ducts, embedded into a desmoplastic stroma. In some areas, the malignant cells are organized into cords (*black arrow*) or single cells (*blue arrow*). The ducts or cords are formed by small cuboidal cells as shown in the insert (60x). (*C*). Cholangiolocarcinoma (20x) displays small malignant ducts, resembling ductular reaction. The malignant ducts are lined by small cuboidal cells as shown in the insert (60x). (*D*). iCCA with ductal plate malformation like features (20x) shows irregular, focally dilated malignant ducts surrounded by fibrous stroma. The malignant cells lining these irregular ducts show nuclear pleomorphism as shown in the insert (60x).

pancreatobiliary differentiation) share the morphology and non-specific (CK7 positive/colloquially"CK7-oma") immunophenotype with iCCAs.[1,15,16] Such tumors frequently metastasize to the liver (mostly pancreatic ductal adenocarcinoma, due to incidence) making the distinction between an iCCA and a metastasis to the liver always challenging. Immunohistochemistry cannot typically resolve the differential, although the loss of SMAD4 expression is more in favor of a metastasis from a pancreatic adenocarcinoma. Nonetheless, loss of SMAD4 can be seen in tumors other than PDAC, including iCCA, and some PDAC retains SMAD4, so this is not a deterministic test.[14,54,55]

Albumin in-situ hybridization (albumin ISH) has been established as a promising biomarker of the hepatic lineage/origin.[56] One study highlighted that a small duct like appearance of an invasive tumor coupled with a positivity for albumin ISH is diagnostic for iCCA over a metastatic adenocarcinoma.[57] According to the same study the utilization of albumin ISH presents with few pitfalls worth mentioning. These include the positivity of pancreatic acinar cell carcinoma and the tendency of large duct type iCCA to show negativity for

albumin ISH.[57] It is also important to note that albumin immunostain is very difficult to interpret due to the background staining of normal cells which could be minimized using the ISH technique instead.[58] Unfortunately, a common phenomenon is when more tumors are subjected to a new test, there is some loss of specificity and sensitivity. This was seen with respect to the albumin ISH, which shows fairly frequent positivity in gallbladder adenocarcinoma and rare positivity in many other tumors.[59]

POORLY DIFFERENTIATED INTRAHEPATIC CHOLANGIOCARCINOMA VERSUS POORLY DIFFERENTIATED HEPATOCELLULAR CARCINOMA

Both iCCA and HCC can present as a poorly differentiated carcinoma and the distinction between these two entities has significant challenges. However, this distinction is still crucial due to the difference in the subsequent therapeutic approach.[60] Since "poorly differentiated" tumors demonstrate little resemblance to their benign counterparts,

Table 2
Gross, histologic, and immunophenotypic comparison of cholangiolocarcinomas to its mimickers: bile duct hamartoma, bile duct adenoma, and biliary adenofibroma

	Gross	Histology	Notes	References
Bile Duct Hamartoma	• Multiple nodules • < 0.5 cm	• Interanastomosing dilated biliary ducts, lined by cuboidal or flat epithelium • May contain inspissated bile or eosinophilic debris • Surrounded by myxomatous or fibrotic stroma	• CK7 + • CK19 +	20,42,43
Bile Duct Adenoma	• Solitary nodule • Subcapsular • < 1 cm	• Uniform benign appearing small caliber bile ducts within a fibrous stroma • No cytological atypia or pushing borders	• CK7 + • CK19 + • *BRAF* V600 E mutations (50%) • Ki67 < 10%, • p53 wild type • p16 + • EZH2 -	20,44–47
Biliary Adenofibroma	• Solitary nodule • Microcystic, • Size is up to 16 cm	• Acinar, microcystic and tubuloglandular elements lined by cuboidal flat or low columnar epithelium • Cells with round nuclei without obvious nucleoli • Fibrous stroma • Possible papillary intraluminal projections with fibrovascular core • Possible nuclear atypia with elongated, penicillate hyperchromatic nuclei, resembling dysplasia	• CK7 + • CK19 +	20,48–51
Cholangiolocarcinoma	• Variable sizes	• Innocent-looking tumor resembling reactive bile ductules • Variable degrees of cytologic atypia, desmoplasia, and single cells infiltration	• CK7 + • CK19 + • Ki67 > 10% • p53 mutated • p16 variable • EZH2+ • CD56+	2,20,26,52,53

morphologic examination is often inconclusive. Small biopsies in which a precursor lesion, or a more differentiated component is absent, amplifies the problem. That said, morphology should not be discounted, since a small focus of bile production by tumor cells confirms the diagnosis of HCC, whereas contrariwise, mucin production is seen only in adenocarcinoma, such as iCCA. Immunohistochemistry can be a helpful addition to the diagnostic armamentarium with some practical considerations worth keeping in mind. In general, a poorly differentiated iCCA should still express CK7 and/or CK19[14–17,61] and will not express any of the hepatocytic lineage markers such as HepPar1 and Arginase.[54,61–65] On the other hand, poorly differentiated HCC rarely express CK7 or CK19 and may continue to express hepatocytic markers such as Arginase,[54,62] although HepPar1 expression diminishes as differentiation gets worse.[54,60] Importantly, the presence of aberrant CK19 expression in HCC has been demonstrated to carry a poorer

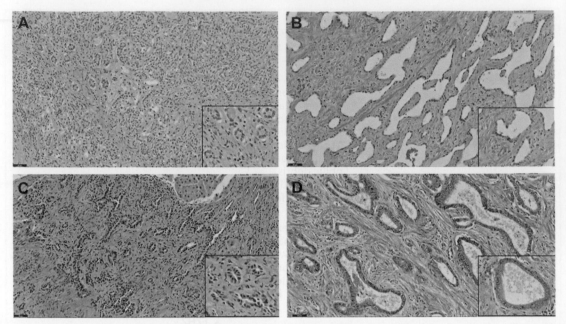

Fig. 3. (*A*). Cholangiolocarcinoma (20x) displays small malignant ducts, resembling ductular reaction. The malignant ducts are lined by small cuboidal cells as shown in the insert (60x). (*B*). Von Meyenburg complex (20x) is comprised by variable sized irregularly shaped bile ducts separated by collagenous stroma. These dilated bile ducts are lined by benign, bland cuboidal to flat cells as seen in insert (60x). (*C*). Bile duct adenoma (20x) displays branching, irregular, non-dilated, and predominantly tubular shaped ducts embedded to a fibrous stroma. The cells lining the irregular ducts are small, cuboidal without cytological atypia as seen in insert (60x). (*D*). Biliary adenofibroma (20x) shows cystic, dilated ducts within a moderately fibrous stroma. The dilated biliary ducts are lined by low columnar to cuboidal epithelium with mildly hyperchromatic nuclei and eosinophilic cytoplasm as seen in the insert (60x).

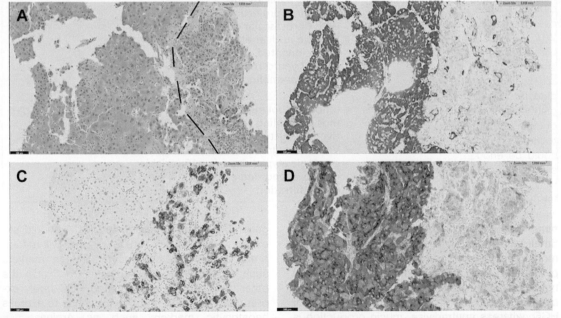

Fig. 4. (*A*). cHCC-CCA (10X) displays blending tumor cells of HCC on the left side and iCCA on the right side of the image. The area of tumor blending is marked by black discontinuous line. (*B*). HepPar-1 immunostain (10X) shows marked reactivity in the HCC area and no reaction in the iCCA cells. (*C*). CK7 (10x) immunostain shows positive staining pattern in the iCCA cells and no reactivity in the HCC area. (*D*). Glypican-3 (10X) is strongly positive in the HCC area and patchy non-reactive, nonspecific (negative) staining is seen in the iCCA area.

prognosis.[66,67] CD10, bile salt export pump (BSEP), and polyclonal CEA are occasionally useful when attempting to classify a poorly differentiated liver tumor as they stain hepatocellular carcinoma with a distinctive "canalicular" pattern.[14,54,63,68,69] Although, the recognition of this canalicular pattern carries significant difficulties, especially in poorly differentiated tumors and may require consultation from an experienced liver pathologist.[14,54] Since BSEP is expressed (practically) only by hepatocytes, it does not require the identification of a canalicular pattern (though this pattern is the most common). The problem with these 3 markers is that very poorly differentiated HCCs do not commonly recapitulate the bile canaliculus. Therefore, the best marker to distinguish poorly differentiated HCC from poorly differentiated iCCA is often glypican 3, which is often positive in poorly differentiated HCC, but only rarely positive in iCCA.[70] Albumin ISH is non-contributory in the scenario since it is a marker of liver primaries and is commonly positive in HCCs and iCCAs alike.[56–58,69]

COMBINED HEPATOCELLULAR-CHOLANGIOCARCINOMA

Another entity to consider in the differential of primary liver carcinoma is combined hepatocellular-cholangiocarcinoma (cHCC-CCA). The pathologic definition of cHCC-CCA has evolved dramatically over the years. However, the last edition of the WHO classification of gastrointestinal and hepatobiliary tumors has simplified this concept. According to the new criteria, cHCC-CCA is a primary liver carcinoma with both hepatocytic and cholangiocytic differentiation in the same tumor. This diagnosis is made regardless of the percentage of each component within the tumor. Immunohistochemistry is confirmatory; however routine H&E could be enough to establish the diagnosis. An example of cHCC-CCA and corresponding immunostains is illustrated in **Fig. 4**.[20,71–73] Furthermore, the presence stem cells or intermediate cells (which are cells that are morphologically in between hepatocytes and cholangiocytes or simultaneously express hepatocytic and cholangiocytic markers) is not required anymore to diagnose cHCC-CCA.[20] Collision tumors (simply a fusion of an HCC and an iCCA) are to be excluded radiologically since they usually exhibit radiological evidence of two separate nodules.[74,75] The presence of all these features is permissive of calling a tumor cHCC-CCA further sub classified as "classical" only to contrast to the other subtype of cHCC-CCA, the intermediate cell carcinoma subtype.

This term (cHCC-CCA, intermediate cell carcinoma subtype or simply intermediate cell carcinoma) is reserved for tumors that are morphologically and immunohistochemically uniform: all the cells are of intermediate morphology between a hepatocyte and a cholangiocyte and all the cells express both hepatocytic and cholangiocytic marker.[20]

CLINICS CARE POINTS

- Differentiating benign peribiliary glands from cholangiocarcinoma on a scant biopsy may be challenging. A panel of immunostains comprising Ki-67, p53, CK7, CK19 and BAP1 may be helpful.

- Tumors arising in the intrahepatic portions of the right and left hepatic ducts may present as hilar masses but should be classified as intrahepatic cholangiocarcinomas. The term perihilar cholangiocarcinoma is reserved for the tumors arising from the extrahepatic portion of the right or left hepatic ducts or the common hepatic duct.

- Cholangiolocarcinoma, a bland subtype of intrahepatic cholangiocarcinoma can be mimicked by 3 benign/preneoplastic lesions: bile duct hamartoma, bile duct adenoma and biliary adenofibroma.

- Albumin-ISH, an established marker of the hepatic lineage/origin may be rarely positive in many other tumors and consequently a diagnostic pitfall.

DISCLOSURE

None.

REFERENCES

1. Bridgewater J, Galle PR, Khan SA, et al. Guidelines for the diagnosis and management of intrahepatic cholangiocarcinoma. J Hepatol 2014;60(Issue 6): 1268–89. ISSN 0168-8278.

2. Aishima S, Oda Y. Pathogenesis and classification of intrahepatic cholangiocarcinoma: different characters of perihilar large duct type versus peripheral small duct type. J Hepatobiliary Pancreat Sci 2015;22:94–100.

3. Chung T, Park YN. Up-to-date pathologic classification and molecular characteristics of intrahepatic cholangiocarcinoma. Front Med 2022;9:857140.

4. Kendall T, Verheij J, Gaudio E, et al. Anatomical, histomorphological and molecular classification of cholangiocarcinoma. Liver Int 2019;39(Suppl 1):7–18.

5. Vijgen S, Terris B, Rubbia-Brandt L. Pathology of intrahepatic cholangiocarcinoma. Hepatobiliary Surg Nutr 2017;6(1):22–34.

6. Jiang K, Al-Diffhala S, Centeno BA. Primary liver cancers-part 1: histopathology, differential diagnoses, and risk stratification. Cancer Control 2018; 25(1). https://doi.org/10.1177/1073274817744625, 1073274817744625.

7. Terada T, Nakanuma Y. Pathological observations of intrahepatic peribiliary glands in 1,000 consecutive autopsy livers. II. A possible source of cholangiocarcinoma. Hepatology 1990;12(1):92–7.

8. Weber A, Schmid RM, Prinz C. Diagnostic approaches for cholangiocarcinoma. World J Gastroenterol 2008;14(26):4131–6.

9. Eloubeidi MA, Chen VK, Jhala NC, et al. Endoscopic ultrasound-guided fine needle aspiration biopsy of suspected cholangiocarcinoma. Clin Gastroenterol Hepatol 2004;2:209–13.

10. Basturk Olca, Farris Alton B, Adsay N Volkan. Chapter 15 - Immunohistology of the Pancreas, Biliary Tract, and Liver. In: David J, editor. Dabbs, diagnostic immunohistochemistry. Third Edition. W.B. Saunders; 2011. p. 541–92, 9781416057666.

11. Khan SA, Thomas HC, Toledano MB, et al. p53 Mutations in human cholangiocarcinoma: a review. Liver Int 2005;25(4):704–16.

12. Furubo S, Harada K, Shimonishi T, et al. Protein expression and genetic alterations of p53 and ras in intrahepatic cholangiocarcinoma. Histopathology 1999;35(3):230–40.

13. Iwamoto KS, Fujii S, Kurata A, et al. p53 mutations in tumor and non-tumor tissues of thorotrast recipients: a model for cellular selection during radiation carcinogenesis in the liver. Carcinogenesis 1999;20(7):1283–91.

14. Choi WT, Ramachandran R, Kakar S. Immunohistochemical approach for the diagnosis of a liver mass on small biopsy specimens. Hum Pathol 2017;63:1–13.

15. Chu P, Wu E, Weiss LM. Cytokeratin 7 and cytokeratin 20 expression in epithelial neoplasms: a survey of 435 cases. Mod Pathol 2000;13(9):962–72.

16. Jain R, Fischer S, Serra S, et al. The use of Cytokeratin 19 (CK19) immunohistochemistry in lesions of the pancreas, gastrointestinal tract, and liver. Appl Immunohistochem Mol Morphol 2010;18(1):9–15.

17. Durnez A, Verslype C, Nevens F, et al. The clinicopathological and prognostic relevance of cytokeratin 7 and 19 expression in hepatocellular carcinoma. A possible progenitor cell origin. Histopathology 2006; 49(2):138–51.

18. Chen XX, Yin Y, Cheng JW, et al. BAP1 acts as a tumor suppressor in intrahepatic cholangiocarcinoma by modulating the ERK1/2 and JNK/c-Jun pathways. Cell Death Dis 2018;9:1036.

19. Carbone M, Yang H, Pass HI, et al. BAP1 and cancer. Nat Rev Cancer 2013;13(3):153–9.

20. Paradis V, Fukayama M, Park YN, et al. editors. Chapter VIII: Tumors of the liver and intrahepatic bile ducts. In: WHO Classification of Tumours Editorial Board. Digestive system tumours. Lyon (France): International Agency for Research on Cancer; 2019. (WHO classification of tumours series, 5th ed; vol. 1): 215-264.

21. Brandi G, Deserti M, Palloni A, et al. Intrahepatic cholangiocarcinoma development in a patient with a novel BAP1 germline mutation and low exposure to asbestos. Cancer Genet 2020;248:57–62.

22. Gupta A, Dixon E. Epidemiology and risk factors: intrahepatic cholangiocarcinoma. Hepatobiliary Surg Nutr 2017;6(2):101–4, 10.21037/hbsn.2017.01.02. PMID: 28503557; PMCID: PMC541127249:57-62. doi: 10.1016/j.cancergen.2020.10.001. Epub 2020 Oct 11. PMID: 33093002.

23. Banales JM, Marin JJG, Lamarca A, et al. Cholangiocarcinoma 2020: the next horizon in mechanisms and management. Nat Rev Gastroenterol Hepatol 2020;17:557–88.

24. Cardinale V, Bragazzi MC, Carpino G, et al. Intrahepatic cholangiocarcinoma: review and update. Hepatoma Res 2018;4:20.

25. Bragazzi MC, Ridola L, Safarikia S, et al. New insights into cholangiocarcinoma: multiple stems and related cell lineages of origin. Ann Gastroenterol 2018;31(1):42–55.

26. Nakanuma Y, Kakuda Y. Pathologic classification of cholangiocarcinoma: New concepts. Best Pract Res Clin Gastroenterol 2015;29(2):277–93.

27. Akita M, Fujikura K, Ajiki T, et al. Dichotomy in intrahepatic cholangiocarcinomas based on histologic similarities to hilar cholangiocarcinomas. Mod Pathol 2017;30(7):986–97.

28. Sigel CS, Drill E, Zhou Y, et al. Intrahepatic Cholangiocarcinomas Have Histologically and Immunophenotypically Distinct Small and Large Duct Patterns. Am J Surg Pathol 2018;42(10):1334–45.

29. Amin MB, Edge S, Greene F, et al. AJCC cancer staging manual. 8th ed. New York, NY: Springer; 2017.

30. Akita M, Sofue K, Fujikura K, et al. Histological and molecular characterization of intrahepatic bile duct cancers suggests an expanded definition of perihilar cholangiocarcinoma. HPB (Oxford) 2019;21(2): 226–34.

31. Tanaka M, Kunita A, Yamagishi M, et al. KRAS mutation in intrahepatic cholangiocarcinoma: Linkage with metastasis-free survival and reduced E-cadherin expression. Liver Int 2022;42(10):2329–40.

32. Merz V, Gaule M, Zecchetto C, et al. Targeting KRAS: the elephant in the room of epithelial cancers. Front Oncol 2021;11:638360.

33. Scheffzek K, Ahmadian MR, Kabsch W, et al. The Ras-RasGAP complex: structural basis for GTPase activation and its loss in oncogenic Ras mutants. Science 1997;277(5324):333–8.

34. Boerner T, Drill E, Pak LM, et al. Genetic determinants of outcome in intrahepatic cholangiocarcinoma. Hepatology 2021;74(3):1429–44.

35. Nakanuma Y, Sato Y, Ikeda H, et al. Intrahepatic cholangiocarcinoma with predominant "ductal plate malformation" pattern: a new subtype. Am J Surg Pathol 2012;36(11):1629–35.

36. Crispo F, Pietrafesa M, Condelli V, et al. IDH1Targeting as a new potential option for intrahepatic cholangiocarcinoma treatment-current state and future perspectives. Molecules 2020;25(16):3754.

37. Hayashi A, Misumi K, Shibahara J, et al. Distinct clinicopathologic and genetic features of 2 histologic subtypes of intrahepatic cholangiocarcinoma. Am J Surg Pathol 2016 Aug;40(8):1021–30.

38. Liau JY, Tsai JH, Yuan RH, et al. Morphological subclassification of intrahepatic cholangiocarcinoma: etiological, clinicopathological, and molecular features. Mod Pathol 2014;27(8):1163–73.

39. Dang L, White D, Gross S, et al. Cancer-associated IDH1 mutations produce 2 hydroxyglutarate. Nature 2009;462:739–44.

40. Saha SK, Parachoniak CA, Ghanta KS, et al. Mutant IDH inhibits HNF-4α to block hepatocyte differentiation and promote biliary cancer. Nature 2014 Sep 4;513(7516): 110–4, [Erratum in: Nature. 2015 Dec 3;528(7580): 152]. PMID: 25043045; PMCID: PMC4499230.

41. Ding N, Che L, Li XL, et al. Oncogenic potential of IDH1R132C mutant in cholangiocarcinoma development in mice. World J Gastroenterol 2016;22(6): 2071–80.

42. Torbenson MS. Hamartomas and malformations of the liver. Semin Diagn Pathol 2019;36(1):39–47.

43. Lev-Toaff AS, Bach AM, Wechsler RJ, et al. The radiologic and pathologic spectrum of biliary hamartomas. AJR Am J Roentgenol 1995;165(2):309–13.

44. Tatsumi R, Ichihara S, Suii H, et al. Bile duct adenoma: imaging features and radiologic-pathologic correlation. Jpn J Radiol 2020;38(6):561–71.

45. Cho C, Rullis I, Rogers LS. Bile duct adenomas as liver nodules. Arch Surg 1978;113(3):272–4.

46. Tsokos CG, Krings G, Yilmaz F, et al. Proliferative index facilitates distinction between benign biliary lesions and intrahepatic cholangiocarcinoma. Hum Pathol 2016;57:61–7.

47. Sasaki M, Matsubara T, Kakuda Y, et al. Immunostaining for polycomb group protein EZH2 and senescent marker p16INK4a may be useful to differentiate cholangiolocellular carcinoma from ductular reaction and bile duct adenoma. Am J Surg Pathol 2014 Mar;38(3):364–9.

48. Varnholt H, Vauthey JN, Dal Cin P, et al. Biliary adenofibroma: a rare neoplasm of bile duct origin with an indolent behavior. Am J Surg Pathol 2003;27(5):693–8.

49. Jacobs MA, Lanciault C, Weinstein S. Incidental biliary adenofibroma with dysplastic features. BJR Case Rep 2015;1(2):20150100.

50. Gurrera A, Alaggio R, Leone G, et al. Biliary adenofibroma of the liver: report of a case and review of the literature. Patholog Res Int 2010;2010: 504584.

51. Arnason T, Borger DR, Corless C, et al. Biliary adenofibroma of liver: morphology, tumor genetics, and outcomes in 6 cases. Am J Surg Pathol 2017; 41(4):499–505.

52. Komuta M, Spee B, Vander Borght S, et al. Clinicopathological study on cholangiolocellular carcinoma suggesting hepatic progenitor cell origin. Hepatology 2008;47:1544–56.

53. Kozaka K, Sasaki M, Fujii T, et al. A subgroup of intrahepatic cholangiocarcinoma with an infiltrating replacement growth pattern and a resemblance to reactive proliferating bile ductules: "bile ductular carcinoma". Histopathology 2007;51:390–400.

54. Takahashi Y, Dungubat E, Kusano H, et al. Application of immunohistochemistry in the pathological diagnosis of liver tumors. Int J Mol Sci 2021; 22(11):5780.

55. Fernández Moro C, Fernandez-Woodbridge A, Alistair D'souza M, et al. Immunohistochemical Typing of Adenocarcinomas of the Pancreatobiliary System Improves Diagnosis and Prognostic Stratification. PLoS One 2016;11(11):e0166067, [Erratum in: PLoS One. 2017 Jan 26;12 (1):e0171283. PMID: 27829047; PMCID: PMC5102456].

56. Bledsoe JR, Shinagare SA, Deshpande V. Difficult Diagnostic Problems in Pancreatobiliary Neoplasia. Arch Pathol Lab Med 2015;139(7):848–57.

57. Brackett DG, Neyaz A, Arora K, et al. Cholangiolar pattern and albumin in situ hybridisation enable a diagnosis of intrahepatic cholangiocarcinoma. J Clin Pathol 2020;73(1):23–9.

58. Ferrone CR, Ting DT, Shahid M, et al. The ability to diagnose intrahepatic cholangiocarcinoma definitively using novel branched DNA-enhanced albumin RNA in situ hybridization technology. Ann Surg Oncol 2016 Jan;23(1):290–6, [Erratum in: Ann Surg Oncol. 2015 Dec;22 Suppl 3:S1604. Erratum in: Ann Surg Oncol. 2015 Dec;22 Suppl 3:S1609. PMID: 25519926; PMCID: PMC4472634].

59. Nasir A, Lehrke HD, Mounajjed T, et al. Albumin in situ hybridization can be positive in adenocarcinomas and other tumors from diverse sites. Am J Clin Pathol 2019;152(2):190–9.

60. Balitzer D, Kakar S. Challenges in diagnosis of hepatocellular carcinoma in cirrhotic liver: a pathologist's perspective. Clin Liver Dis 2021;17(4):249–54.

61. Wee A. Diagnostic utility of immunohistochemistry in hepatocellular carcinoma, its variants and their mimics. Appl Immunohistochem Mol Morphol 2006; 14(3):266–72.

62. Zimmerman RL, Burke MA, Young NA, et al. Diagnostic value of hepatocyte paraffin 1 antibody to discriminate hepatocellular carcinoma from

metastatic carcinoma in fine-needle aspiration biopsies of the liver. Cancer 2001;93(4):288–91.

63. Nguyen T, Phillips D, Jain D, et al. Comparison of 5 Immunohistochemical Markers of Hepatocellular Differentiation for the Diagnosis of Hepatocellular Carcinoma. Arch Pathol Lab Med 2015;139(8): 1028–34.

64. Yan BC, Gong C, Song J, et al. Arginase-1: a new immunohistochemical marker of hepatocytes and hepatocellular neoplasms. Am J Surg Pathol 2010; 34(8):1147–54.

65. Wang HL, Kim CJ, Koo J, et al. Practical immunohistochemistry in neoplastic pathology of the gastrointestinal tract, liver, biliary tract, and pancreas. Arch Pathol Lab Med 2017;141(9):1155–80.

66. Uenishi T, Kubo S, Yamamoto T, et al. Cytokeratin 19 expression in hepatocellular carcinoma predicts early postoperative recurrence. Cancer Sci 2003; 94(10):851–7.

67. Wu PC, Fang JW, Lau VK, et al. Classification of hepatocellular carcinoma according to hepatocellular and biliary differentiation markers. Clinical and biological implications. Am J Pathol 1996;149(4): 1167–75.

68. Ahuja A, Gupta N, Kalra N, et al. Role of CD10 immunochemistry in differentiating hepatocellular carcinoma from metastatic carcinoma of the liver. Cytopathology 2008;19(4):229–35.

69. Lagana SM, Salomao M, Remotti HE, et al. Bile salt export pump: a sensitive and specific immunohistochemical marker of hepatocellular carcinoma. Histopathology 2015;66(4):598–602.

70. Lagana SM, Salomao M, Bao F, et al. Utility of an immunohistochemical panel consisting of glypican-3, heat-shock protein-70, and glutamine synthetase in the distinction of low-grade hepatocellular carcinoma from hepatocellular adenoma. Appl Immunohistochem Mol Morphol 2013;21(2):170–6.

71. Brunt E, Aishima S, Clavien PA, et al. cHCC-CCA: Consensus terminology for primary liver carcinomas with both hepatocytic and cholangiocytic differentiation. Hepatology 2018;68(1):113–26.

72. Stavraka C, Rush H, Ross P. Combined hepatocellular cholangiocarcinoma (cHCC-CC): an update of genetics, molecular biology, and therapeutic interventions. J Hepatocell Carcinoma 2018;6:11–21.

73. Yeh MM. Pathology of combined hepatocellular-cholangiocarcinoma. J Gastroenterol Hepatol 2010; 25(9):1485–92.

74. Al Hamoudi W, Khalaf H, Allam N, et al. Coincidental occurrence of hepatocellular carcinoma and cholangiocarcinoma (collision tumors) after liver transplantation: a case report. Hepat Mon 2012;12(10 HCC):e5871.

75. Komuta M, Yeh MM. A review on the update of combined hepatocellular cholangiocarcinoma. Semin Liver Dis 2020;40(2):124–30.

Mesenchymal Neoplasms of the Liver

David J. Papke Jr, MD, PhD

KEYWORDS

- Mesenchymal hamartoma of the liver • Undifferentiated embryonal sarcoma of the liver
- Calcifying nested stromal-epithelial tumor • Anastomosing hemangioma
- Hepatic small vessel neoplasm • Epithelioid hemangioendothelioma • Hepatic angiosarcoma
- Inflammatory pseudotumor-like follicular dendritic cell sarcoma

Key points

- Mesenchymal hamartoma and undifferentiated embryonal sarcoma of the liver are related tumor types that both harbor chromosome 19q13.3/13.4 structural alterations; *TP53* alterations are common in undifferentiated embryonal sarcoma and absent in mesenchymal hamartoma.

- Calcifying nested stromal-epithelial tumor is a rare primary hepatic neoplasm that shows epithelial (but not hepatocellular) differentiation, nested architecture, and *CTNNB1* and *TERT* promoter alterations.

- Anastomosing hemangioma and hepatic small vessel neoplasm (HSVN) are rare benign vascular tumors that harbor *GNAQ*, *GNA11*, and *GNA14* mutations. HSVN shows infiltrative growth but the lack of nuclear atypia or endothelial multilayering separates it from angiosarcoma.

- Epithelioid hemangioendothelioma frequently presents with multifocal hepatic masses and harbors *WWTR1::CAMTA1* or, rarely, *YAP1::TFE3* fusion. Keratin expression is a diagnostic pitfall for misdiagnosis of carcinoma, and atypical examples can resemble angiosarcoma.

- In the liver, metastases are more common than primary malignancies; metastatic sarcomatoid carcinoma and metastatic melanoma should be considered in the differential diagnosis for sarcomatoid malignancies.

ABSTRACT

Mesenchymal neoplasms of the liver can be diagnostically challenging, particularly on core needle biopsies. Here, I discuss recent updates in neoplasms that are specific to the liver (mesenchymal hamartoma, undifferentiated embryonal sarcoma, calcifying nested stromal-epithelial tumor), vascular tumors of the liver (anastomosing hemangioma, hepatic small vessel neoplasm, epithelioid hemangioendothelioma, angiosarcoma), and other tumor types that can occur primarily in the liver (PEComa/angiomyolipoma, inflammatory pseudotumor-like follicular dendritic cell sarcoma, EBV-associated smooth muscle tumor, inflammatory myofibroblastic tumor, malignant rhabdoid tumor). Lastly, I discuss metastatic sarcomas to the liver, as well as pitfalls presented by metastatic melanoma and sarcomatoid carcinoma.

OVERVIEW

Mesenchymal neoplasms of the liver can be challenging to diagnose, in part because diagnostically helpful architectural features can be poorly represented in core needle biopsies. The rarity of primary mesenchymal neoplasms also contributes to their diagnostic challenge. Primary mesenchymal neoplasms specific to the liver include mesenchymal hamartoma of the liver (MHL), undifferentiated embryonal sarcoma of the liver (UESL), and calcifying nested stromal-epithelial tumor (CNSET). I will discuss the diagnosis of these

Department of Pathology, Brigham and Women's Hospital, Harvard Medical School, 75 Francis Street, Boston, MA 02115, USA
E-mail address: dpapke@partners.org

Surgical Pathology 16 (2023) 609–634
https://doi.org/10.1016/j.path.2023.04.013
1875-9181/23/© 2023 Elsevier Inc. All rights reserved.

tumor types, as well as recent studies that have elucidated their clinical behavior and underlying tumor biology.

The spectrum of vascular tumors includes anastomosing hemangioma (benign), hepatic small vessel neoplasm (HSVN; a benign but sometimes locally aggressive tumor), epithelioid hemangioendothelioma (EHE; a sarcoma that often has a protracted clinical course), and hepatic angiosarcoma (a definitionally high-grade, aggressive sarcoma). Despite their disparate clinical courses, these tumor types can be challenging to distinguish on core biopsies. Herein, I will discuss useful histopathologic features to distinguish these tumor types, as well as their clinical behavior and recent updates in our understanding of their pathogenesis.

Finally, I will discuss other mesenchymal tumors that can primarily involve the liver, including perivascular epithelioid cell tumor (PEComa)/angiomyolipoma, inflammatory pseudotumor-like follicular dendritic cell sarcoma (FDCS), Epstein Barr virus (EBV)-associated smooth muscle tumor, inflammatory myofibroblastic tumor (IMT), and malignant rhabdoid tumor (MRT). Because most malignant neoplasms in the liver are metastases,[1] I will also discuss metastatic melanoma and sarcomatoid carcinoma, both of which have the potential to be misdiagnosed as sarcoma.

PRIMARY MESENCHYMAL NEOPLASMS UNIQUE TO THE LIVER

Primary mesenchymal neoplasms that are specific to the liver are uncommon and include MHL, UESL, and CNSET (Table 1).

MESENCHYMAL HAMARTOMA AND UNDIFFERENTIATED EMBRYONAL SARCOMA OF THE LIVER

MHL is a benign tumor type that typically occurs in patients aged younger than 2 years and is generally cured by surgical resection.[2] MHL usually presents as a solitary mass, which can sometimes be large and have a prominent cystic component.[3,4] Histologically, it is composed of an admixture of benign bile ducts and haphazardly arranged, bland spindle cells in a variably myxoid to collagenous stroma (Fig. 1).

MHL is characterized by recurrent alterations of chromosome 19q13.3/13.4,[5,6] including t(11;19) (q11;q13.3/13.4) involving MALAT1 on chromosome 11.[7] These chromosomal alterations are present in the spindle cells but not the admixed bile ducts, suggesting that the latter are a nonneoplastic component of the lesion.[7] A recent

case report implicated DICER1 alterations in MHL[8]; however, the tumors in this report are unusual cystic lesions that do not seem to meet morphologic criteria for MHL and might instead represent distinctive DICER1-associated hepatic neoplasms.[9,10]

UESL is an aggressive malignancy that occurs in children and young adults, with a median age at presentation of around 5 to 10 years.[11] UESL tends to present as a large, sometimes painful mass. Although in initial studies UESL was associated with high mortality rate,[11] subsequent studies have shown that patients with surgically resectable disease achieve long-term disease-free survival with combined surgery/chemotherapy in most cases.[12–15] Histologically, UESL shows markedly pleomorphic neoplastic cells, some of which show spindle cell morphology. Characteristically, there are tumor giant cells that show prominent cytoplasmic hyaline globules (Fig. 2A). The diagnosis is based largely on morphology because UESL shows a nonspecific immunophenotype including expression of desmin and keratins in about 50% of cases each (Fig. 2B–C).[16] The differential diagnosis primarily includes other pleomorphic sarcomas but the rarity of pleomorphic sarcomas in young patients makes differential diagnostic considerations such as metastatic dedifferentiated liposarcoma (DDLPS) much less likely. A recent report of a rhabdoid tumor of the liver harboring t(11;19) raises the possibility that the morphologic spectrum of UESL might be wider than previously recognized, although more examples need to be studied to make this determination.[17]

There are examples of UESL ex-MHL, strongly suggesting that these tumor types share a common biology.[15] Consistent with this notion, UESL was found to harbor just the same chromosome 19 alterations as MHL.[7] This chromosome 19q13.3 to 13.4 locus contains chromosome 19 micro-RNA cluster (C19MC), the largest known human micro-RNA (miRNA) cluster that codes for dozens of miRNAs.[18] C19MC is primate-specific,[18] and it represents an imprinted locus, in which expression of the maternal allele is silenced while the paternal allele is expressed during placental development.[19] An alternate, unusual genetic mechanism drives another subset of MHL: "androgenetic-biparental mosaicism," in which tumor cells harbor 2 copies of the paternal allele, instead of 1 copy each of maternal and paternal alleles.[20] In this subset of cases, one allele is demethylated and expressed in the absence of a structural rearrangement, whereas the other remains methylated and silenced. C19MC expression has been implicated in

Table 1
List of primary hepatic mesenchymal neoplasms with genetic and immunohistochemical features

Neoplasm(s)	Genetic Alteration (Prevalence)	IHC Markers (Sensitivity)
MHL	19q13.3/13.4 alterations (100%)[a]	No specific markers
UESL	• 19q13.3/13.4 alterations (80%–100%) • TP53 alterations (90%) • Complex copy number alterations (100%)	• No specific markers • Keratins, desmin (50% each)
CNSET	• CTNNB1 alterations (100%) • TERT promoter mutations (100%)	β-catenin (100%)
Anastomosing hemangioma HSVN	• GNAQ mutations • GNA11 mutations • GNA14 mutations	• No specific markers • Ki-67 < 10%
EHE	WWTR1::CAMTA1 (90%) YAP1::TFE3 (5%)	CAMTA1 (~100% for CAMTA1 fusions) TFE3 positive, YAP1 loss (~100% for YAP1::TFE3 fusion)
Primary angiosarcoma	• MAPK pathway alterations (50%) • TP53 inactivating alterations (20%–30%) • KDR and/or PLCG1 alterations (25%) • CIC alterations (5%–10%)[b]	p53 mutant pattern (~20–30%)
PEComa/angiomyolipoma	TSC1/TSC2 alterations (90%) TFE3 rearrangements (5%–10%)	• HMB-45/melan-A (80%–90% each) • SMA/desmin (95% positive for ≥1 marker) TFE3 (correlates with fusions)
Inflammatory pseudotumor-like follicular dendritic cell sarcoma	Not yet well defined	• CD21, CD35 (90% each) • EBV RNA ISH (100%)
EBV-associated smooth muscle neoplasm	Not yet well defined	• SMA, desmin (~100%) • EBV RNA ISH (100%)
IMT	• ALK1 fusions (50%–60%) • ROS1 fusions (~5%)	ALK, ROS1 (correlate with fusions)
Malignant rhabdoid tumor	SMARCB1 inactivating alterations (~100%)	INI1 loss (~100%)
Solitary fibrous tumor	NAB2::STAT6 (>95%)	STAT6, CD34 (~95% each)
Embryonal rhabdomyosarcoma	• Chromosome 11p15.5 loss of heterozygosity • Nonspecific mutations	Desmin, myogenin, myo-D1 (~100%)

Abbreviations: IHC, immunohistochemistry; SMA, smooth muscle actin; ISH, in situ hybridization.
[a] DICER1 alterations have been reported in lesions bearing some resemblance to mesenchymal hamartoma.
[b] 30% of CIC-rearranged round cell sarcomas express CD31 and 50% express ERG; therefore, some reported angiosarcomas with CIC rearrangement might instead represent CIC-rearranged round cell sarcomas.

tumorigenesis of other hepatocellular neoplasms, including hepatocellular carcinoma, possibly because its miRNAs inhibit tumor suppressor genes and thus promote tumorigenesis.[21,22]

Because MHL and UESL are likely related neoplasms that harbor common C19MC alterations, studies have investigated the genetic features that might explain their disparate clinical behavior

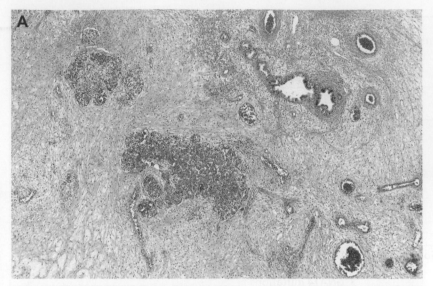

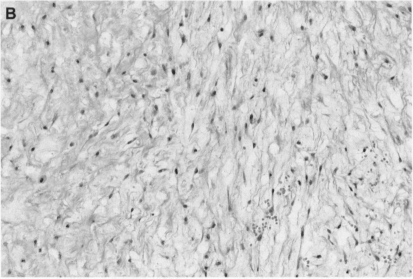

Fig. 1. MHL. (*A*) Mesenchymal hamartoma shows a proliferation of bland spindle cells, with haphazardly admixed benign bile ducts and small lobules of hepatocytes. It has been shown that the spindle cells are neoplastic, whereas the bile ducts are not. (*B*) On higher power, the spindle cells show pale eosinophilic cytoplasm and tapered nuclei. There is no cytologic atypia.

and/or progression from MHL to UESL. Published examples of UESL occurring in the setting of Li-Fraumeni syndrome implicated *TP53* alterations,[23] and additional studies demonstrated complex karyotypes in UESL.[15,24] A recent molecular genetic study of 13 UESL by Setty and colleagues systematically investigated this question; these researchers identified C19MC structural alterations in 10 of 13 tumors, *TP53* mutations/copy number loss in 12, and complex copy number alterations in all 13.[25] The authors also demonstrated C19MC miRNA overexpression in all 13 tumors. Ultimately, this study and others considered together have shown that MHL and UESL exist on a biologic spectrum, and that UESL has complex copy number alterations and *TP53* inactivation that genetically distinguish it from MHL.

CALCIFYING NESTED STROMAL-EPITHELIAL TUMOR

CNSET is a primary liver tumor that was first described in 2001,[26] and described subsequently mostly in small case series and isolated case reports. Literature surveys in 2019 identified 38 unique published examples, which occurred in young patients (median age: 14 years; range: 2–34 years), 70% of whom were female.[27,28] Some patients presented with Cushing syndrome,[29,30] and some tumors occurred in association with Beckwith-Wiedemann syndrome,[31,32] but otherwise presentations were nonspecific. Morphologically, CNSET shows nests of neoplastic epithelioid cells with palely eosinophilic cytoplasm and ovoid nuclei with small nucleoli (**Fig.** 3A–B). The nests

Fig. 2. UESL. (*A*) UESL is an overtly malignant, highly pleomorphic sarcoma. Neoplastic cells show intracytoplasmic hyaline globules, a characteristic feature. (*B*, *C*) IHC in UESL. UESL is essentially a morphologic diagnosis. It has a nonspecific immunophenotype; about half express desmin (*B*), and about half express keratins (*C*, pan-keratin).

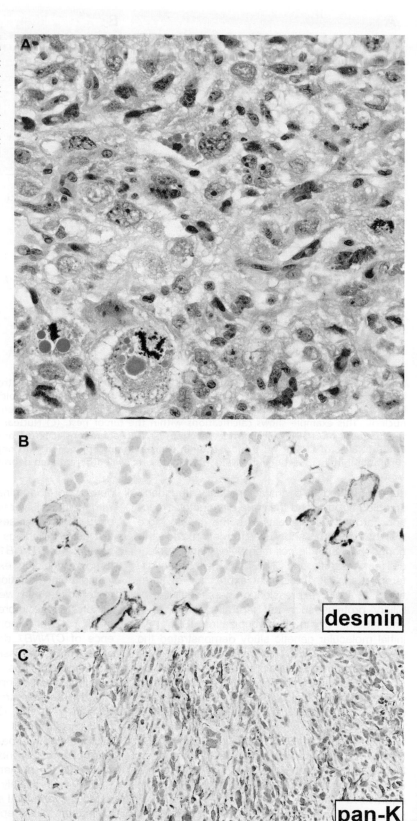

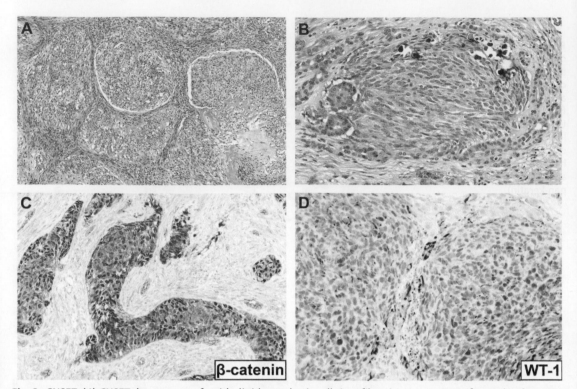

Fig. 3. CNSET. (*A*) CNSET shows nests of epithelioid neoplastic cells in a fibrotic stroma. Bone formation is present in just more than half of tumors. There are multiple foci of dense hyaline osteoid matrix in this example. (*B*) On higher power, the neoplastic cells show monomorphic ovoid nuclei with open chromatin and small, distinct nucleoli. This example shows calcifications within the tumor nest. (*C*) Nuclear β-catenin expression confirms the diagnosis of CNSET, which harbors recurrent *CTNNB1* alterations. (*D*) Nuclear WT-1 expression is also present in about 80% of CNSET. WT-1 and β-catenin expression, in conjunction with negativity for synaptophysin and chromogranin, help distinguish CNSET from metastatic well-differentiated neuroendocrine tumor.

are embedded in a characteristically abundant, spindled stroma, and there are bile ductular reactions around tumor nests in some cases. More than half of tumors show bone formation, and a minority show spindle cell morphology and/or clear cell features. Although CNSET shows epithelial differentiation, with consistent expression of keratins,[29] it lacks expression of hepatocellular or biliary proteins such as HepPar-1, arginase-1, and albumin (by in situ hybridization; ISH).[33] An initial molecular genetic study demonstrated the presence of *CTNNB1* exon 3 deletions in 2 sequenced tumors.[34] Consistent with these findings, CNSET uniformly shows nuclear expression of β-catenin, and it also shows nuclear expression of WT-1 in about 80% of cases (**Fig. 3**C–D).[27,34,35]

Until recently, there were only rare reports of metastasizing CNSET,[36,37] and only about 10% to 15% of tumors were known to have recurred locally.[27,35] A recent series with long-term follow-up demonstrated that CNSET might be more aggressive than previously thought.[33] In this series, 4 of 7 patients with follow-up developed lung metastases, and 2 of these 4 patients also

developed abdominal metastases. One patient with multifocal liver tumors at presentation developed lung metastases and died of disease. Molecular genetic findings in this series confirmed the presence of *CTNNB1* alterations in all sequenced tumors, including exon 3/4 deletions and activating point mutations. Additionally, *TERT* promoter mutations were found in all sequenced tumors. Mitoses more than 5/10 high-power fields, multifocal liver tumors at presentation, and presence of *CTNNB1* deletions all were associated with a more aggressive clinical courses, although these associations need further corroboration given the small number of cases in this series.

With its nested architecture and desmoplastic-appearing stroma, CNSET presents a pitfall for the misdiagnosis of carcinoma or well-differentiated neuroendocrine tumor, especially in examples that do not show bone formation (**Table 2**). Of the primary hepatocellular neoplasms, CNSET most closely resembles hepatoblastoma, particularly the fetal subtype. Both are composed of monomorphic epithelioid cells, and both of these neoplasms express nuclear β-catenin.[38]

Table 2
Pitfalls for the misdiagnosis of carcinoma

Pitfalls for Misdiagnosis of Conventional Carcinoma			
Neoplasm	Diagnostic pitfall	Reasons for pitfall	Clues and tests to avoid pitfall
CNSET	Metastatic carcinoma	• Keratin expression • Nested architecture	• Monomorphic cytomorphology • β-catenin positivity
	Hepatoblastoma	• Keratin expression • Nested architecture	• Negativity for hepato-cellular markers
	Metastatic well-differentiated neuroendocrine tumor	• Keratin expression • Nested architecture	• Negativity for neuroen-docrine markers
EHE	Metastatic carcinoma	• Keratin expression • Epithelioid morphology	• Sinusoidal growth pattern • Positivity for vascular markers
Angiosarcoma	Carcinoma	• Keratin expression • Epithelioid morphology	• Sinusoidal growth pattern • Positivity for vascular markers
PEComa	Hepatocellular carcinoma	• Granular cytoplasm • Epithelioid morphology	• Unusually low mitotic activity • Keratin negativity in most cases
Malignant rhabdoid tumor	Carcinoma, hepatoblastoma	• Keratin expression • Epithelioid morphology	• Unusually young age • INI1 loss • Negativity for hepato-cellular markers
DSRCT	Carcinoma	• Keratin positivity • Nested architecture • Epithelioid morphology	• Unusually young age for carcinoma • Expression of desmin
Pitfalls for misdiagnosis of sarcomatoid carcinoma			
Neoplasm	Diagnostic pitfall	Reason for pitfall	Test to avoid pitfall
Metastatic leiomyosarcoma	Metastatic sarcomatoid carcinoma	• Keratin positivity	• Desmin usually positive
Metastatic melanoma	Metastatic sarcomatoid carcinoma	• Keratin positivity (rare)	• Diffuse SOX10, S100 positivity • History of melanoma is helpful

However, hepatoblastoma does not have the dense fibrous stroma of CNSET, and it also expresses HepPar-1, arginase-1, and albumin (the latter by ISH), markers that can distinguish it from CNSET.[39,40] Another differential diagnostic consideration is hepatocellular carcinoma, which is distinguished from CNSET by the expression of HepPar-1 and arginase-1; although hepatocellular carcinoma can lose expression of these markers,[41] this loss generally occurs in poorly differentiated tumors that would not show the monomorphic appearance of CNSET. Finally, CNSET shows some morphologic overlap with metastatic well-differentiated neuroendocrine tumor, which could be a diagnostic pitfall particularly in cases of multifocal CNSET. These tumor types are easily distinguished by immunohistochemistry (IHC) because CNSET is consistently negative for chromogranin and synaptophysin while well-differentiated neuroendocrine tumors are consistently positive (see **Table 2**).

VASCULAR NEOPLASMS

Primary vascular neoplasms of the liver can be diagnostically challenging, particularly on core needle biopsies in which architectural features are not apparent. Benign hemangiomas are the most common mesenchymal tumors of the liver, with an estimated population prevalence of 2.5%,[42] and these include sclerosed hemangioma, cavernous hemangioma, and the more recently described anastomosing hemangioma and HSVN. Of these benign hemangiomas, anastomosing hemangioma and HSVN are the only ones that present a diagnostic pitfall for the misdiagnosis of angiosarcoma. Here, I will discuss these 2 benign tumor types, along with EHE and angiosarcoma (see **Table 1**).

ANASTOMOSING HEMANGIOMA AND HEPATIC SMALL VESSEL NEOPLASM

Anastomosing hemangioma was initially described in a series of 6 tumors of the genitourinary tract,[43] and subsequently it has been described to occur in the retroperitoneum, paraspinal soft tissue, and abdominal organs including the liver.[44–46] Anastomosing hemangioma is a benign vascular tumor that shows complex, anastomosing vascular channels lined by bland endothelial cells (**Fig. 4**A). In contrast to angiosarcoma, the endothelial cells in anastomosing hemangioma are monolayered, and the tumor does not demonstrate infiltrative growth into hepatic parenchyma. Fibrin thrombi are commonly present. About half of tumors show extramedullary hematopoiesis, and about half show intracytoplasmic hyaline globules in neoplastic endothelial cells. IHC for vascular markers is useful to highlight the architecture of the lesion and to confirm the lack of endothelial multilayering (**Fig. 4**B). Anastomosing hemangioma harbors the same activating alterations that are present in other benign hemangioma types, including in GNAQ, GNA11, and GNA14.[47–49]

HSVN was originally described to have uncertain biologic potential,[50] but with longer clinical follow-up, it is now thought to represent a benign but sometimes locally aggressive vascular neoplasm.[51] Similar to anastomosing hemangioma, HSVN shows complex anastomosing vascular channels surfaced by a monolayer of endothelial cells that lack nuclear atypia. However, in contrast to anastomosing hemangioma, HSVN also shows infiltrative growth into adjacent hepatic parenchyma (**Fig. 4**C), which can make it challenging to distinguish from angiosarcoma. This differential diagnosis is one of the few instances in soft tissue pathology where Ki-67 IHC has diagnostic utility; in one recent series, HSVN consistently showed a Ki-67 proliferative index of less than 10%, whereas only angiosarcoma showed a higher Ki-67 proliferative index.[50] However, the converse is not true, and

so a low Ki-67 does not exclude the diagnosis of angiosarcoma. Similar to anastomosing hemangioma and kaposiform hemangioendothelioma, HSVN harbors mutations in GNAQ and GNA14, and it lacks TP53 alterations[51]; therefore, p53 IHC also has utility in distinguishing HSVN from angiosarcoma, the latter of which shows TP53 alterations in ~20 to 30% of tumors.[52,53]

EPITHELIOID HEMANGIOENDOTHELIOMA

Although EHE was initially described as a tumor of intermediate biologic potential,[54] it is now known to be a sarcoma, the prognosis of which depends on the involved body site(s).[55–57] EHE of the liver presents with multifocal hepatic disease in about 75% of patients,[57] and it presents with involvement of extrahepatic body sites in about 40% of patients.[58,59] In long-term follow-up, most patients with hepatic EHE die of disease, with roughly 40% overall survival at 5 years of follow-up.[57,59]

There are 2 main morphologic variants of EHE, each of which has distinctive clinicopathologic features. About 90% of EHE harbor WWTR1::CAMTA1 fusions.[60–62] CAMTA1-rearranged EHE shows mildly atypical neoplastic cells that are embedded singly and in small cords in a characteristic myxohyaline stroma (**Fig. 5**A). At its interface with background hepatic parenchyma, EHE shows a sinusoidal pattern of growth (**Fig. 5**B). EHE also shows plugging of native portal tract vessels with tumor cells, which is a helpful diagnostic clue when present. CAMTA1 IHC is highly sensitive and specific for EHE harboring CAMTA1 fusion, with strong and diffuse nuclear expression in essentially all such cases (**Fig. 5**C).[63,64]

About 5% of EHE harbor alternate YAP1::TFE3 fusions,[65] and this subtype of EHE can rarely occur in the liver.[66,67] EHE with YAP1::TFE3 fusion shows distinctive morphology, with nests of epithelioid endothelial cells showing voluminous, glassy cytoplasm and frank vasoformation (**Fig. 5**D). Recent studies have shown that this subtype of EHE has a clinical course distinct from CAMTA1-rearranged EHE, with a higher frequency of multifocal disease and metastasis (compared with CAMTA1-rearranged EHE of all sites) but a significantly higher 5-year progression-free survival of 85% to 90%.[68,69] IHC directed against the C-terminus of YAP1 demonstrates the loss of expression in YAP1::TFE3-rearranged EHE (**Fig. 5**E),[70] and TFE3 IHC shows strong and diffuse nuclear expression.[65] Although it is sensitive, TFE3 IHC is somewhat nonspecific,[61,71] such that only strong and diffuse TFE3 expression in the correct morphologic context should be used to support the diagnosis

Fig. 4. Anastomosing hemangioma and HSVN. (*A*) Anastomosing hemangioma is composed of complexly anastomosing vascular channels that lack endothelial multilayering or nuclear atypia. Extramedullary hematopoiesis is a common feature, exemplified here by a megakaryocyte (*arrow*). (*B*) IHC for CD31 (shown), SMA, and/or ERG can be useful to highlight the lack of endothelial multilayering. In this hepatic anastomosing hemangioma, CD31 highlights densely packed vessels with monolayers of endothelial cells. (*C*) Although HSVN bears close resemblance to anastomosing hemangioma, it is distinguished by its infiltrative interface with adjacent hepatic parenchyma. Here, this HSVN can be seen infiltrating around a native portal tract.

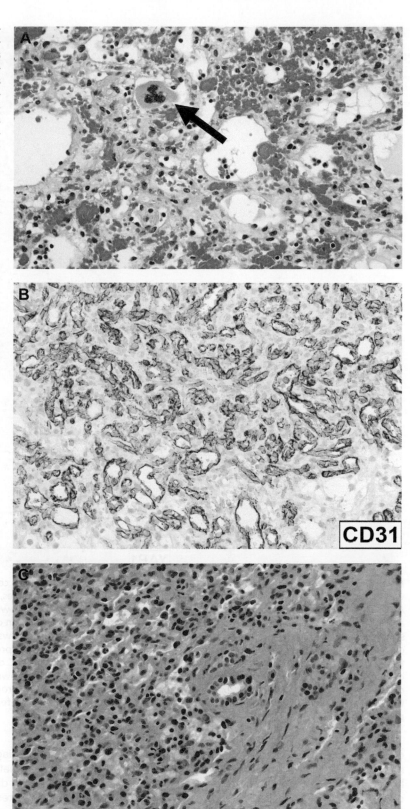

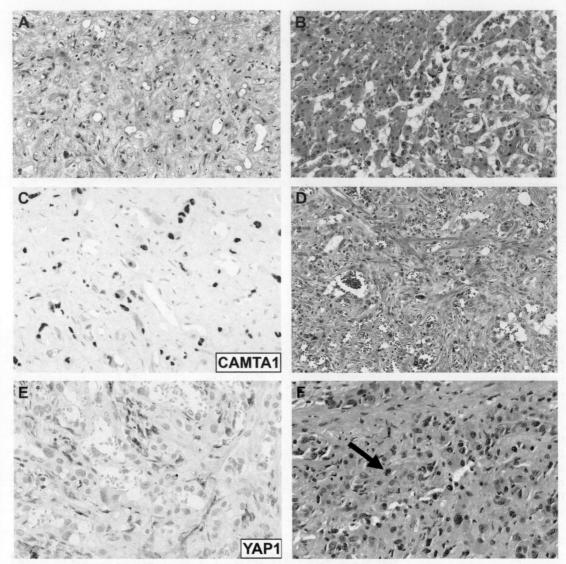

Fig. 5. EHE. (*A*) EHE with *WWTR1::CAMTA1* fusion shows neoplastic endothelial cells scattered singly and in cords within a characteristic myxohyaline stroma. Some cells show cytoplasmic vacuoles, a useful diagnostic feature. (*B*) At the interface between tumor and background hepatic parenchyma, EHE shows an infiltrative growth pattern along sinusoids that would be very unusual for carcinoma. (*C*) Nuclear expression of CAMTA1 by IHC is highly sensitive and specific for the diagnosis of EHE. (*D*) EHE with *YAP1::TFE3* fusion shows nests of epithelioid neoplastic cells with voluminous cytoplasm, round nuclei with vesicular chromatin, and prominent nucleoli. There is also frank vasoformation, in contrast to EHE with *WWTR1::CAMTA1* fusion. (*E*) IHC demonstrates loss of expression of the C-terminus of YAP1, consistent with *YAP1::TFE3* fusion. TFE3 IHC (not shown) shows strong and diffuse nuclear staining, and both stains can be used to confirm the diagnosis in the appropriate morphologic context. (*F*) Marked cytologic atypia and increased mitotic activity (*arrow*) are high-risk features associated with inferior progression-free survival.

of EHE with *YAP1::TFE3* fusion. Given its distinctive morphology, clinical course, and genetics, it seems likely that EHE with *YAP1::TFE3* fusion represents a diagnostic entity distinct from *CAMTA1*-rearranged EHE, although in the most recent WHO classification, these tumor types share a common classification.[72]

The differential diagnosis of EHE includes carcinoma (especially metastatic carcinoma in patients with multifocal liver disease) and epithelioid angiosarcoma. EHE expresses keratins in up to 60% of cases,[73] presenting a potential pitfall for the misdiagnosis of carcinoma (see **Table 2**). However, the sinusoidal growth and myxohyaline stroma of EHE would be unusual for carcinoma, and these features should prompt consideration of a vascular neoplasm. Epithelioid angiosarcoma is another diagnostic consideration, particularly in examples of EHE with marked cytologic atypia (see later discussion). Because CAMTA1 IHC is highly specific for EHE,[64] I have a low threshold for performing CAMTA1 IHC to rule out EHE before diagnosing epithelioid angiosarcoma in the liver.

Recent studies have shown that increased mitotic activity, large tumor size, nuclear atypia, and pleural involvement are associated with decreased survival.[68,74,75] Shibayama and colleagues proposed a risk stratification model, in which tumors were stratified into low-risk, intermediate-risk, and high-risk groups based on tumor size and atypical histologic features (defined as tumor necrosis, >1 mitosis/2 mm^2, and/or marked nuclear atypia) (**Fig. 5**F).[76] In this model, low-risk, intermediate-risk, and high-risk tumors showed 5-year overall survival rates of 100%, 81.8%, and 16.9%, respectively.[76] Only 2 of 31 patients with liver involvement in this series had high-risk tumors, suggesting that high-risk liver disease is uncommon. Given that these atypical histologic features have been associated with worse prognosis in multiple studies, it is important to state their presence if they are identified.

Recent work has elucidated our understanding of the tumor biology of EHE and has pointed to potential treatment strategies. *WWTR1* encodes TAZ, and both YAP1 and TAZ are downstream effectors of the Hippo pathway that regulates cell proliferation.[77] In the protein resulting from *WWTR1::CAMTA1* fusion, the CAMTA1 component promotes translocation of the fusion protein into the nucleus, where the TAZ component can then serve as a transcription factor.[78] Expression of the *WWTR1::CAMTA1* fusion gene in a mouse model is sufficient to drive the development of EHE,[79] and the fusion proteins in both *CAMTA1*-rearranged and *YAP1*-rearranged EHE subtypes have been shown to drive oncogenic transcriptional programs.[80] These programs include the expression of connective tissue growth factor,[81] a protein that binds integrins that are thought to promote invasion and metastasis.[82,83] Integrin signaling depends on the Ras-Mitogen-activated protein kinase (MAPK) pathway,[84] and a recent in vitro study demonstrated that inhibition of this pathway with sorafenib and MAPK kinase (MEK) inhibitors decreased tumor cell colony formation.[81] These studies provide a biologic basis for recent clinical trials using the MEK inhibitor trametinib in patients with metastatic or unresectable EHE; more time is needed to determine whether this treatment is effective in preventing disease progression.

HEPATIC ANGIOSARCOMA

Hepatic angiosarcoma is a highly aggressive malignancy, with a dismal median survival of under 6 months.[85] Most hepatic angiosarcomas arise de novo, with a median age at presentation of 65 years and a slight male predominance,[86] although the age range is wide and includes children.[87] Rarely, hepatic angiosarcoma can arise due to exposure to toxins including arsenic and vinyl chloride.[88–91] Hepatic angiosarcoma shows a variety of growth patterns, and most commonly, it forms a discrete mass.[92] Less commonly, it diffusely infiltrates the liver sinusoids, a subtle growth pattern that can be hard to recognize (**Fig. 6**A–B). When hepatic angiosarcoma forms a discrete mass, it typically forms complexly anastomosing vascular channels, with cytologic atypia, endothelial multilayering, and infiltration of hepatic parenchyma (**Fig. 6**C–E). Occasional examples show spindle cell or epithelioid morphology without evident vasoformation, in which case the glassy cytoplasm is a useful diagnostic clue. It is uncommon for angiosarcoma to show prominent nuclear pleomorphism. Even morphologically low-grade appearing angiosarcomas have a high risk of distant metastasis, and so angiosarcoma is definitionally high-grade.[93] IHC demonstrates expression of CD31 and ERG in nearly all cases, whereas the sensitivity of CD34 is only ~60% to 70%.[94] CD31 IHC is particularly useful to highlight endothelial multilayering (**Fig. 6**F).

The differential diagnosis of hepatic angiosarcoma is broad and depends on the tumor morphology. Morphologically bland examples show histologic overlap with benign vascular tumors such as anastomosing hemangioma and HSVN. However, in contrast to these benign tumor types, angiosarcoma shows endothelial multilayering. There are no immunohistochemical stains that reliably distinguish angiosarcoma from these benign tumor types, although a Ki-67 proliferation index greater than 10% or a p53 mutant staining pattern would strongly favor the diagnosis of angiosarcoma in this differential.[50] The differential diagnosis also includes EHE, which can show marked cytologic atypia in some cases; CAMTA1 IHC is essentially always negative in angiosarcoma, and therefore, this marker is useful to rule out EHE with marked cytologic atypia.[63,64] Keratins are expressed in around 30% of angiosarcomas, especially ones with epithelioid morphology, presenting a potential diagnostic pitfall (see **Table 2**).[95] Diagnostic clues for angiosarcoma include the presence of glassy cytoplasm, cytoplasmic vacuoles, and infiltrative growth through hepatic sinusoids, all of which would be unusual for carcinoma. IHC for

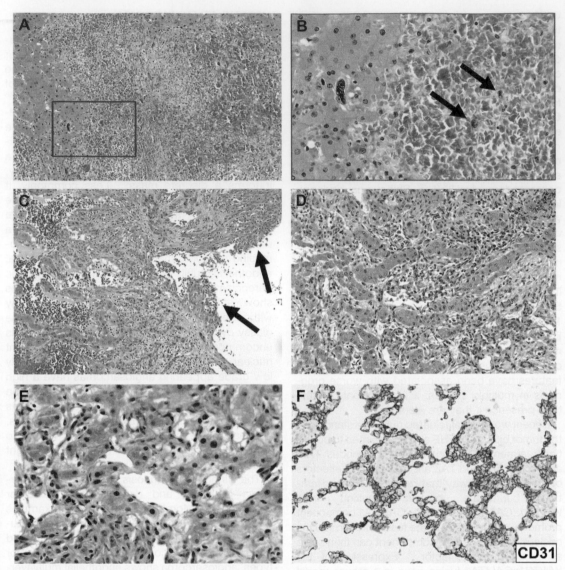

Fig. 6. Hepatic angiosarcoma. (*A, B*) Hepatic angiosarcoma showing hemorrhage and sinusoidal growth. (*A*) This hepatic angiosarcoma showed multiple scattered hemorrhagic foci at low power. (*B*) This higher power image of the region boxed in A shows that there are rare, atypical cells in the hemorrhage (*arrows*), as well as a markedly atypical cell infiltrating adjacent hepatic sinusoids. (*C*) This hepatic angiosarcoma shows prominent endothelial multilayering (*arrows*). (*D, E*) Dissecting growth through hepatic sinusoids is characteristic and provides a useful diagnostic clue. (*F*) IHC for CD31 highlights endothelial cells that are multilayered and that are wrapping around residual hepatocytes.

CD31 and ERG can resolve this differential diagnosis, with the caveat that weak ERG positivity is nonspecific and should be interpreted with caution.[96] Given the clinical implications of the diagnosis of angiosarcoma, if there is diagnostic uncertainty, then it is important to advise repeat biopsy.

The genetic features of angiosarcoma have been partially elucidated in recent studies. *MYC* amplification is characteristic of radiation-associated angiosarcoma but only present in a minor subset of primary angiosarcoma.[97,98] Instead, primary angiosarcoma shows MAPK pathway alterations in about 50% of tumors and *TP53* and/or *CDKN2A* alterations in 20% to 30%.[53] *KDR* and/or *PLCG1*, both involved in vascular endothelial growth factor signaling, are altered in about 25% of angiosarcomas, including both primary and secondary tumors.[99–101] Although angiosarcoma was originally reported to show complex copy number alterations in most cases,[102] more recent study identified this finding in only 25% of cases.[103] A small subset of angiosarcomas harbor

CIC alterations, including mutations and rearrangements[100]; these tumors show epithelioid morphology, younger than average age at presentation, and more aggressive clinical behavior.[100] However, it was shown recently that CIC-rearranged round cell sarcomas can express ERG in half of cases and CD31 in about a third; none of these tumors showed vasoformation, and DNA methylation profiling showed that these tumors clustered with CIC-rearranged round cell sarcomas and not angiosarcoma.[104] Therefore, it seems that a subset of CIC-rearranged round cell sarcomas likely express vascular markers and present a pitfall for misdiagnosis of epithelioid angiosarcoma.

OTHER MESENCHYMAL NEOPLASMS THAT CAN PRIMARILY OCCUR IN THE LIVER

There are several other mesenchymal neoplasms that can occur primarily in the liver, including PEComa/angiomyolipoma, inflammatory pseudotumor-like FDCS, EBV-associated smooth muscle tumor (EBV-SMT), IMT, and MRT (see Table 1). In this section, I will briefly survey these neoplasms, which are rare and have distinctive features that facilitate their recognition.

PERIVASCULAR EPITHELIOID CELL TUMOR/ ANGIOMYOLIPOMA

The concept of PEComa was elucidated in the 1990s, when it was determined that angiomyolipoma, pulmonary lymphangiomyomatosis, clear cell "sugar" tumor of the lung, and tumors now termed epithelioid PEComa all share ultrastructural and immunohistochemical characteristics.[105–108] We now know that both sporadic and tuberous sclerosis-associated tumors in the PEComa family harbor mammalian target of rapamycin (mTOR) pathway alterations in most cases, most commonly in TSC1 and TSC2.[109,110] A minor subset of PEComas harbor TFE3 rearrangements.[111,112]

Hepatic PEComa and angiomyolipoma both tend to occur in middle-aged adults, with a marked female predominance.[113] Angiomyolipoma shows a mixture of adipose tissue, blood vessels, and epithelioid cells (Fig. 7A). In PEComa, the perivascular epithelioid cells predominate, and sometimes, there are no evident adipocytes in the tumor. The neoplastic cells of PEComa show granular to clear cytoplasm and vesicular nuclei with prominent, melanocyte-like nuclei (Fig. 7B). Usually, smooth muscle actin (SMA) and desmin are expressed strongly but only in scattered cells, a staining pattern that would be unusual for a smooth muscle neoplasm (Fig. 7C). IHC also demonstrates expression of melanosomal proteins HMB-45 and/or melan-A in most tumors (Fig. 7D). PEComas harboring TFE3 translocations show epithelioid morphology with prominent clear cell features, and they show nuclear expression of TFE3.[112] The morphologic differential diagnosis of epithelioid PEComa includes hepatocellular carcinoma, metastatic clear cell renal or adrenocortical carcinoma, and metastatic melanoma (see Table 1). IHC is useful to resolve the differential diagnosis of carcinoma; although PEComa rarely expresses keratins, it does not generally show the strong and diffuse expression seen in carcinoma.[114] Similarly, although PEComa does express melanocytic markers such as HMB-45 and melan-A, it does not express SOX10,[115] which is strongly and diffusely positive in metastatic melanoma and therefore distinguishes these tumor types.

It can be challenging to predict the behavior of PEComa based on morphologic features. In a study of PEComas of soft tissue and the gynecologic tract, worrisome features include significant mitotic activity (>1 mitoses per 50 HPF), high nuclear grade, size greater than 8 cm, and/or necrosis; tumors showing at least 2 worrisome features were considered malignant.[114] Although these criteria have not been validated in hepatic tumors, the presence of significant nuclear atypia or mitotic activity should be noted because there are rare reports of malignant PEComa of the liver giving rise to distant metastases.[116,117]

FOLLICULAR DENDRITIC CELL SARCOMA

FDCS is a rare mesenchymal neoplasm that occurs in lymph nodes, soft tissue, and viscera. Conventional FDCS occurs across a wide age range, with a peak age at presentation of around 50 years and no sex predilection. It is composed of overtly malignant-appearing, epithelioid to spindled neoplastic cells that show characteristic whorled architecture and prominent admixed lymphocytes. Conventional FDCS is exceedingly rare in the liver, with only isolated case reports in the literature.[118] In general, FDCS is an aggressive sarcoma, and up to half of patients die of disease in long-term follow-up.[119]

There is an EBV-driven variant of FDCS, termed "inflammatory pseudotumor-like FDCS" (IPL-FDCS). Although IPL-FDCS is less common than conventional FDCS in general, it has a predilection for the liver and is much more common at this body site than conventional FDCS.[120,121] IPL-DFCS has a female predominance with a median age at presentation of 45 years, and it is most common in East Asia, possibly reflecting endemic

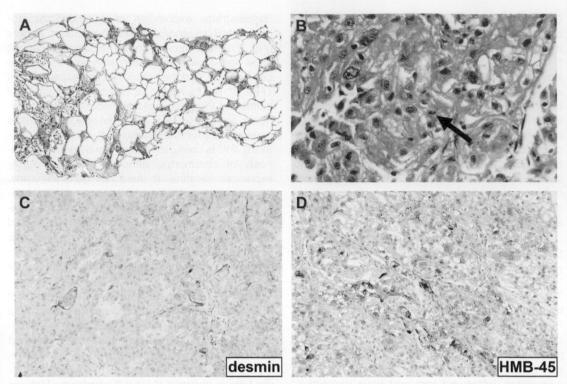

Fig. 7. PEComa/angiomyolipoma. (A) This angiomyolipoma of the liver is dominated by the adipocytic component and shows just scattered epithelioid neoplastic cells and small blood vessels. (B) This malignant PEComa
of the liver shows marked nuclear atypia and mitotic activity (arrow). The neoplastic cells have prominent nucleoli
that resemble those of malignant melanoma. Malignant PEComas of the liver are extremely rare. (C, D) IHC in
angiomyolipoma/PEComa. (C). Angiomyolipoma and PEComa express SMA and desmin (shown), characteristically
showing strong positivity in scattered cells. (D) Expression of HMB-45 (shown) and melan-A is also characteristic.

EBV infection in this region.[122] Histologically, IPL-
DFCS shows the whorled architecture and lymphocytic inflammation of conventional FDCS but
in contrast, it shows a more polymorphous
neoplastic cell population, with less severe cytologic atypia and more fibrotic stroma (Fig. 8A).
Similar to conventional FDCS, IPL-FDCS expresses of CD21 and CD35 in ~90% of cases
each (Fig. 8B).[123] FDCS has also been shown to
express D2-40, SSTR2A, and PD-L1 in about half
of cases each, although there is no systematic
study of these antibodies in IPL-FDCS.[119,124]
Along with the IHC markers positive in conventional FDCS, ISH for EBV RNA can be used to
confirm the diagnosis (Fig. 8C). EMA expression
is seen in ~40% of FDCS but keratins are usually
negative and help distinguish FDCS from carcinoma.[123] The differential diagnosis also includes
IMT, but IMT is not as prominently whorled as
IPL-FDCS, nor does it express CD21, CD35, or
EBV RNA (ISH). Overall, IPL-FDCS has a better
prognosis than conventional FDCS, with a roughly
30% local recurrence rate and only rare reports of
metastasis to date.[122]

EPSTEIN BARR VIRUS-ASSOCIATED SMOOTH MUSCLE TUMOR

EBV-SMT is rare and occurs in severely immunosuppressed patients, generally in the setting of acquired immunodeficiency syndrome or organ
transplantation.[125,126] These tumors are frequently
multicentric, and the liver is a common site of
involvement.[127] Microscopically, EBV-SMT has a
distinctive morphology, with somewhat primitive-
appearing smooth muscle cells that show brightly
eosinophilic cytoplasm and distinct cell borders.
Often there are admixed nodules or whorls of
smaller neoplastic cells. EBV-SMT usually lacks
cytologic atypia, and high mitotic activity is uncommon. IHC demonstrates the expression of smooth
muscle markers, and EBV RNA ISH confirms the
diagnosis. EBV-SMT is generally treated with surgery combined, if possible, with the treatment of
the underlying cause of immunosuppression.[128]
Patients with EBV-SMT have a mortality rate of
15% to 40%, depending on the patient population,
although some of this high mortality is due to other
sequelae of immunosuppression.[127,128] Patients

Fig. 8. IPL-FDCS. (*A*) Histologically, this IPL-FDCS of the liver shows whorls of neoplastic cells with large nuclei and prominent admixed lymphocytes. It shows somewhat more haphazard architecture and less nuclear atypia than conventional FDCS. (*B*) IHC demonstrates the expression of follicular dendritic cell markers, including CD21 (shown), CD23, and CD35; CD21 IHC highlights the whorled architecture. Follicular dendritic cells can also express desmin and keratins, presenting a potential diagnostic pitfall. (*C*) ISH for Epstein-Barr viral RNA is positive, confirming the diagnosis.

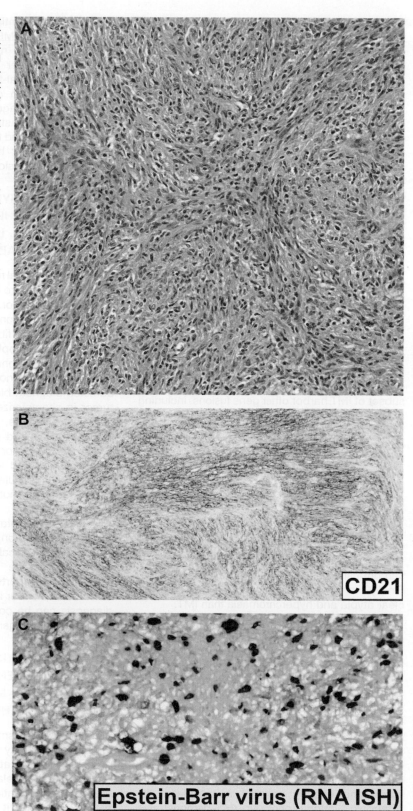

who are able to recover immune function have a very good prognosis,[128] and tumors can spontaneously resolve if the underlying immunosuppression is reversed.[129,130]

INFLAMMATORY MYOFIBROBLASTIC TUMOR

IMT is a rare mesenchymal neoplasm that commonly occurs in children and young adults, with a minority of cases occurring in older adults.[131,132] IMT is recognized to rarely occur in the liver.[133] Histologically, it is composed of fascicles of spindle cells with vesicular nuclei and prominent nucleoli. The stroma is variably myxoid to collagenous, and, characteristically, there is prominent admixed inflammation composed of plasma cells, neutrophils, and/or lymphocytes. IHC demonstrates the expression of SMA and sometimes desmin; similar to other tumors with myofibroblastic differentiation, about 15% of IMT express keratins.[134] ALK fusions are present in about 50% to 60% of IMT, and tumors with these fusions show strong and diffuse expression of ALK by IHC.[132] ALK fusions are more common in younger patients, and in older patients, the diagnosis is often based on morphology.[131] A minor subset of IMT harbor other gene fusions, including in ROS1.

The differential diagnosis of IMT includes inflammatory pseudotumor, metastatic leiomyosarcoma, and, possibly, sarcomatoid carcinoma. Inflammatory pseudotumors (discussed in detail in another article) show a much less organized proliferation of fibroblasts/myofibroblasts, and there is frequently an associated ductular reaction.[135] Leiomyosarcoma shows brightly eosinophilic cytoplasm and distinct cell borders, neither of which are features of IMT, and generally leiomyosarcoma shows significantly more nuclear atypia. Finally, sarcomatoid carcinoma shows more nuclear atypia and hyperchromasia than IMT.

MALIGNANT RHABDOID TUMOR

MRT is a rare, highly aggressive sarcoma of infancy and early childhood, with most patients presenting under 1 year of age. Although MRT usually occurs in the kidney or perinephric adipose tissue, rarely it can present primarily in the liver.[136,137] About 60% of patients with MRT of the liver present with metastatic disease, and 90% of patients die of disease.[138] Morphologically, MRT shows sheets of neoplastic cells with eccentric, vesicular nuclei and brightly eosinophilic cytoplasm (ie, "rhabdoid" cytomorphology). IHC demonstrates the loss of expression of integrase interactor 1 (INI1),[139] consistent with SMARCB1 inactivation

identified in essentially all cases.[140,141] About 60% of extrarenal MRT express keratins but they are consistently negative for desmin and CD34,[142] the latter of which helps distinguish MRT from proximal-type epithelioid sarcoma.[143] Keratin expression could present a diagnostic pitfall for the misdiagnosis of hepatocellular carcinoma or hepatoblastoma (see Table 2) but MRT can be distinguished by its rhabdoid cytomorphology, negativity for hepatocellular markers, and loss of INI1 expression.[137]

OTHER MESENCHYMAL NEOPLASMS THAT CAN OCCUR IN THE LIVER: SOLITARY FIBROUS TUMOR, LEIOMYOSARCOMA, AND EMBRYONAL RHABDOMYOSARCOMA

Other mesenchymal neoplasms that can occur primarily in the liver are exceedingly rare and include solitary fibrous tumor, primary hepatic leiomyosarcoma, and embryonal rhabdomyosarcoma (see Table 1). Solitary fibrous tumor shows haphazardly arranged neoplastic cells, which are ovoid to spindled in morphology. The stroma is characteristically collagenous, and there are usually admixed staghorn blood vessels. Solitary fibrous tumor is characterized by NAB2::STAT6 fusions in ~95% of cases,[144,145] and IHC for STAT6 is highly sensitive and specific for the diagnosis.[146] The liver is a common site of metastasis for solitary fibrous tumor, and so this possibility should be considered, particularly in patients with a potentially spurious remote history of a "fibroma" or "meningioma."

Because metastatic leiomyosarcoma is so much more common in the liver than primary leiomyosarcoma, clinical exclusion of a primary elsewhere should be recommended. There are isolated case reports of embryonal rhabdomyosarcoma of the liver in children and adults[147]; this diagnosis can be confirmed by IHC for desmin, myo-D1, and myogenin.

SECONDARY MALIGNANCIES OF THE LIVER: PITFALLS, CHALLENGES, AND GENERAL APPROACHES TO SARCOMATOID NEOPLASMS IN THE LIVER

Metastatic neoplasms to the liver are more common than primary hepatic malignancies.[1] In particular, metastatic sarcomatoid carcinoma and metastatic melanoma can mimic sarcoma, presenting a potential diagnostic pitfall (see Table 2); therefore, it is important to consider a broad differential diagnosis for sarcomatoid neoplasms and to rule out sarcomatoid carcinoma

Fig. 9. Metastatic sarcomatoid carcinoma. (*A*) Sarcomatoid carcinoma usually shows mixed epithelioid and spindle cell morphology, including scattered cells with pleomorphic and hyperchromatic nuclei. Collagenous stroma is a common feature of sarcomatoid carcinoma. (*B*) CAM5.2 IHC demonstrates diffuse positivity. IHC for broad-spectrum keratins is helpful when positive but some sarcomatoid carcinomas can lose expression of keratins. A clinical history of primary carcinoma elsewhere is helpful to raise the diagnostic possibility of metastatic, keratin-negative sarcomatoid carcinoma.

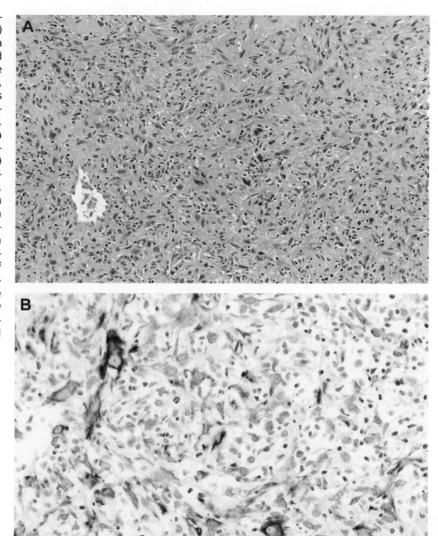

and melanoma. Metastatic sarcomatoid carcinoma typically occurs in older adults and shows overtly malignant, mixed epithelioid and spindle cell morphology, with scattered cells showing hyperchromatic nuclei and nuclear pleomorphism (Fig. 9A). Often times patients present with widely metastatic disease, such that the primary site cannot be determined; given the dismal prognosis, with a median survival of under 1 year, determination of primary site has limited clinical utility in most cases.[148] IHC for broad-spectrum keratins can be helpful to support the diagnosis (Fig. 9B). Sarcomatoid carcinomas often lose the expression of transcription factors useful for determining lineage, except for sarcomatoid renal or pulmonary carcinoma that sometimes retain

the expression of PAX8 or TTF-1, respectively. In general, most sarcomatoid carcinomas in the liver are metastases because primary sarcomatoid carcinoma of the liver is exceedingly uncommon.[149]

Metastatic melanoma can show predominantly spindle cell morphology and can express desmin,[150] presenting a pitfall for misdiagnosis of leiomyosarcoma (Fig. 10A). In most cases, melanoma shows strong and diffuse expression of both SOX10 and S-100 protein,[151] and thus these markers are very useful screens when working up a sarcomatoid neoplasm in the liver (Fig. 10B). The strong and diffuse expression of SOX10 and S-100 protein is also useful to distinguish melanoma from malignant peripheral nerve

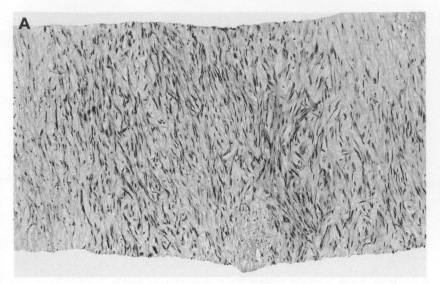

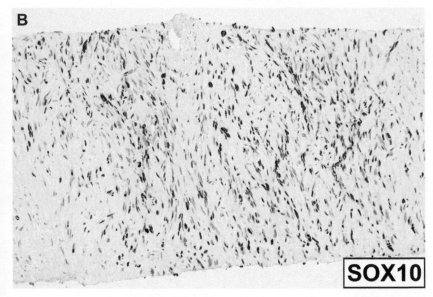

SOX10

Fig. 10. Metastatic melanoma. (A) This metastatic melanoma is a fascicular spindle cell neoplasm with eosinophilic cytoplasm, features that raise the differential diagnosis of leiomyosarcoma. Melanoma sometimes presents with widespread metastatic disease, including liver metastases, and in about 5% of patients there is no identifiable primary tumor on subsequent clinical workup. (B) IHC for SOX10 (pictured) and S-100 protein demonstrates strong and diffuse expression, an extent of expression that is essentially never seen in MPNST.

sheath tumor (MPNST) because the latter never shows diffuse expression of these proteins and commonly lacks expression of both of them.[152] IHC against the trimethylated histone H3 K27 residue (H3K27me3) shows loss in ~50% of MPNST, including ~80% of high-grade examples[153]; whereas it is useful to support the diagnosis of MPNST, H3K27me3 IHC should only be used in the appropriate context because loss is also common in melanoma.[154] Melanoma can sometimes lose the expression of SOX10 and S-100 protein, in which case it is frequently misdiagnosed as a sarcoma[155]; in such cases, the clinical history of melanoma is critical, and mutation-specific antibodies for BRAF V600E and NRAS Q61R can be helpful in some cases.

Leiomyosarcoma commonly metastasizes to the liver. Morphologically, leiomyosarcoma shows fascicles of neoplastic cells with brightly eosinophilic cytoplasm, distinct cell borders, and elongated nuclei with blunt ends (Fig 11A). Leiomyosarcoma expresses keratins and EMA in about 40% of cases each, presenting a pitfall for the misdiagnosis of metastatic sarcomatoid carcinoma (see Table 2).[156] Although SMA expression is nonspecific within this differential diagnosis, IHC for desmin is helpful because desmin expression in sarcomatoid carcinoma is exceptionally rare.

Gastrointestinal stromal tumor (GIST) also frequently gives rise to liver metastases but there is nearly always a clinical history of a primary

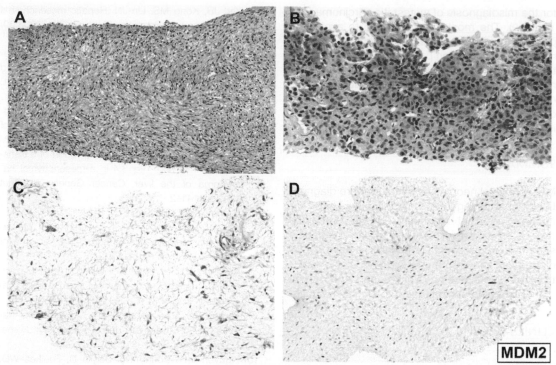

Fig. 11. Secondary sarcomas of the liver. (*A*) Metastatic leiomyosarcoma. This metastatic leiomyosarcoma shows fascicles of spindle cells with brightly eosinophilic cytoplasm and atypical nuclei. This patient had multiple liver masses but no known primary at the time of biopsy. (*B*) Metastatic GIST. This metastatic epithelioid GIST shows relatively uniform cytomorphology, a helpful diagnostic clue. It would be unusual for a patient to present with metastatic GIST in the liver without an evident mass in the luminal gastrointestinal tract. (*C, D*) DDLPS. DDLPS can present with a reported clinical history of multiple liver masses. However, re-review of the imaging generally demonstrates an associated well-differentiated component in the retroperitoneum. (*C*) Histologically DDLPS can show a wide range of morphologic patterns, which generally show at least scattered nuclear pleomorphism and/or nuclear hyperchromasia. In this example, the DDLPS is a myxoid spindle cell neoplasm, with scattered pleomorphic and hyperchromatic nuclei. (*D*) IHC for MDM2 (shown) and/or CDK4 highlights neoplastic nuclei, confirming the diagnosis of DDLPS.

tumor of the luminal gastrointestinal tract. Morphologically, GIST typically shows a monomorphic proliferation of spindled or epithelioid cells with palely eosinophilic cytoplasm and, sometimes, paranuclear cytoplasmic vacuoles (**Fig 11**B). IHC for KIT and DOG1 is helpful because only ~3% of GISTs are negative for both markers.[157]

Occasionally, DDLPS can seem clinically to be a hepatic mass or, in some cases, multiple hepatic masses. Microscopically, DDLPS shows a wide range of morphologic patterns, and most show nuclear pleomorphism (**Fig. 11**C–D). Nearly all examples of DDLPS show amplification chromosome 12q15, including *MDM2* and, in most cases, *CDK4*.[158] IHC shows expression of MDM2 and CDK4 in 85% to 95% of tumors each.[159–161] Because *STAT6* is located on chromosome 12q and coamplified in ~10% to 15% of cases, it can present a potential diagnostic pitfall for the

misdiagnosis of solitary fibrous tumor.[162] Careful examination of imaging studies with an expert musculoskeletal radiologist is helpful to confirm the presence of an associated well-differentiated component. In my practice, I perform IHC for MDM2 and CDK4 in my last round of stains of pleomorphic tumors of the liver, as a screen to exclude DDLPS.

Finally, desmoplastic small round cell tumor (DSRCT) is a round cell sarcoma with *EWSR1::WT1* fusion that commonly presents with widely metastatic disease, including with hepatic involvement in about a third of patients.[163,164] DSRCT has a median age at presentation of around 20 to 25 years, with a striking predilection for men, and it usually shows round cell morphology with characteristic desmoplastic stroma. However, there are occasional examples with more epithelioid morphology,[165] and most DSRCT express keratins, presenting a pitfall for the misdiagnosis of metastatic carcinoma (see **Table 2**). The most important clue to avoid this pitfall is the clinical context of a highly aggressive malignancy in a young patient. IHC can help avoid this pitfall because DSRCT expresses desmin,[164] a marker that is essentially always negative in carcinoma. The diagnosis can be confirmed by IHC directed against the C-terminus of WT-1, which is retained in the fusion protein.[166]

SUMMARY

Mesenchymal neoplasms of the liver are diagnostically challenging due to their rarity. There are multiple potential diagnostic pitfalls: sarcomas can be mistaken for carcinoma, and metastatic sarcomatoid carcinoma or melanoma can be misdiagnosed as sarcoma. Awareness of the spectrum of diagnostic possibilities and appropriate use of IHC help avoid falling into diagnostic traps.

CLINICS CARE POINTS

- Metastatic sarcomas are more common than primary hepatic sarcomas.

- Metastatic melanoma and metastatic sarcomatoid carcinoma present diagnostic pitfalls for sarcoma.

- In contrast to benign vascular tumor types, hepatic angiosarcoma demonstrates nuclear atypia and endothelial multilayering.

- Epithelioid hemangioendothelioma and hepatic angiosarcoma commonly express keratins and present a pitfall for the misdiagnosis of metastatic carcinoma.

DISCLOSURE

The author reports no conflicts of interest.

ACKNOWLEDGMENTS

I gratefully acknowledge Dr Christopher Fletcher for providing cases for photography.

REFERENCES

1. Goodman ZD. Neoplasms of the liver. Mod Pathol 2007;20(Suppl 1):S49–60.
2. Martins-Filho SN, Putra J. Hepatic mesenchymal hamartoma and undifferentiated embryonal sarcoma of the liver: a pathologic review. Hepatic Oncology 2020;7:HEP19.
3. Yen JB, Kong MS, Lin JN. Hepatic mesenchymal hamartoma. J Paediatr Child Health 2003;39:632–4.
4. Maqbool H, Mushtaq S, Hassan U, et al. Case series of mesenchymal hamartoma: a rare childhood hepatic neoplasm. J Gastrointest Cancer 2020;51:1030–3.
5. Speleman F, de Telder V, de Potter KR, et al. Cytogenetic analysis of a mesenchymal hamartoma of the liver. Cancer Genet Cytogenet 1989;40:29–32.
6. Mascarello JT, Krous HF. Second report of a translocation involving 19q13.4 in a mesenchymal hamartoma of the liver. Cancer Genet Cytogenet 1992;58:141–2.
7. Mathews J, Duncavage EJ, Pfeifer JD. Characterization of translocations in mesenchymal hamartoma and undifferentiated embryonal sarcoma of the liver. Exp Mol Pathol 2013;95:319–24.
8. Apellaniz-Ruiz M, Segni M, Kettwig M, et al. Mesenchymal hamartoma of the liver and DICER1 syndrome. N Engl J Med 2019;380:1834–42.
9. Vargas SO, Perez-Atayde AR. Mesenchymal hamartoma of the liver and DICER1 syndrome. N Engl J Med 2019;381:586–7.
10. Nguyen V-H, Bouron-Dal Soglio D, Foulkes WD. Mesenchymal hamartoma of the liver and DICER1 syndrome. Reply. N Engl J Med 2019;381:587.
11. Stocker JT, Ishak KG. Undifferentiated (embryonal) sarcoma of the liver: report of 31 cases. Cancer 1978;42:336–48.
12. Techavichit P, Masand PM, Himes RW, et al. Undifferentiated embryonal sarcoma of the liver (UESL): A single-center experience and review of the literature. J Pediatr Hematol Oncol 2016;38:261–8.
13. Mathias MD, Ambati SR, Chou AJ, et al. A single-center experience with undifferentiated embryonal sarcoma of the liver. Pediatr Blood Cancer 2016;63:2246–8.
14. Ismail H, Dembowska-Bagińska B, Broniszczak D, et al. Treatment of undifferentiated embryonal sarcoma of the liver in children - Single center experience. J Pediatr Surg 2013;48:2202–6.
15. Shehata BM, Gupta NA, Katzenstein HM, et al. Undifferentiated embryonal sarcoma of the liver is associated with mesenchymal hamartoma and multiple chromosomal abnormalities: A review of eleven cases. Pediatr Dev Pathol 2011;14:111–6.
16. Zheng JM, Tao X, Xu AM, et al. Primary and recurrent embryonal sarcoma of the liver: Clinicopathological and immunohistochemical analysis. Histopathology 2007;51:195–203.
17. Papke DJ, Fisch AS, Ranganathan S, et al. Undifferentiated embryonal sarcoma of the liver with rhabdoid morphology mimicking carcinoma: Expanding the morphologic spectrum or a distinct variant? Pediatr Dev Pathol 2021;24:564–9.

18. Bentwich I, Avniel A, Karov Y, et al. Identification of hundreds of conserved and nonconserved human microRNAs. Nat Genet 2005;37:766–70.

19. Noguer-Dance M, Abu-Amero S, Al-Khtib M, et al. The primate-specific microRNA gene cluster (C19MC) is imprinted in the placenta. Hum Mol Genet 2010;19:3566–82.

20. Keller RB, Demellawy DE, Quaglia A, et al. Methylation status of the chromosome arm 19q microRNA cluster in sporadic and androgenetic-biparental mosaicism-associated hepatic mesenchymal hamartoma. Pediatr Dev Pathol 2015;18:218–27.

21. Fornari F, Milazzo M, Chieco P, et al. In hepatocellular carcinoma miR-519d is up-regulated by p53 and DNA hypomethylation and targets CDKN1A/p21, PTEN, AKT3 and TIMP2. J Pathol 2012;227:275–85.

22. Flor I, Bullerdiek J. The dark side of a success story: microRNAs of the C19MC cluster in human tumours. J Pathol 2012;227:270–4.

23. Lack EE, Schloo BL, Azumi N, et al. Undifferentiated (embryonal) sarcoma of the liver. Clinical and pathologic study of 16 cases with emphasis on immunohistochemical features. Am J Surg Pathol 1991;15:1–16.

24. Sowery RD, Jensen C, Morrison KB, et al. Comparative genomic hybridization detects multiple chromosomal amplifications and deletions in undifferentiated embryonal sarcoma of the liver. Cancer Genet Cytogenet 2001;126:128–33.

25. Setty BA, Jinesh GG, Arnold M, et al. The genomic landscape of undifferentiated embryonal sarcoma of the liver is typified by C19MC structural rearrangement and overexpression combined with TP53 mutation or loss. PLoS Genet 2020;16(4): e1008642.

26. Ishak KG, Goodman ZD, Stocker JT. Miscellaneous malignant tumors (Chapter 11). In: Rosai J, Sobin L, editors. Tumors of the liver and Intrahepatic bile ducts. Washington, D.C.: Armed Forces Institute of Pathology; 2001. p. 276–8.

27. Benedict M, Zhang X. Calcifying nested stromal-epithelial tumor of the liver an update and literature review. Arch Pathol Lab Med 2019;143:264–8.

28. Geramizadeh B. Nested stromal-epithelial tumor of the liver: A review. Gastrointest Tumors 2019;6:1–10.

29. Heerema-McKenney A, Leuschner I, Smith N, et al. Nested stromal epithelial tumor of the liver: Six cases of a distinctive pediatric neoplasm with frequent calcifications and association with Cushing syndrome. Am J Surg Pathol 2005;29:10–20.

30. Weeda VD, De Rouver PR, Bras H, et al. Cushing syndrome as presenting symptom of calcifying nested stromal-epithelial tumor of the liver in an adolescent boy: A case report. J Med Case Rep 2016;10:4–7.

31. Malowany JI, Merritt NH, Chan NG, et al. Nested stromal epithelial tumor of the liver in Beckwith-Wiedemann syndrome. Pediatr Dev Pathol 2013; 16:312–7.

32. Khoshnam N, Robinson H, Clay MR, et al. Calcifying nested stromal-epithelial tumor (CNSET) of the liver in Beckwith-Wiedemann syndrome. Eur J Med Genet 2017;60:136–9.

33. Papke DJ, Dong F, Zhang X, et al. Calcifying nested stromal–epithelial tumor: a clinicopathologic and molecular genetic study of eight cases highlighting metastatic potential and recurrent CTNNB1 and TERT promoter alterations. Mod Pathol 2021; 34:1696–703.

34. Assmann G, Kappler R, Zeindl-Eberhart E, et al. β-Catenin mutations in 2 nested stromal epithelial tumors of the liver - A neoplasia with defective mesenchymal-epithelial transition. Hum Pathol 2012;43:1815–27.

35. Makhlouf HR, Abdul-Al HM, Wang G, et al. Calcifying nested stromal-epithelial tumors of the liver. Am J Surg Pathol 2009;33:976–83.

36. Brodsky SV, Sandoval C, Sharma N, et al. Recurrent nested stromal epithelial tumor of the liver with extrahepatic metastasis: case report and review of literature. Pediatr Dev 2008;11:469–73.

37. Hommann M, Kaemmerer D, Daffner W, et al. Nested stromal epithelial tumor of the liver-liver transplantation and follow-up. J Gastrointest Cancer 2011;42:292–5.

38. Curia MC, Zuckermann M, De Lellis L, et al. Sporadic childhood hepatoblastomas show activation of β-catenin, mismatch repair defects and p53 mutations. Mod Pathol 2008;21:7–14.

39. López-Terrada D, Alaggio R, De Dávila MT, et al. Towards an international pediatric liver tumor consensus classification: Proceedings of the Los Angeles COG liver tumors symposium. Mod Pathol 2014;27:472–91.

40. Chen DA, Koehne De Gonzalez A, Fazlollahi L, et al. In situ hybridisation for albumin RNA in paediatric liver cancers compared with common immunohistochemical markers. J Clin Pathol 2021;74: 98–101.

41. Yan BC, Gong C, Song J, et al. Arginase-1: A new immunohistochemical marker of hepatocytes and hepatocellular neoplasms. Am J Surg Pathol 2010;34:1147–54.

42. Mocchegiani F, Vincenzi P, Coletta M, et al. Prevalence and clinical outcome of hepatic haemangioma with specific reference to the risk of rupture: A large retrospective cross-sectional study. Dig Liver Dis 2016;48:309–14.

43. Montgomery E, Epstein JI. Anastomosing hemangioma of the genitourinary tract A lesion mimicking angiosarcoma. Am J Surg Pathol 2009;33:1364–9.

44. John I, Folpe AL. Anastomosing hemangiomas arising in unusual locations: A clinicopathologic study of 17 soft tissue cases showing a predilection

for the paraspinal region. Am J Surg Pathol 2016; 40:1084–9.

45. Lin J, Bigge J, Ulbright TM, et al. Anastomosing hemangioma of the liver and gastrointestinal tract an unusual variant histologically mimicking angiosarcoma. Am J Surg Pathol 2013;37:1761–5.

46. Lunn B, Yasir S, Lam-Himlin D, et al. Anastomosing hemangioma of the liver: A case series. Abdominal Radiology 2019;44:2781–7.

47. Bean GR, Joseph NM, Gill RM, et al. Recurrent GNAQ mutations in anastomosing hemangiomas. Mod Pathol 2017;30:722–7.

48. Bean GR, Joseph NM, Folpe AL, et al. Recurrent GNA14 mutations in anastomosing haemangiomas. Histopathology 2018;73:354–7.

49. Liau JY, Tsai JH, Lan J, et al. GNA11 joins GNAQ and GNA14 as a recurrently mutated gene in anastomosing hemangioma. Virchows Arch 2020;476: 475–81.

50. Gill RM, Buelow B, Mather C, et al. Hepatic small vessel neoplasm, a rare infiltrative vascular neoplasm of uncertain malignant potential. Hum Pathol 2016;54:143–51.

51. Joseph NM, Brunt EM, Marginean C, et al. Frequent GNAQ and GNA14 Mutations in Hepatic Small Vessel Neoplasm. Am J Surg Pathol 2018; 42:1201–7.

52. Behjati S, Tarpey PS, Sheldon H, et al. Recurrent PTPRB and PLCG1 mutations in angiosarcoma. Nat Genet 2014;46:376–9.

53. Murali R, Chandramohan R, Möller I, et al. Targeted massively parallel sequencing of angiosarcomas reveals frequent activation of the mitogen activated protein kinase pathway. Oncotarget 2015;6:36041–52.

54. Weiss SW, Enzinger FM. Epithelioid hemangioendothelioma a vascular tumor often mistaken for a carcinoma. Cancer 1982;50:970–81.

55. Kleer CG, Unni KK, McLeod RA. Epithelioid hemangioendothelioma of bone. Am J Surg Pathol 1996;20:1301–11.

56. Mentzel T, Beham A, Calonje E, et al. Epithelioid Hhemangioendothelioma of skin and soft tissues: Clinicopathologic and immunohistochemical study of 30 cases. Am J Surg Pathol 1997;21:363–74.

57. Makhlouf HR, Ishak KG, Goodman ZD. Epithelioid hemangioendothelioma of the liver: A clinicopathologic study of 137 cases. Cancer 1999;85:562–82.

58. Lau K, Massad M, Pollak C, et al. Clinical patterns and outcome in epithelioid hemangioendothelioma with or without pulmonary involvement: Insights from an internet registry in the study of a rare cancer. Chest 2011;140:1312–8.

59. Mehrabi A, Kashfi A, Fonouni H, et al. Primary malignant hepatic epithelioid hemangioendothelioma: A comprehensive review of the literature with emphasis on the surgical therapy. Cancer 2006; 107:2108–21.

60. Mendlick MR, Nelson M, Pickering D, et al. Translocation t(1;3)(p36.3;q25) is a nonrandom aberration in epithelioid hemangioendothelioma. Am J Surg Pathol 2001;25:684–7.

61. Flucke U, Vogels RJC, de Saint Aubain Somerhausen N, et al. Epithelioid Hemangioendothelioma: Clinicopathologic, immunohistochemical, and molecular genetic analysis of 39 cases. Diagn Pathol 2014;9:1–12.

62. Tanas MR, Sboner A, Oliveira AM, et al. Identification of a disease-defining gene fusion in epithelioid hemangioendothelioma. Sci Transl Med 2011; 3(98):98ra82.

63. Shibuya R, Matsuyama A, Shiba E, et al. CAMTA1 is a useful immunohistochemical marker for diagnosing epithelioid haemangioendothelioma. Histopathology 2015;67:827–35.

64. Doyle LA, Fletcher CDM, Hornick JL. Nuclear expression of CAMTA1 distinguishes epithelioid hemangioendothelioma from histologic mimics. Am J Surg Pathol 2016;40:94–102.

65. Antonescu C, Le Loarer F, Mosquera J, et al. Novel YAP1-TFE3 fusion defines a distinct subset of epithelioid hemangioendothelioma. Genes Chromosomes Cancer 2013;52:775–84.

66. Kuo FY, Huang HY, Chen CL, et al. TFE3-rearranged hepatic epithelioid hemangioendothelioma—a case report with immunohistochemical and molecular study. APMIS 2017;125:849–53.

67. Lotfalla MM, Folpe AL, Fritchie KJ, et al. Hepatic YAP1-TFE3 rearranged epithelioid hemangioendothelioma. Case Reports in Gastrointestinal Medicine 2019;2019:1–5.

68. Rosenbaum E, Jadeja B, Xu B, et al. Prognostic stratification of clinical and molecular epithelioid hemangioendothelioma subsets. Mod Pathol 2020;33:591–602.

69. Dermawan JK, Azzato EM, Billings SD, et al. YAP1-TFE3-fused hemangioendothelioma: a multi-institutional clinicopathologic study of 24 genetically-confirmed cases. Mod Pathol 2021;34: 2211–21.

70. Anderson WJ, Fletcher CDM, Hornick JL. Loss of expression of YAP1 C-terminus as an ancillary marker for epithelioid hemangioendothelioma variant with YAP1-TFE3 fusion and other YAP1-related vascular neoplasms. Mod Pathol 2021;1: 13–8.

71. Lee SJ, Yang WI, Chung W-S, et al. Epithelioid hemangioendotheliomas with TFE3 gene translocations are compossible with CAMTA1 gene rearrangements. Oncotarget 2016;7:7480–8.

72. Rubin BP, Deyrup AT, Doyle LA. Epithelioid haemangioendothelioma. In: WHO Classification of Tumours Editorial Board, editor. WHO classification of Tumours: soft tissue and bone Tumours. 5th edition. Lyon (France): IARC Press; 2020. p. 172–5.

73. Lee HE, Torbenson MS, Wu T-T, et al. Aberrant keratin expression is common in primary hepatic malignant vascular tumors: A potential diagnostic pitfall. Ann Diagn Pathol 2020;49:151589.

74. Deyrup AT, Tighiouart M, Montag AG, et al. Epithelioid hemangioendothelioma of soft tissue: A proposal for risk stratification based on 49 cases. Am J Surg Pathol 2008;32:924–7.

75. Anderson T, Zhang L, Hameed M, et al. Thoracic epithelioid malignant vascular tumors: A clinicopathologic study of 52 cases with emphasis on pathologic grading and molecular studies of WWTR1-CAMTA1 fusions. Am J Surg Pathol 2015; 39:132–9.

76. Shibayama T, Makise N, Motoi T, et al. Clinicopathologic characterization of epithelioid hemangioendothelioma in a series of 62 cases: A proposal of risk stratification and identification of a synaptophysin-positive aggressive subset. Am J Surg Pathol 2021;45:616–26.

77. Chen YA, Lu CY, Cheng TY, et al. WW domain-containing proteins YAP and TAZ in the hippo pathway as key regulators in stemness maintenance, tissue homeostasis, and tumorigenesis. Front Oncol 2019;9:60.

78. Tanas MR, Ma S, Jadaan FO, et al. Mechanism of action of a WWTR1(TAZ)-CAMTA1 fusion oncoprotein. Oncogene 2016;35:929–38.

79. Seavey CN, Pobbati AV, Hallett A, et al. WWTR1(TAZ)-CAMTA1 gene fusion is sufficient to dysregulate YAP/TAZ signaling and drive epithelioid hemangioendothelioma tumorigenesis. Genes and Development 2021;35:512–27.

80. Merritt N, Garcia K, Rajendran D, et al. TAZ-CAMTA1 and YAP-TFE3 alter the TAZ/YAP transcriptome by recruiting the ATAC histone acetyltransferase complex. Elife 2021;10:e62857.

81. Ma S, Kanai R, Pobbati AV, et al. The TAZ-CAMTA1 fusion protein promotes tumorigenesis via connective tissue growth factor and Ras–MAPK signaling in epithelioid hemangioendothelioma. Clin Cancer Res 2022;28:3116–26.

82. Jacobson A, Cunningham JL. Connective tissue growth factor in tumor pathogenesis. Fibrogenesis Tissue Repair 2012;5:S8.

83. Trikha M, Timar J, Lundy SK, et al. The high affinity aIIbfi3 integrin is involved in invasion of human melanoma cells. Cancer Res 1997;57:2522–8.

84. Shattil SJ, Kim C, Ginsberg MH. The final steps of integrin activation: The end game. Nat Rev Mol Cell Biol 2010;11:288–300.

85. Wilson GC, Lluis N, Nalesnik MA, et al. Hepatic angiosarcoma: A multi-institutional, international experience with 44 cases. Ann Surg Oncol 2019; 26:576–82.

86. Martínez C, Lai JK, Ramai D, et al. Cancer registry study of malignant hepatic vascular tumors: Hepatic angiosarcomas and hepatic epithelioid hemangioendotheliomas. Cancer Med 2021;10: 8883–90.

87. Selby DM, Stocker JT, Ishak KG. Angiosarcoma of the liver in childhood: A clinicopathologic and follow-up study of 10 cases. Pediatr Pathol 1992; 12:485–98.

88. Regelson W, Kim U, Ospina J, et al. Hemangioendothelial sarcoma of liver from chronic arsenic intoxication by Fowler's solution. Cancer 1968;21: 514–22.

89. Creech JL, Johnson MN. Angiosarcoma of liver in the manufacture of polyvinyl chloride. J Occup Med 1974;16:150–1.

90. Makk L. Liver damage and angiosarcoma in vinyl chloride workers. A systematic detection program. JAMA, J Am Med Assoc 1974;230:64–8.

91. Centeno JA, Mullick FG, Martinez L, et al. Pathology related to chronic arsenic exposure. Environmental Health Perspectives 2002;110:883–6.

92. Yasir S, Torbenson MS. Angiosarcoma of the liver: Clinicopathologic features and morphologic patterns. Am J Surg Pathol 2019;43:581–90.

93. Nascimento AF, Raut CP, Fletcher CDM. Primary angiosarcoma of the breast: Clinicopathologic analysis of 49 cases, suggesting that grade is not prognostic. Am J Surg Pathol 2008;32:1896–904.

94. Sullivan HC, Edgar MA, Cohen C, et al. The utility of ERG, CD31 and CD34 in the cytological diagnosis of angiosarcoma: An analysis of 25 cases. J Clin Pathol 2015;68:44–50.

95. Miettinen M, Fetsch JF. Distribution of keratins in normal endothelial cells and a spectrum of vascular tumors: Implications in tumor diagnosis. Hum Pathol 2000;31:1062–7.

96. Minner S, Luebke AM, Kluth M, et al. High level of Ets-related gene expression has high specificity for prostate cancer: a tissue microarray study of 11,483 cancers: High specificity of ERG expression for prostate cancer. Histopathology 2012;61: 445–53.

97. Manner J, Radlwimmer B, Hohenberger P, et al. MYC high level gene amplification is a distinctive feature of angiosarcomas after irradiation or chronic lymphedema. Am J Pathol 2010;176:34–9.

98. Guo Tianhua, Zhang Lei, Chang Ning-en, et al. Consistent MYC and FLT4 gene amplification in radiation-induced angiosarcoma but not in other radiation-associated atypical vascular lesions. Genes Chromosomes Cancer 2011;50:25–33.

99. Antonescu CR, Yoshida A, Guo T, et al. KDR activating mutations in human angiosarcomas are sensitive to specific kinase inhibitors. Cancer Res 2009;69:7175–9.

100. Huang S, Zhang L, Sung Y, et al. Recurrent CIC gene abnormalities in angiosarcomas: A molecular study of 120 cases with concurrent investigation of

PLCG1, KDR, MYC, and FLT4 gene alterations. Am J Surg Pathol 2016;40:645–55.

101. Beca F, Krings G, Chen YY, et al. Primary mammary angiosarcomas harbor frequent mutations in KDR and PIK3CA and show evidence of distinct pathogenesis. Mod Pathol 2020;33:1518–26.

102. Antonescu C. Malignant vascular tumors-an update. Mod Pathol 2014;27:30–8.

103. Verbeke SLJ, de Jong D, Bertoni F, et al. Array CGH analysis identifies two distinct subgroups of primary angiosarcoma of bone. Genes, Chromosomes & Cancer 2015;54:72–81.

104. Kojima N, Arai Y, Satomi K, et al. Co-expression of ERG and CD31 in a subset of CIC-rearranged sarcoma: A potential diagnostic pitfall. Mod Pathol 2022;35:1439–48.

105. Bonetti F, Pea M, Martignoni G, et al. Cellular heterogeneity in lymphangiomyomatosis of the lung. Hum Pathol 1991;22:727–8.

106. Bonetti F, Pea M, Martignoni G, et al. PEC and sugar. Am J Surg Pathol 1992;16:307–8.

107. Bonetti F, Chiodera PL, Pea M, et al. Transbronchial biopsy in lymphangiomyomatosis of the lung. HMB45 for diagnosis. Am J Surg Pathol 1993;17:1092–102.

108. Pea M, Martignoni G, Zamboni G, et al. Perivascular epithelioid cell. Am J Surg Pathol 1996;20:1149–53.

109. Crino PB, Henske EP. The tuberous sclerosis complex. N Engl J Med 2006;355(13):1345–56.

110. Kenerson H, Folpe AL, Takayama TK, et al. Activation of the mTOR pathway in sporadic angiomyolipomas and other perivascular epithelioid cell neoplasms. Hum Pathol 2007;38:1361–71.

111. Tanaka M, Kato K, Gomi K, et al. Perivascular epithelioid cell tumor with SFPQ/PSF-TFE3 gene fusion in a patient with advanced neuroblastoma. Am J Surg Pathol 2009;33:1416–20.

112. Argani P, Aulmann S, Illei PB, et al. A distinctive subset of PEComas harbors TFE3 gene fusions. Am J Surg Pathol 2010;34:1395–406.

113. Tsui WM, Colombari R, Portmann BC, et al. Hepatic angiomyolipoma: A clinicopathologic study of 30 cases and delineation of unusual morphologic variants. Am J Surg Pathol 1999;23:34–48.

114. Folpe AL, Mentzel T, Lehr H-A, et al. Perivascular epithelioid cell neoplasms of soft tissue and gynecologic origin: A clinicopathologic study of 26 cases and review of the literature. Am J Surg Pathol 2005;29:1558–75.

115. Miettinen M, McCue PA, Sarlomo-Rikala M, et al. Sox10 – A marker for not only Schwannian and melanocytic neoplasms but also myoepithelial cell tumors of soft tissue. A systematic analysis of 5134 tumors. Am J Surg Pathol 2015;39:826–35.

116. Dalle S, De Vos R, van Damme B, et al. Malignant angiomyolipoma of the liver: A hitherto unreported variant. Histopathology 2000;36:443–50.

117. Parfitt JR, Bella AJ, Izawa JI, et al. Malignant neoplasm of perivascular epithelioid cells of the liver. Arch Pathol Lab Med 2006;130:1219–22.

118. Torres U, Hawkins WG, Antonescu CR, et al. Hepatic follicular dendritic cell sarcoma without Epstein-Barr Virus expression. Arch Pathol Lab Med 2005;129:1480–3.

119. Agaimy A, Michal M, Hadravsky L, et al. Follicular dendritic cell sarcoma: Clinicopathologic study of 15 cases with emphasis on novel expression of MDM2, somatostatin receptor 2A, and PD-L1. Ann Diagn Pathol 2016;23:21–8.

120. Shek TW, Ho FC, Ng IO, et al. Follicular dendritic cell tumor of the liver. Evidence for an Epstein-Barr Virus-related clonal proliferation of follicular dendritic cells. Am J Surg Pathol 1996;20:313–24.

121. Selves J, Meggetto F, Brousset P, et al. Inflammatory pseudotumor of the liver. Evidence for follicular dendritic reticulum cell proliferation associated with clonal Epstein-Barr Virus. Am J Surg Pathol 1996;20:747–53.

122. Bai L-Y, Kwang W-K, Chiang I-P, et al. Follicular dendritic cell tumor of the liver associated with Epstein–Barr Virus. Jpn J Clin Oncol 2006;36:249–53.

123. Fonseca R, Yamakawa M, Nakamura S, et al. Follicular dendritic cell sarcoma and interdigitating reticulum cell sarcoma: A review. Am J Hematol 1998;59:161–7.

124. Xu J, Sun HH, Fletcher CDM, et al. Expression of programmed cell death 1 ligands (PD-L1 and PD-L2) in histiocytic and dendritic cell disorders. Am J Surg Pathol 2016;40:443–53.

125. Chadwick EG, Connor EJ, Hanson IC, et al. Tumors of smooth-muscle origin in HIV-infected children. JAMA 1990;263:3182–4.

126. Lee ES, Locker J, Nalesnik M, et al. The association of Epstein–Barr virus with smooth-muscle tumors occurring after organ transplantation. N Engl J Med 1995;332:19–25.

127. Deyrup AT, Lee VK, Hill CE, et al. Epstein-Barr Virus-associated smooth muscle tumors are distinctive mesenchymal tumors reflecting multiple infection events. Am J Surg Pathol 2006;30:8.

128. Issarachaikul R, Shuangshoti S, Suankratay C. Epstein-Barr Virus-associated smooth muscle tumors in AIDS patients: A largest case (series). Intern Med 2014;53:2391–6.

129. Ara T, Endo T, Goto H, et al. Antiretroviral therapy achieved metabolic complete remission of hepatic AIDS related Epstein-Barr virus-associated smooth muscle tumor. Antivir Ther 2022;27, 135965352211268.

130. Chong YB, Lu P-L, Ma Y-C, et al. Epstein-Barr Virus-associated smooth muscle tumor and its correlation with CD4 levels in a patient with HIV infection. Front Cell Infect Microbiol 2022;12:725342.

131. Coffin CM, Hornick JL, Fletcher CDM. Inflammatory myofibroblastic tumor: Comparison of clinicopathologic, histologic, and immunohistochemical features including

ALK expression in atypical and aggressive cases. Am J Surg Pathol 2007;31:12.

132. Antonescu CR, Suurmeijer AJ, Zhang L, et al. Molecular characterization of inflammatory myofibroblastic tumors with frequent ALK and ROS1 fusions and rare novel RET gene rearrangement. Am J Surg Pathol 2015;39:957–67.

133. Coffin CM, Watterson J, Priest JR, et al. Extrapulmonary inflammatory myofibroblastic tumor (inflammatory pseudotumor). A clinicopathologic and immunohistochemical study of 84 cases. Am J Surg Pathol 1995;19:859–72.

134. Qiu X, Montgomery E, Sun B. Inflammatory myofibroblastic tumor and low-grade myofibroblastic sarcoma: a comparative study of clinicopathologic features and further observations on the immunohistochemical profile of myofibroblasts. Hum Pathol 2008;39:846–56.

135. Arora KS, Anderson MA, Neyaz A, et al. Fibrohistiocytic variant of hepatic pseudotumor: An antibiotic responsive tumefactive lesion. Am J Surg Pathol 2021;45:1314–23.

136. Gonzalez-Crussi F, Goldschmidt RA, Hsueh W, et al. Infantile sarcoma with intracytoplasmic filamentous inclusions: distinctive tumor of possible histiocytic origin. Cancer 1982;49:2365–75.

137. Fazlollahi L, Hsiao SJ, Kochhar M, et al. Malignant rhabdoid tumor, an aggressive tumor often misclassified as small cell variant of hepatoblastoma. Cancers 2019;11:1992.

138. Trobaugh-Lotrario AD, Finegold MJ, Feusner JH. Rhabdoid tumors of the liver: Rare, aggressive, and poorly responsive to standard cytotoxic chemotherapy. Pediatr Blood Cancer 2011;57:423–8.

139. Hoot AC, Russo P, Judkins AR, et al. Immunohistochemical analysis of hSNF5/INI1 distinguishes renal and extra-renal malignant rhabdoid tumors from other pediatric soft tissue tumors. Am J Surg Pathol 2004;28:1485–91.

140. Versteege I, Sévenet N, Lange J, et al. Truncating mutations of hSNF5/INI1 in aggressive paediatric cancer. Nature 1998;394:203–6.

141. Biegel JA, Zhou JY, Rorke LB, et al. Germ-line and acquired mutations of INI1 in atypical teratoid and rhabdoid tumors. Cancer Res 1999;59:74–9.

142. Fanburg-Smith JC, Hengge M, Hengge UR, et al. Extrarenal rhabdoid tumors of soft tissue: A clinicopathologic and immunohistochemical study of 18 cases. Ann Diagn Pathol 1998;2:351–62.

143. Guillou L, Wadden C, Coindre JM, et al. "Proximal-type" epithelioid sarcoma, a distinctive aggressive neoplasm showing rhabdoid features. Clinicopathologic, immunohistochemical, and ultrastructural study of a series. Am J Surg Pathol 1997;21:130–46.

144. Chmielecki J, Crago AM, Rosenberg M, et al. Whole-exome sequencing identifies a recurrent NAB2-STAT6 fusion in solitary fibrous tumors. Nat Genet 2013;45:131–2.

145. Robinson DR, Wu Y-M, Kalyana-Sundaram S, et al. Identification of recurrent NAB2-STAT6 gene fusions in solitary fibrous tumor by integrative sequencing. Nat Genet 2013;45:180–5.

146. Doyle LA, Vivero M, Fletcher CDM, et al. Nuclear expression of STAT6 distinguishes solitary fibrous tumor from histologic mimics. Mod Pathol 2014;27:390–5.

147. Arora A, Jaiswal R, Anand N, et al. Primary embryonal rhabdomyosarcoma of the liver. BMJ Case Rep 2016;2016, bcr2016218292.

148. Huey RW, Makawita S, Xiao L, et al. Sarcomatoid carcinoma presenting as cancers of unknown primary: A clinicopathological portrait. BMC Cancer 2019;19:965.

149. Wege H, Schulze K, von Felden J, et al. Rare variants of primary liver cancer: Fibrolamellar, combined, and sarcomatoid hepatocellular carcinomas. Eur J Med Genet 2021;64:104313.

150. Agaimy A, Specht K, Stoehr R, et al. Metastatic malignant melanoma with complete loss of differentiation markers (undifferentiated/dedifferentiated melanoma): Analysis of 14 patients emphasizing phenotypic plasticity and the value of molecular testing as surrogate diagnostic marker. Am J Surg Pathol 2016;40:181–91.

151. Nonaka D, Chiriboga L, Rubin BP. Sox10: A pan-Schwannian and melanocytic marker. Am J Surg Pathol 2008;32:1291–8.

152. Karamchandani JR, Nielsen TO, Van De Rijn M, et al. Sox10 and s100 in the diagnosis of soft-tissue neoplasms. Appl Immunohistochem Mol Morphol AIMM 2012;20:445–50.

153. Schaefer IM, Fletcher CDM, Hornick JL. Loss of H3K27 trimethylation distinguishes malignant peripheral nerve sheath tumors from histologic mimics. Mod Pathol 2016;29:4–13.

154. Le Guellec S, Macagno N, Velasco V, et al. Loss of H3K27 trimethylation is not suitable for distinguishing malignant peripheral nerve sheath tumor from melanoma: A study of 387 cases including mimicking lesions. Mod Pathol 2017;30:1677–87.

155. Agaimy A, Stoehr R, Hornung A, et al. Dedifferentiated and undifferentiated melanomas: Report of 35 new cases with literature review and proposal of diagnostic criteria. Am J Surg Pathol 2021;45:240–54.

156. Iwata J, Fletcher CDM. Immunohistochemical detection of cytokeratin and epithelial membrane antigen in leiomyosarcoma: A systematic study of 100 cases. Pathol Int 2000;50:7–14.

157. Papke DJ, Forgó E, Charville GW, et al. PDGFRA immunohistochemistry predicts PDGFRA mutations in gastrointestinal stromal tumors. Am J Surg Pathol 2022;46:3–10.

158. Creytens D, Van Gorp J, Speel EJ, et al. Character-ization of the 12q amplicons in lipomatous soft tis-sue tumors by multiplex ligation-dependent probe amplification-based copy number analysis. Anti-cancer Res 2015;35:1835–42.

159. Pilotti S, Della Torre G, Mezzelani A, et al. The expression of MDM2/CDK4 gene product in the dif-ferential diagnosis of well differentiated liposar-coma and large deep-seated lipoma. Br J Cancer 2000;82:1271–5.

160. Binh MBN, Sastre-Garau X, Guillou L, et al. MDM2 and CDK4 immunostainings are useful adjuncts in diagnosing well-differentiated and dedifferentiated liposarcoma subtypes: a comparative analysis of 559 soft tissue neoplasms with genetic data. Am J Surg Pathol 2005;29:1340–7.

161. Thway K, Flora R, Shah C, et al. Diagnostic utility of p16, CDK4, and MDM2 as an immunohisto-chemical panel in distinguishing well-differentiated and dedifferentiated liposarcomas from other adipocytic tumors. Am J Surg Pathol 2012;36:462–9.

162. Doyle LA, Tao D, Mariño-Enríquez A. STAT6 is amplified in a subset of dedifferentiated liposar-coma. Mod Pathol 2014;27:1231–7.

163. Gerald WL, Ladanyi M, De Alava E, et al. Clinical, pathologic, and molecular spectrum of tumors associated with t(11;22)(p13;q12): Desmoplastic small round-cell tumor and its variants. J Clin Oncol 1998;16:3028–36.

164. Lae ME, Roche PC, Jin L, et al. Desmoplastic small round cell tumor: A clinicopathologic, immunohis-tochemical, and molecular study of 32 tumors. Am J Surg Pathol 2002;26:823–35.

165. Pasquinelli G, Montanaro L, Martinelli GN. Desmo-plastic small round-cell tumor: A case report on the large cell variant with immunohistochemical, ultra-structural, and molecular genetic analysis. Ultra-struct Pathol 2000;24:333–7.

166. Barnoud R, Sabourin JC, Pasquier D, et al. Immu-nohistochemical expression of WT1 by desmoplas-tic small round cell tumor: A comparative study with other small round cell tumors. Am J Surg Pathol 2000;24:830–6.

Moving?

Make sure your subscription moves with you!

To notify us of your new address, find your **Clinics Account Number** (located on your mailing label above your name), and contact customer service at:

Email: journalscustomerservice-usa@elsevier.com

800-654-2452 (subscribers in the U.S. & Canada)
314-447-8871 (subscribers outside of the U.S. & Canada)

Fax number: 314-447-8029

Elsevier Health Sciences Division
Subscription Customer Service
3251 Riverport Lane
Maryland Heights, MO 63043

*To ensure uninterrupted delivery of your subscription, please notify us at least 4 weeks in advance of move.

Printed and bound by CPI Group (UK) Ltd, Croydon, CR0 4YY

03/10/2024

01040362-0020